# PET-CT-MRI Applications of Musculoskeletal Disorders, Part II

*Editors*

ALI GHOLAMREZANEZHAD
ALI GUERMAZI
ALI SALAVATI
ABASS ALAVI

# PET CLINICS

www.pet.theclinics.com

*Consulting Editor*
ABASS ALAVI

January 2019 • Volume 14 • Number 1

**ELSEVIER**

1600 John F. Kennedy Boulevard • Suite 1800 • Philadelphia, Pennsylvania, 19103-2899

http://www.pet.theclinics.com

**PET CLINICS Volume 14, Number 1**
**January 2019 ISSN 1556-8598, ISBN-13: 978-0-323-65485-2**

Editor: John Vassallo (j.vassallo@elsevier.com)
Developmental Editor: Casey Potter

### Photocopying

Single photocopies of single articles may be made for personal use as allowed by national copyright laws. Permission of the Publisher and payment of a fee is required for all other photocopying, including multiple or systematic copying, copying for advertising or promotional purposes, resale, and all forms of document delivery. Special rates are available for educational institutions that wish to make photocopies for non-profit educational classroom use. For information on how to seek permission visit www.elsevier.com/permissions or call: (+44) 1865 843830 (UK)/(+1) 215 239 3804 (USA).

### Derivative Works

Subscribers may reproduce tables of contents or prepare lists of articles including abstracts for internal circulation within their institutions. Permission of the Publisher is required for resale or distribution outside the institution. Permission of the Publisher is required for all other derivative works, including compilations and translations (please consult www.elsevier.com/permissions).

### Electronic Storage or Usage

Permission of the Publisher is required to store or use electronically any material contained in this periodical, including any article or part of an article (please consult www.elsevier.com/permissions). Except as outlined above, no part of this publication may be reproduced, stored in a retrieval system or transmitted in any form or by any means, electronic, mechanical, photocopying, recording or otherwise, without prior written permission of the Publisher.

### Notice

No responsibility is assumed by the Publisher for any injury and/or damage to persons or property as a matter of products liability, negligence or otherwise, or from any use or operation of any methods, products, instructions or ideas contained in the material herein. Because of rapid advances in the medical sciences, in particular, independent verification of diagnoses and drug dosages should be made. Although all advertising material is expected to conform to ethical (medical) standards, inclusion in this publication does not constitute a guarantee or endorsement of the quality or value of such product or of the claims made of it by its manufacturer.

*PET Clinics* (ISSN 1556-8598) is published quarterly by Elsevier Inc., 360 Park Avenue South, New York, NY 10010-1710. Months of issue are January, April, July, and October. Periodicals postage paid at New York, NY, and additional mailing offices. Subscription prices per year are $240.00 (US individuals), $396.00 (US institutions), $100.00 (US students), $279.00 (Canadian individuals), $446.00 (Canadian institutions), $140.00 (Canadian students), $275.00 (foreign individuals), $446.00 (foreign institutions), and $140.00 (foreign students). To receive student and resident rate, orders must be accompanied by name of affiliated institution, date of term, and the signature of program/residency coordinator on institution letterhead. Orders will be billed at individual rate until proof of status is received. Foreign air speed delivery is included in all Clinics subscription prices. All prices are subject to change without notice. POSTMASTER: Send address changes to PET Clinics, Elsevier Health Sciences Division, Subscription Customer Service, 3251 Riverport Lane, Maryland Heights, MO 63043. **Customer Service: 1-800-654-2452 (U.S. and Canada); 314-447-8871 (outside U.S. and Canada). Fax: 314-447-8029. E-mail: journalscustomerservice-usa@elsevier.com (for print support); journalsonlinesupport-usa@elsevier.com (for online support).**

*Reprints.* For copies of 100 or more of articles in this publication, please contact the Commercial Reprints Department, Elsevier Inc., 360 Park Avenue South, New York, NY 10010-1710. Tel.: 212-633-3874; Fax: 212-633-3820; E-mail: reprints@elsevier.com.

PET Clinics is covered in MEDLINE/PubMed (Index Medicus).

# Contributors

## CONSULTING EDITOR

**ABASS ALAVI, MD, MD (Hon), PhD (Hon), DSc (Hon)**
Professor of Radiology and Neurology, Department of Radiology, Division of Nuclear Medicine, Hospital of the University of Pennsylvania, University of Pennsylvania Perelman School of Medicine, Philadelphia, Pennsylvania, USA

## EDITORS

**ALI GHOLAMREZANEZHAD, MD**
University Hospitals Cleveland Medical Center, Cleveland, Ohio, USA

**ALI GUERMAZI, MD, PhD**
Professor of Radiology, Boston University School of Medicine, Boston, Massachusetts, USA

**ALI SALAVATI, MD, MPH**
Department of Radiology, University of Minnesota, Minneapolis, Minnesota, USA

**ABASS ALAVI, MD, MD (Hon), PhD (Hon), DSc (Hon)**
Professor of Radiology and Neurology, Department of Radiology, Division of Nuclear Medicine, Hospital of the University of Pennsylvania, University of Pennsylvania Perelman School of Medicine, Philadelphia, Pennsylvania, USA

## AUTHORS

**ABDULLAH AL-ZAGHAL, MD**
Department of Radiology, Hospital of University of Pennsylvania, Philadelphia, Pennsylvania, USA

**ABASS ALAVI, MD, MD (Hon), PhD (Hon), DSc (Hon)**
Professor of Radiology and Neurology, Department of Radiology, Division of Nuclear Medicine, Hospital of the University of Pennsylvania, University of Pennsylvania Perelman School of Medicine, Philadelphia, Pennsylvania, USA

**ANDREA ANGELINI, MD, PhD**
Department of Orthopedics and Orthopedic Oncology, University of Padova, Padova, Italy

**MAJID ASSADI, MD, FASNC**
The Persian Gulf Nuclear Medicine Research Center, Bushehr University of Medical Sciences, Bushehr, Iran

**ALECXIH G. AUSTIN, BS**
Department of Radiology, University of Pennsylvania, Philadelphia, Pennsylvania, USA

**CYRUS AYUBCHA, MD**
Department of Radiology, Hospital of
University of Pennsylvania, Philadelphia,
Pennsylvania, USA

**TOBIAS BÄUERLE, MD**
Institute of Radiology, University Medical
Center Erlangen, Erlangen, Germany

**SANDIP BASU, MBBS (HONS), DRM, DNB,
MNAMS**
Radiation Medicine Centre, Bhabha Atomic
Research Centre, Tata Memorial Centre
Annexe, Homi Bhabha National Institute,
Mumbai, Maharashtra, India

**ALI BATOULI, MD**
Fellow, Department of Neuroradiology, Oregon
Health and Science University, Portland,
Oregon, USA

**STEPHEN M. BROSKI, MD**
Assistant Professor, Department of Radiology,
Division of Nuclear Medicine, Mayo Clinic,
Rochester, Minnesota, USA

**PAOLO CASTELLUCCI, MD**
Nuclear Medicine, Azienda Ospedaliero-
Universitaria di Bologna, University of Bologna,
Bologna, Italy

**FRANCESCO CECI, MD, PhD**
Department of Molecular and Medical
Pharmacology, Ahmanson Translational
Imaging Division, University of California, Los
Angeles (UCLA), Los Angeles, California, USA;
Nuclear Medicine, Azienda Ospedaliero-
Universitaria di Bologna, University of Bologna,
Bologna, Italy

**STEPHAN ELLMANN, MD**
Institute of Radiology, University Medical
Center Erlangen, Erlangen, Germany

**ALI GHOLAMREZANEZHAD, MD, FEBNM,
DABR**
Department of Diagnostic Radiology, Keck
School of Medicine of USC, University of
Southern California (USC), Los Angeles,
California, USA

**GARRY E. GOLD, MD**
Departments of Radiology, Bioengineering and
Orthopaedic Surgery, Stanford University,
Stanford, California, USA

**ALI GUERMAZI, MD, PhD**
Professor of Radiology and Medicine,
Department of Radiology, University of
Erlangen-Nuremberg, Erlangen, Germany;
Department of Radiology, Quantitative Imaging
Center, Boston University School of Medicine,
Boston, Massachusetts, USA

**DOUGLAS J. HARRISON, MD, MS**
Assistant Professor, Department of Pediatrics,
The University of Texas MD Anderson Cancer
Center, Houston, Texas, USA

**DAICHI HAYASHI, MD, PhD**
Research Assistant Professor, Department of
Radiology, Quantitative Imaging Center,
Boston University School of Medicine, Boston,
Massachusetts, USA

**HOSSEIN JADVAR, MD, PhD, MPH, MBA**
Associate Professor, Departments of Nuclear
Medicine and Radiology, Keck School of
Medicine of USC, University of Southern
California, Los Angeles, California,
USA

**PEGAH JAHANGIRI, MD**
Division of Nuclear Medicine, Hospital of
University of Pennsylvania, Philadelphia,
Pennsylvania, USA

**VENKATA S. JONNAKUTI, BS**
Department of Radiology, University of
Pennsylvania, Philadelphia, Pennsylvania, USA

**AYSE T. KENDI, MD**
Associate Professor, Department of Radiology,
Division of Nuclear Medicine, Mayo Clinic,
Rochester, Minnesota, USA

**HEDIEH KHALATBARI, MD, MBA**
Assistant Professor of Pediatric Radiology,
Department of Radiology, University of
Washington School of Medicine, Seattle
Children's Hospital, Seattle, Washington,
USA

**FELIKS KOGAN, PhD**
Department of Radiology, Stanford University,
Stanford, California, USA

**SOHEIL KOORAKI, MD**
Department of Radiology, Shariati Hospital,
Tehran University of Medical Sciences, Tehran,
Iran

**ESHA KOTHEKAR, MD**
Department of Radiology, Hospital of
University of Pennsylvania, Philadelphia,
Pennsylvania, USA

**TORSTEN KUWERT, MD**
Clinic of Nuclear Medicine, University Medical
Center Erlangen, Erlangen, Germany

**NEHA KWATRA, MD**
Staff Radiologist, Instructor, Department of
Radiology, Division of Nuclear Medicine and
Molecular Imaging, Boston Children's Hospital,
Harvard Medical School, Boston,
Massachusetts, USA

**GEORGE MATCUK, MD**
Associate Professor, Department of Diagnostic
Radiology, Keck School of Medicine of USC,
University of Southern California, Los Angeles,
California, USA

**MOHAMMAD HOSEIN NAJAFI, MD**
Department of Cardiology, Tehran Medical
Unit, Azad University, Tehran, Iran

**MARGUERITE T. PARISI, MD, MS**
Professor of Pediatric Radiology, Departments
of Radiology and Pediatrics, University of
Washington School of Medicine, Seattle
Children's Hospital, Seattle, Washington,
USA

**ALOK PAWASKAR, MBBS, DRM, DNB**
Consultant and Head, Nuclear Medicine
Department, Oncolife Cancer Centre, Satara,
Maharashtra, India; Radiation Medicine
Centre, Bhabha Atomic Research Centre, Tata
Memorial Centre Annexe, Mumbai,
Maharashtra, India

**DAVID PETROV, MD**
Resident, Department of Radiology, Allegheny
Health Network, Pittsburgh, Pennsylvania,
USA

**CHAMITH S. RAJAPAKSE, PhD**
Department of Radiology, University of
Pennsylvania, Philadelphia, Pennsylvania, USA

**WILLIAM Y. RAYNOR, BS**
Department of Radiology, University of
Pennsylvania, Drexel University College of
Medicine, Philadelphia, Pennsylvania,
USA

**CATHERINE C. REILLY, BS**
Department of Radiology, University of
Pennsylvania, Philadelphia, Pennsylvania, USA

**PHILIPP RITT, PhD**
Clinic of Nuclear Medicine, University Medical
Center Erlangen, Erlangen, Germany

**FRANK W. ROEMER, MD**
Associate Professor of Radiology, Department
of Radiology, Stony Brook Medicine, Stony
Brook, New York, USA; Institute of Radiology,
University Medical Center Erlangen, Erlangen,
Germany

**SCOTT RUDKIN, MD**
Resident, Department of Radiology, Allegheny
Health Network, Pittsburgh, Pennsylvania,
USA

**CHRISTIAN SCHMIDKONZ, MD**
Clinic of Nuclear Medicine, University Medical
Center Erlangen, Erlangen, Germany

**SIAVASH MEHDIZADEH SERAJ, MD**
Department of Radiology, University of
Pennsylvania, Philadelphia, Pennsylvania, USA

**BARRY L. SHULKIN, MD, MBA**
Chief, Division of Nuclear Medicine,
Department of Diagnostic Imaging, St. Jude
Children's Research Hospital, Memphis,
Tennessee, USA

**RATHAN M. SUBRAMANIAM, MD, PhD,
MPH**
Professor, Department of Radiology, Division
of Nuclear Medicine, Harold Simmons
Comprehensive Cancer Center, The University
of Texas Southwestern Medical Center, Dallas,
Texas, USA

**MICHAEL UDER, MD**
Institute of Radiology, University Medical
Center Erlangen, Erlangen, Germany

**ERIK VELEZ, MD**
Department of Diagnostic Radiology, Keck
School of Medicine of USC, University of
Southern California (USC), Los Angeles,
California, USA

**THOMAS J. WERNER, MSE**
Department of Radiology, University of
Pennsylvania, Philadelphia, Pennsylvania, USA

**JAMES S. YODER, BS**
Department of Radiology, Stanford University, Stanford, California, USA

**JASON R. YOUNG, MD**
Division of Nuclear Medicine, Department of Radiology, Mayo Clinic, Rochester, Minnesota, USA

**MAHDI ZIRAKCHIAN ZADEH, MD, MHM**
Department of Radiology, Children's Hospital of Philadelphia, University of Pennsylvania, Philadelphia, Pennsylvania, USA

**HONGMING ZHUANG, MD, PhD**
Radiology, University of Pennsylvania, Philadelphia, Pennsylvania, USA

# Contents

> Although computed tomography (CT) and MR imaging alone have been used extensively to evaluate various musculoskeletal disorders, hybrid imaging modalities of PET-CT and PET–MR imaging were recently developed, combining the advantages of each method: molecular information from PET and anatomical information from CT or MR imaging. Furthermore, different radiotracers can be used in PET to uncover different disease mechanisms. In this article, potential applications of PET-CT and PET–MR imaging for benign musculoskeletal disorders are organized by benign cell proliferation/dysplasia, diabetic foot complications, joint prostheses, degeneration, inflammation, and trauma, metabolic bone disorders, and pain (acute and chronic) and peripheral nerve imaging.

> Radiography remains the first-line imaging tool to characterize structural changes of osteoarthritis (OA) in both clinical and research settings, but MRI continues to play a large role in OA research. Compositional MRI enables evaluation of the biochemical properties of joint tissues, allowing assessment of early "premorphologic" changes that cannot be depicted on conventional MRI Hybrid PET-CT and PET–MRI allow integration of high-resolution structural information on CT and MRI with metabolic information obtained from PET related to OA disease process. We describe OA imaging by means of conventional radiography, MRI PET-CT, and PET–MRI.

> An imbalance in bone remodeling results in many metabolic bone diseases, such as osteoporosis. fluorine-18 sodium fluoride PET imaging allows the assessment of bone remodeling process in a anatomy specific manner. On the other hand structural imaging modalities such as MRI can now generate high resolution images of bone including the trabecular and cortical microstructure. Molecular (functional) imaging with PET in conjunction with structural imaging has the potential to improve the way metabolic bone diseases are managed in the clinic.

> In vivo molecular imaging detects biologic processes at molecular level and provides diagnostic information at an earlier time point during disease onset or repair.

It offers definite advantage over anatomic imaging in terms of improved sensitivity and ability to quantify. Radionuclide molecular imaging has been widely used in clinical practice. This article discusses the role of radionuclide imaging in various infective and inflammatory diseases affecting musculoskeletal system with a focus on PET. It appears that, as more data become available, combined PET/MR imaging could emerge as a front runner in the imaging of musculoskeletal infection and inflammation.

Over the last decade, major advances have been made in PET imaging, including the introduction of hybrid PET/computed tomography and PET/MR imaging systems, facilitating a better understanding of the pathophysiology underlying a vast array of human diseases. PET has not only remained the clinical standard for most oncological disorders but also emerged as a potentially viable modality in nononcological disorders, including many musculoskeletal pathologies.

2-Deoxy-2-[$^{18}$F]fluoroglucose (FDG) uptake in muscle is influenced by many normal physiologic processes and can also indicate pathology. Variability in physiologic uptake can be reduced with proper patient preparation, allowing for a better determination of abnormal activity. Although malignant diseases, such as rhabdomyosarcoma and skeletal muscle metastasis, are clear applications of FDG-PET/CT, there may be additional applications in infection and benign inflammatory disorders that warrant further research.

PET has been founded as a useful technique in the staging, restaging, prognostication, and treatment planning for numerus cancers, with an incremental application in precision oncology. This paper summarized the current state-of-the-art application of PET/CT in the management of patients with peripheral nerve tumors. Furthermore, the potential clinical uses of emerging themes and technological advances are reviewed, consisting hybrid PET/MR imaging and alternative radiotracers for the application in peripheral nerve oncology.

Knowledge of the PET imaging findings of osseous spinal neoplasms is essential, because they are common incidental findings on PET scans done for staging of unrelated primary malignancies. Additionally, PET can help differentiate lesions that are not clearly defined by anatomic modalities alone. PET can also be used for follow-up of aggressive tumors to assess response to treatment, often proving superior to CT or MR imaging alone for this purpose. This review discusses the role of PET/CT and PET/MR imaging in the diagnosis and management of primary benign and malignant osseous tumors of the spine.

A number of PET agents are useful for evaluation of skeletal metastatic disease, and have significant advantages over 99mTc-MDP scintigraphy, including superior diagnostic accuracy, higher spatial resolution, and shorter imaging times- often with the ability to depict soft tissue local recurrence and metastasis in the same examination. While these agents have excellent diagnostic utility, they are not 100% specific for skeletal metastasis, and so normal patterns of biodistribution, benign osseous lesions that may demonstrate radiotracer uptake, and the significance of morphologic changes on CT such as osteolysis or osteosclerosis must be kept in mind to ensure accurate interpretation.

Bone metastases are a common source of osseous malignancy in the skeleton and affect up to 70% of all cancer patients. Hybrid imaging modalities including positron emission tomography (PET)/computed tomography (CT) and PET/MRI play an increasing role for the detection and follow-up of metastatic disease, especially in monitoring treatment response upon local or systemic therapy. This review summarizes current applications of PET/CT and PET/MRI in the clinical setting for imaging of metastases.

Conventional modalities, such as bone scintigraphy, are commonly used to assess osseous abnormalities in skeletal metastasis. Fluorine-18 ($^{18}$F)-sodium fluoride (NaF) PET similarly portrays osteoblastic activity but with improved spatial and contrast resolution and more accurate anatomic localization. However, these modalities rely on indirect evidence for tumor activity. PET imaging with $^{18}$F-fluorodeoxyglucose (FDG) and tumor-specific tracers may have an increased role by directly portraying the metabolic activity of cancer cells, which are often seeded in bone marrow and cause osseous disease after initial latency. This article describes the utility and limitations of these modalities in assessing skeletal metastases.

The use of PET/computed tomography (CT) for the evaluation and management of children, adolescents, and young adults continues to expand. The principal tracer used is 18F-fluorodeoxyglucose and the principal indication is oncology, particularly musculoskeletal neoplasms. The purpose of this article is to review the common applications of PET/CT for imaging of musculoskeletal issues in pediatrics and to introduce the use of PET/CT for nononcologic issues, such as infectious/inflammatory disorders, and review the use of 18F–sodium fluoride in trauma and sports-related injuries.

We aimed to review the latest cutting-edge trends in emerging techniques of musculoskeletal imaging. This study reviews the current status and the preliminary studies of Magnetic Resonance Fingerprinting (MRF), Ultrashort Echo Time (UTE) sequence, Positron Emission Tomography (PET)/MR and Dual-Energy CT scan (DECT) in various oncologic and non-oncologic conditions of the musculoskeletal system. The current application, current and future research trends and limitations of each imaging technique were discussed. There are substantial potentials in MRF, UTE, PET/MR and DECT for characterization of various musculoskeletal disorders. Further dedicated studies in various fields are necessary.

Fluorodeoxyglucose positron emission tomography/computed tomography (18F-FDG-PET/CT) is the imaging method of choice in sarcoma patients. PET may help in diagnosis, grading, staging, biopsy guidance, monitoring response to therapy, restaging for recurrence, and prognosis. 18F-FDG-PET/MRI combines the higher tissue contrast of MRI in the study of soft-tissue lesions and the peculiarities of PET imaging that allow the characterization of tissues. The use of 18F-FDG-PET/MRI in these patients has reduces the radiation dose, which is of great importance, particularly in children. Data support the routine use of 18F-FDG-PET either using CT or MRI in patients with sarcoma.

# PET CLINICS

SERIES OF RELATED INTEREST

*MRI Clinics of North America*
Available at: MRI.theclinics.com
*Neuroimaging Clinics of North America*
Available at: Neuroimaging.theclinics.com
*Radiologic Clinics of North America*
Available at: Radiologic.theclinics.com

**THE CLINICS ARE AVAILABLE ONLINE!**
Access your subscription at:
www.theclinics.com

## PROGRAM OBJECTIVE

The goal of the *PET Clinics* is to keep practicing radiologists and radiology residents up to date with current clinical practice in positron emission tomography by providing timely articles reviewing the state of the art in patient care.

## TARGET AUDIENCE

Practicing radiologists, radiology residents, and other health care professionals who provide patient care utilizing radiologic findings.

## LEARNING OBJECTIVES

Upon completion of this activity, participants will be able to:
1. Review applications of PET in the evaluation of spine and joint disorders.
2. Discuss current and future applications of PET-CT-MRI in assessing muscle disorders and in musculoskeletal disorders.
3. Recognize the role of PET-CT-MRI in the diagnostic management of primary and secondary spinal neoplastic disease.

## ACCREDITATION

The Elsevier Office of Continuing Medical Education (EOCME) is accredited by the Accreditation Council for Continuing Medical Education (ACCME) to provide continuing medical education for physicians.

The EOCME designates this enduring material for a maximum of 15 *AMA PRA Category 1 Credit*(s)™. Physicians should claim only the credit commensurate with the extent of their participation in the activity.

All other health care professionals requesting continuing education credit for this enduring material will be issued a certificate of participation.

## DISCLOSURE OF CONFLICTS OF INTEREST

The EOCME assesses conflict of interest with its instructors, faculty, planners, and other individuals who are in a position to control the content of CME activities. All relevant conflicts of interest that are identified are thoroughly vetted by EOCME for fair balance, scientific objectivity, and patient care recommendations. EOCME is committed to providing its learners with CME activities that promote improvements or quality in healthcare and not a specific proprietary business or a commercial interest.

**The planning committee, staff, authors and editors listed below have identified no financial relationships or relationships to products or devices they or their spouse/life partner have with commercial interest related to the content of this CME activity:**

Abass Alavi, MD, MD(Hon), PhD(Hon), DSc(Hon); Abdullah Al-Zaghal, MD; Andrea Angelini, MD, PhD; Majid Assadi, MD, FASNC; Alecxih G. Austin, BS; Cyrus Ayubcha; Sandip Basu, MBBS(Hon), DRM, DNB; Tobias Bäuerle, MD; Ali Batouli, MD; Stephen M. Broski, MD; Paolo Castellucci, MD; Francesco Ceci, MD, PhD; Stephen Ellmann, MD; Ali Gholamrezanezhad, MD, FEBNM, DABR; Garry E. Gold, MD; Douglas J. Harrison, MD, MS; Hossein Jadvar, MD, PhD, MPH, MBA; Pegah Jahangiri; Venkata S. Jonnakuti, BS; Ayse T. Kendi, MD; Alison Kemp; Hedieh Khalatbari, MD, MBA; Feliks Kogan, PhD; Soheil Kooraki, MD; Esha Kothekar, MD; Torsten Kuwert, MD; Neha Kwatra, MD; George Matcuk, MD; Mohammad Hosein Najafi, MD; Marguerite T. Parisi, MD, MS; Alok Pawaskar, MBBS, DRM, DNB; David Petrov, MD; Chamith S. Rajapakse, PhD; William Y. Raynor, BS; Catherine C. Reilly, BS; Philip Ritt, PhD; Frank W. Roemer, MD; Scott Rudkin, MD; Ali Salavati, MD, MPH; Christian Schmidkonz, MD; Siavash Mehdizadeh Seraj, MD; Barry L. Shulkin, MD, MBA; Michael Uder, MD; John Vassallo; Erik Velez, MD; Vignesh Viswanathan; Thomas J. Werner, MSE; Jason R. Young, MD; Mahdi Zirakchian Zadeh, MD, MHM; Hongming Zhuang, MD, PhD.

**The planning committee, staff, authors and editors listed below have identified financial relationships or relationships to products or devices they or their spouse/life partner have with commercial interest related to the content of this CME activity:**

**Ali Guermazi, MD, PhD:** owns stock in Boston Imaging Core Lab, LLC and is a consultant/advisor for Merck KGaA, Kolon TissueGene, Inc., OrthoTrophix, Inc., AstraZeneca, and Genzyme Corporation
**Daichi Hayashi, MD, PhD:** owns stock in Boston Imaging Core Lab, LLC
**Rathan M. Subramaniam, MD, PhD, MPH:** is a consultant/advisor for Blue Earth Diagnostics Limited
**James S. Yoder, BS:** receives research support from GE Electric Company

## UNAPPROVED/OFF-LABEL USE DISCLOSURE

The EOCME requires CME faculty to disclose to the participants:
1. When products or procedures being discussed are off-label, unlabelled, experimental, and/or investigational (not US Food and Drug Administration [FDA] approved); and
2. Any limitations on the information presented, such as data that are preliminary or that represent ongoing research, interim analyses, and/or unsupported opinions. Faculty may discuss information about pharmaceutical agents that is outside of FDA-approved labelling. This information is intended solely for CME and is not intended to promote off-label use of these medications. If you have any questions, contact the medical affairs department of the manufacturer for the most recent prescribing information.

**TO ENROLL**

To enroll in the *PET Clinics* Continuing Medical Education program, call customer service at 1-800-654-2452 or sign up online at http://www.theclinics.com/home/cme. The CME program is available to subscribers for an additional annual fee of USD $235.

**METHOD OF PARTICIPATION**

In order to claim credit, participants must complete the following:

1. Complete enrolment as indicated above.
2. Read the activity.
3. Complete the CME Test and Evaluation. Participants must achieve a score of 70% on the test. All CME Tests and Evaluations must be completed online.

**CME INQUIRIES/SPECIAL NEEDS**

For all CME inquiries or special needs, please contact elsevierCME@elsevier.com

# Preface

# PET-Computed Tomography and PET-MR Imaging and Their Applications in the Twenty-First Century

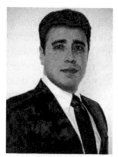

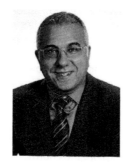

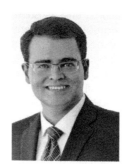

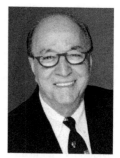

Ali Gholamrezanezhad, MD

Ali Guermazi, MD, PhD

Ali Salavati, MD, MPH

Abass Alavi, MD, MD (Hon), PhD (Hon), DSc (Hon)

*Editors*

Since the discovery of x-ray by Roentgen in 1895, planar radiography has remained a major imaging technique in assessing skeletal abnormalities with reasonable success. However, poor contrast between diseased sites and the background results in low sensitivity of this modality in detecting early disease and monitoring its course over time. The introduction of computed tomography (CT) in 1971 by Hounsfield further enhanced the role of x-ray-based disease assessment, and as such, XCT has played an important role in the day-to-day management of musculoskeletal (MSK) disorders. Since the early 1980s, when the first MR imaging instruments were introduced for human studies, the impact of imaging for examining soft tissue abnormalities in MSK disorders has been substantially enhanced. Currently, XCT and MR imaging are the main imaging modalities available in this domain but suffer from many deficiencies that need to be addressed by employing more advanced approaches. Since the early 1970s, 99m-Technitium (Tc)-labeled phosphates have been extensively used to detect benign and malignant disorders of the skeletal system. These radiotracers allow planar and tomographic imaging (SPECT [single-photon emission computed tomography]), but the quality of images generated is somewhat suboptimal for detection of the affected sites and quantification of the disease activity.

Fluorine18-sodium fluoride (18F-NaF), a positron-emitting tracer, was initially used in the early 1960s as a bone-seeking tracer but was abandoned soon after the introduction of 99m-Tc-labeled phosphates because of the limited availability of this compound and appropriate instruments. However, over the past four decades, with the introduction of PET imaging as a viable and successful molecular diagnostic modality, there is a resurgence of interest in using novel tracers in many domains, including the MSK system. This has resulted in the reintroduction of 18F-NaF for examining osseous abnormalities at the molecular level throughout the body. Furthermore, the introduction of 18F-fluorodeoxyglucose (FDG) in 1976 by the University of Pennsylvania investigators has allowed detection and monitoring of the course of a multitude of diseases and disorders, including those of soft tissue organs and the MSK system. Despite heavy emphasis being placed on FDG-PET for detection and characterization of various malignancies, increasingly, FDG is used for detection of infection and inflammation in many organs. The introduction of PET/CT in

PET Clin 14 (2019) xv–xvii
https://doi.org/10.1016/j.cpet.2018.09.001
1556-8598/19/© 2018 Published by Elsevier Inc.

pet.theclinics.com

2001 and PET/MR imaging in the past decade, as two advanced imaging modalities that combine both molecular and structural aspects, has substantially enhanced the role of PET-based technology and is expected to revolutionize the disciplines of Orthopedics and Rheumatology.

Following the experience that has been gained by the introduction of these new technologies to medical imaging, it has become apparent that structural imaging alone is insensitive and nonspecific for many clinical applications, and as such, leads to undertreatment or overtreatment of many human maladies. By now, it has become apparent that PET is substantially more sensitive and specific than either CT or MR imaging in many organ disease entities, and therefore, it will play a major role in the future practice of medicine. Combining structural imaging with PET allows precise localization of molecular abnormalities and also quantification of disease activity. Accurate quantification provided by PET is another major asset of this modality and has become an essential element for measuring response to therapeutic interventions.

Originally, FDG was introduced as a molecular probe to examine central nervous system dysfunction due to Alzheimer disease, head injury, seizure disorders, and miscellaneous neuropsychiatric diseases. Since the 1980s, when whole body imaging with PET became feasible, FDG-PET has been primarily used to manage a multitude of malignant disorders and has truly revolutionized the discipline of medical, radiation, and surgical oncology over the years. Currently, the main indication for performing FDG-PET imaging deals with diagnosis, staging, assessment of response, and detection of recurrence in most suspected or proven malignancies. However, in the past two decades, it has become quite apparent that FDG is the tracer of choice for detecting inflammation due to infection or other underlying pathologic processes. Unfortunately, because of the limited experience and published data in this domain, no medical insurance coverage reimbursement exists for adopting FDG-PET imaging in the day-to-day practice of medicine. Therefore, there is a dire need to validate and provide convincing evidence for its validity and routine use in in the future.

Recently, 18F-NaF was approved as an acceptable procedure for detecting metastasis to the skeletal system, and it provides the main clinical indication for its use in medicine. However, there is some controversy about the validity of detecting metastasis by this approach. Since cancer cells spread to the red marrow space in the skeleton, FDG-PET imaging can effectively determine evidence of metastatic disease in the skeleton with high sensitivity and specificity. In contrast, skeletal imaging with radiotracers including 18F-NaF is of limited value because of poor sensitivity and specificity. We believe performing FDG-PET will obviate using either conventional or non-FDG-PET-based techniques for detection and monitoring of metastasis to the skeleton. Therefore, it is very timely for the scientific community to explore the role of 18F-NaF for assessing a variety of benign disorders and enhance the role of medical imaging numerous disorders of the skeletal system. In addition, 18F-NaF is a powerful tracer for detection of calcification in either the skeleton or soft tissues, including in the atherosclerotic plaques in the major and coronary arteries.

Since PET allows molecular imaging of underlying biological phenomena in many human disorders, its uses in medicine, including those related to disorders of the MSK system, are limitless. Research applications of PET-based molecular imaging provide a great opportunity for scientists to explore the enormous potential of this imaging modality in assessment of MSK disorders by utilizing various novel tracers that are being tested in the rest of the body. In these two issues, we have invited world MSK experts in PET/CT/MR imaging to provide the most up-to-date and latest information about their respective domains of expertise in MSK disorders. This comprehensive review allows clinicians and scientists to realize the vast potential of this new powerful approach, and in the long run, this will substantially benefit many patients with disabling diseases and disorders of this system. We hope these two issues of *PET Clinics* encourage future studies to collect the data needed to demonstrate the excellence of PET/CT/MR imaging in the evaluation of MSK disorders. The articles in these two issues illustrate what we know about the role of PET in the MSK system and where there are gaps and holes that should be filled, and also to help recognize opportunities and benefits.

The second issue of *PET Clinics* on MSK disorders provides a detailed overview of the basic principles and technical and methodological considerations of the performance of PET/CT/MR imaging for MSK applications in a practical manner and mainly focuses on benign pathologies. This will in particular help orthopedic surgeons and rheumatologists without deep knowledge of nuclear medicine and PET technology make a foundation for successive reading and have a better understanding of the technique and the acquisition protocols. Articles also cover the application of PET/CT/MR imaging with FDG and other radiopharmaceuticals in various clinical settings. These include applications of PET in primary benign soft tissue tumors of extremities and also osteoporosis, infection, and inflammation. There are several articles centered around the role of PET imaging of the MSK system in the context of competing imaging modalities, including spectral and dual-energy CT, dynamic contrast-enhanced MR imaging, contrast-enhanced CT imaging (including iodine overlay image), and also quantitative imaging.

Ali Gholamrezanezhad, MD
Keck School of Medicine, University of Southern California (USC)
1520 San Pablo Street
Los Angeles, CA 90033, USA

Ali Guermazi, MD, PhD
Boston University School of Medicine
Boston Medical Centre
820 Harrison Avenue, FGH Building, 3rd Floor
Boston, MA 02118, USA

Ali Salavati, MD, MPH
Department of Radiology
University of Minnesota
420 Delaware Street Southeast
Minneapolis, MN 55455, USA

Abass Alavi, MD, MD (Hon), PhD (Hon), DSc (Hon)
Department of Radiology
Hospital of the University of Pennsylvania
3400 Spruce Street
Philadelphia, PA 19104, USA

*E-mail addresses:*
Ali.Gholamrezanezhad@UHhospitals.org
(A. Gholamrezanezhad)
Ali.Guermazi@bmc.org (A. Guermazi)
salavati@gmail.com (A. Salavati)
Abass.Alavi@uphs.upenn.edu (A. Alavi)

# Applications of PET–Computed Tomography–Magnetic Resonance in the Management of Benign Musculoskeletal Disorders

James S. Yoder, BS[a], Feliks Kogan, PhD[a],
Garry E. Gold, MD[a,b,c],*

## KEYWORDS

- Positron emission tomography–computed tomography (PET-CT)
- Positron emission tomography–MR imaging (PET–MR imaging) • Musculoskeletal disorders
- Imaging

## KEY POINTS

- Musculoskeletal disorders' etiologies and mechanisms can be complex where molecular changes precede structural changes.
- Earlier detection and further understanding of musculoskeletal disorders is needed for better treatment and prevention.
- Hybrid imaging systems (PET-CT and PET–MR imaging) can combine molecular information from PET with anatomic information from CT or MR imaging.
- PET-CT and PET–MR imaging have been used for imaging musculoskeletal disorders with success.
- Both hybrid modalities have the potential to be applied to more musculoskeletal disorders.

## INTRODUCTION

The advancement of different imaging modalities has allowed further understanding of the musculoskeletal system and its disorders. Imaging methods, such as radiography, ultrasound, computed tomography (CT), MR imaging, and PET, have different benefits depending on the anatomy and pathophysiology being examined. For example, CT imaging gives detailed structure of cortical and trabecular bone. MR imaging provides soft tissue contrast so that bone marrow, muscles, tendons, ligaments, cartilage, and fat can be assessed. Therefore, both CT and MR imaging provide the needed anatomic detail for musculoskeletal assessment. PET imaging provides functional information that CT and MR imaging cannot through positron-emitting radiotracers, but it is inferior to CT and MR imaging with regard to spatial resolution.[1] Given the complicated manifestation and processes of musculoskeletal disorders, a single imaging method may not be sufficient for understanding a given disorder. Furthermore, there has been a need for earlier detection of musculoskeletal disorders so that

Disclosure Statement: The authors receive research support from (GE Healthcare, Waukesha, Wisconsin).
[a] Department of Radiology, Stanford University, Stanford, CA, USA; [b] Department of Bioengineering, Stanford University, Stanford, CA, USA; [c] Department of Orthopaedic Surgery, Stanford University, Stanford, CA, USA
* Corresponding author. Department of Radiology, Stanford University, 1201 Welch Road, Stanford, CA 94305.
E-mail address: gold@stanford.edu

PET Clin 14 (2019) 1–15
https://doi.org/10.1016/j.cpet.2018.08.001

treatment and prevention plans can be more effective.

The introduction of hybrid imaging systems, such as PET-CT and PET–MR imaging, allow for the fusion of the advantages for each single imaging modality so that the complex diseases and disorders of the musculoskeletal system can be better understood. In this review, we give background information on hybrid PET-CT and PET–MR imaging and how these hybrid modalities can be applied to various musculoskeletal disorders.

## PET–COMPUTED TOMOGRAPHY AND PET–MR IMAGING

PET-CT scanners have been used in clinical medicine since the early 2000s and combine the molecular information from PET with the high resolution of CT.[2,3] PET-CT has the appeal of obtaining detailed images of the bone and its associated molecular information, which can be useful in musculoskeletal disorders. The radiotracer provides information on glucose or bone metabolism, whereas the CT provides anatomic localization and detailed bony structure.

PET–MR imaging systems have been more recently introduced and attempt to combine the advantages that each of the single imaging modalities present for musculoskeletal imaging, much like PET-CT scanners.[4,5] PET–MR imaging uses lower radiation doses when compared with PET-CT because the CT exposure component is eliminated, which is important when considering how these modalities can be applied to patient populations.[6] Furthermore, MR imaging is a favorable modality compared with CT for numerous musculoskeletal disorders because of the superior soft tissue contrast of MR imaging and how prominent soft tissue is in musculoskeletal disorders.

## PET TRACERS

Two most commonly used radiotracers for PET imaging for musculoskeletal disorders are $^{18}$F-fluorodeoxyglucose ($^{18}$F-FDG) and $^{18}$F-sodium fluoride ($^{18}$F-NaF). $^{18}$F-FDG is the most extensively used PET radiotracer in clinical practice[7,8] due to it being an analog of glucose. The use of $^{18}$F-FDG for musculoskeletal disorders is appealing because tumors, activated inflammatory cells, and sites of infection have high metabolic needs and could potentially be marked with high intensity signals on PET images.[9]

On the other hand, $^{18}$F-NaF is useful for the imaging of bony disorders because bone tissue is continuously remodeling and the $^{18}$F ions can exchange with the hydroxyl ions (-OH) on the surface of hydroxyapatite to form fluoroapatite,[10,11] which is one of the main components of bone. Therefore, $^{18}$F-NaF uptake on PET images can help to elucidate blood flow as well as osteolytic and osteoblastic activity[12,13] for bone breakdown or formation, respectively. As for musculoskeletal disorders, $^{18}$F-NaF can be useful for the assessment of metabolic bone diseases, bone graft viability, fracture healing, osteonecrosis, and tumors.

Various tissues take up these PET tracers, and interpretation of the PET signals is necessary. Although there are different ways to quantify PET tracer uptake, the most commonly used way is via standard uptake value (SUV), which is the tissue activity concentration normalized by the fraction of the injected dose/unit weight.

## APPLICATIONS

The following sections describe various applications of PET-CT and PET–MR imaging to different categories of benign musculoskeletal disorders. The categories include benign cell proliferation/dysplasia, diabetic foot complications, joint prostheses, inflammation, metabolic bone disorders, and pain (acute and chronic) and peripheral nerve imaging.

## BENIGN CELL PROLIFERATION/DYSPLASIA

PET-CT and PET–MR imaging has shown promise in the imaging of primary, benign tumors of the musculoskeletal system. Tumors of the musculoskeletal system may be present in the bone, bone marrow, cartilage, or other types of soft tissue sarcomas. Like most disorders of the musculoskeletal system, radiographs or CT have been used for a longer period for imaging, whereas the value of MR imaging has only recently been utilized. Radiography and CT have been valuable imaging modalities in the detection of subtle matrix calcifications and hence can be useful in confirming the diagnosis of a bone-forming or cartilage-forming tumor.[14–18]

On the other hand, MR imaging alone is generally accepted as the most sensitive imaging method for defining the extent of bone tumors, but it is thought to be less specific than x-ray based techniques in differential diagnosis.[19] MR imaging is useful for the evaluation of primary tumors that originate from anatomic sites that are not optimally evaluated with CT, such as connective tissue, soft tissue, and bone marrow, due to the soft tissue contrast providing high spatial resolution definition of tumor volume and staging.[20,21] The feasibility of MR imaging–based bone marrow segmentation by using software techniques for quantitative calculation of pure red marrow metabolism at FDG PET has been reported,[22] which could be useful in the clinical evaluation of benign bone marrow disorders.

FDG PET can be used to examine red marrow activity and to detect involvement in benign processes, such as chronic anemia and myelofibrosis, because these processes lead to increased hematopoiesis and reconversion of yellow to red marrow.[1] The advantage of using FDG PET is that it can detect metabolically active lesions, whereas CT can provide spatial information regarding the bone marrow. A disadvantage of using FDG PET to image bone marrow happens when a patient is undergoing granulocyte colony-stimulating factor therapy, which causes a physiologic response of increased metabolic processes in the bone marrow. The increased FDG uptake in the bone marrow can mimic diffuse metastatic disease, so caution needs to be applied if PET imaging is being used to image bone marrow.

Myelofibrosis is a hematopoietic stem cell neoplasm characterized by bone marrow inflammation, reactive bone marrow fibrosis, and extramedullary hematopoiesis. One study used $^{18}$F-FDG PET-CT to noninvasively visualize and quantify the extent and activity of bone marrow involvement in patients with myelofibrosis (**Fig. 1**).[23] The investigators concluded that the intensity of bone marrow $^{18}$F-FDG uptake decreases as bone marrow fibrosis increases, and $^{18}$F-FDG PET-CT is a promising technique for the quantitation of bone marrow inflammation in myelofibrosis. Further studies are needed to assess $^{18}$F-NaF PET and possible PET–MR imaging for myelofibrosis.

Fibrous dysplasia is a benign disorder in which fibrous tissue replaces bone. One of the issues with imaging fibrous dysplasia is that it may show an increase in FDG uptake and therefore mimic malignant bone involvement in FDG PET. Being able to distinguish fibrous dysplasia from malignant tumors or lymphoma is important for patients and clinicians. A case study that used combined FDG PET-CT scanning on a patient with known fibrous dysplasia found an elevation in the uptake of FDG in numerous locations that were identified as fibrous dysplasia by CT.[24] The investigators concluded that FDG PET coregistered with CT might help to distinguish fibrous dysplasia from osseous malignancies. Furthermore, because fibrous dysplasia is characterized by changes in bone remodeling, or the loss of bone, $^{18}$F-NaF PET imaging with CT or MR imaging might help to assess the severity of the disease and track patients' responses to bisphosphonate therapy.

Because $^{18}$F-NaF PET imaging is not specific for malignant tumors and can accumulate in benign osseous abnormalities, hybrid imaging via PET-CT or PET–MR imaging can help to differentiate tumors with accuracy better than PET alone. For example, one study compared $^{18}$F-NaF PET-CT with PET alone and found the specificity for lesions to be 97% and 72%, respectively, and for patients to be 88% and 56%, respectively.[25]

## DIABETIC FOOT COMPLICATIONS

Diabetes can lead to a number of complications in the foot, including vascular disease, Charcot neuropathy, soft tissue infection, and osteomyelitis.[26] It can be challenging to form a definitive diagnosis from MR imaging because signal abnormalities in the bone and bone marrow can be nonspecific to the different diseases. PET–MR imaging has the potential to differentiate between each of these diseases so that the patient can be optimally treated and further damage can be halted.

For example, Basu and colleagues[27] found that there was a significant difference in FDG uptake in an uncomplicated diabetic foot, a foot with Charcot neuroarthropathy, and a foot with osteomyelitis. The sensitivity and accuracy for diagnosis of Charcot neuroarthropathy were 100% and 93.8% for FDG PET, and 76.9% and 75.0% for MR imaging. Additionally, in a patient population with a complicated diabetic foot, FDG PET had a sensitivity, specificity, and accuracy of 81%, 93%, and 90% for osteomyelitis diagnosis, and 91%, 78%, and 81%, respectively, for MR imaging (**Fig. 2**).[28] These results demonstrate that FDG PET and MR imaging can differentiate between Charcot neuroarthropathy and osteomyelitis, but more research is needed to investigate if PET–MR imaging hybrid imaging can increase the sensitivity, specificity, and accuracy of diagnosing patients within the diabetic foot population.

## JOINT PROSTHESES

Joint replacement can be commonly accompanied with postoperative pain. Aseptic loosening or infection can cause this pain, and it is a clinical challenge to differentiate between these 2 causes of pain.[29] CT and MR imaging are used for patients who have pain related to arthroplasty, but the images from CT and MR imaging can be inconclusive due to the metal artifacts from the prosthesis. Recent methods have been shown to improve MR imaging around joint replacements.[30]

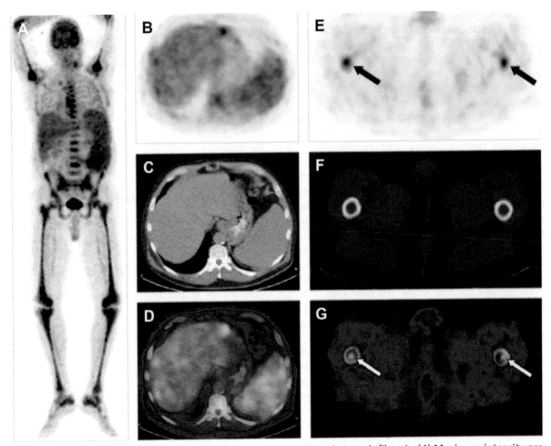

**Fig. 1.** PET-CT images of 60-year-old man with histopathological grade I myelofibrosis. (*A*) Maximum intensity projection image with high ¹⁸F-FDG uptake in the spleen and bone marrow extending into the small bones of the feet. (*B*) Transaxial PET, (*C*) CT, and (*D*) PET-CT show splenic uptake. (*E*) Transaxial PET, (*F*) CT, and (*G*) PET-CT images show femoral bone marrow uptake (*arrows*). The increased ¹⁸F-FDG uptake in this patient with histopathological grade I myelofibrosis indicates an early and highly active state of the disease. (*Reprinted by permission from* Springer Nature. From Derlin T, Alchalby H, Bannas P, et al. Assessment of bone marrow inflammation in patients with myelofibrosis: an 18F-fluorodeoxyglucose PET/CT study. Eur J Nucl Med Mol Imaging 2015;42:696.)

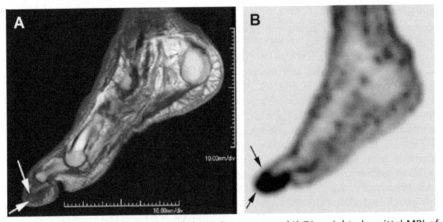

**Fig. 2.** Diabetic male presented with an ulcer of the right great toe. (*A*) T1-weighted sagittal MRI of right foot with loss of signal intensity in great toe (*white arrows*), suggestive of osteomyelitis. (*B*) PET with increased FDG uptake at the corresponding site of abnormality (*black arrows*). The PET scan further confirmed the diagnosis of osteomyelitis in the great toe. (*Reprinted by permission from* Springer Nature. From Nawaz A, Torigian DA, Siegelman ES, et al. Diagnostic performance of FDG-PET, MRI, and plain film radiography (PFR) for the diagnosis of osteomyelitis in the diabetic foot. Mol Imaging Biol 2010;12(3):337.)

FDG PET has a potential role in detecting infections in hip and knee prostheses because the imaging modality is not affected by metal artifacts. Chryssikos and colleagues[31] performed a study on patients with hip prostheses and pain. PET images were suggestive of septic loosening if increased FDG uptake was found at the stem-prosthesis interface, whereas uptake adjacent to the prosthesis neck was interpreted as a nonspecific reaction. Twenty-eight of 35 positive studies were confirmed as infected, whereas 87 of 92 negative studies were confirmed aseptic. The sensitivity, specificity, positive predictive value, and negative predictive value of FDG PET were 85%, 93%, 80%, and 95%, respectively. Furthermore, a study involving 38 hip prostheses and 36 knee prostheses found the sensitivity, specificity, and accuracy of FDG PET for detecting infection were 90.0%, 89.3%, and 89.5%, respectively, for hip prostheses, and 90.9%, 72.0%, and 77.8%, respectively, for knee prostheses.[32] These studies demonstrate how FDG PET can be used to accurately diagnose and differentiate septic and aseptic causes of pain in hip and knee prostheses. Combining these PET techniques with methods for multispectral MR imaging[33] may provide an effective way of diagnosing total joint infection without an invasive fluid aspiration and correcting for distortions from metal artifacts. There have been studies using PET–MR imaging and PET-CT-MR imaging that have had success in metal artifact correction[34,35] so using PET-CT or PET–MR imaging to image prostheses is possible and continues to be researched.

F-NaF PET can also be used to measure bone blood flow and bone viability when determining if a joint replacement is necessary or has been successful. Schiepers and colleagues[36] found that a decrease in blood flow or a decrease in $^{18}$F-NaF uptake predicted the need for joint arthroplasty. Furthermore, 2 studies that investigated the uptake of $^{18}$F-NaF in the bone graft used in hip arthroplasties found that the uptake in the allograft was similar to the adjacent cortical bone immediately after surgery. However, the uptake decreased in the allograft compared with the adjacent cortical bone (9 months to 5 years postsurgery), which indicated normal bony incorporation.[37,38]

## DEGENERATION, INFLAMMATION, AND TRAUMA

The metabolic information of PET and the anatomic differentiation from MR imaging are complementary for the evaluation of various arthritides and for treatment monitoring. Musculoskeletal disorders involving degeneration, inflammation, and trauma have the potential to be identified through FDG PET because activated inflamed cells have higher metabolic activity and through $^{18}$F-NaF PET because some of these disorders involve bone remodeling. The combination of PET and MR imaging has promise in these musculoskeletal disorders because there is a need for biomarkers to detect these diseases at a reversible stage before tissue loss and degeneration.

## Osteoarthritis

Osteoarthritis (OA) is a disease of the entire joint, which affects tissues such as bone, cartilage, menisci, ligaments, and synovial tissue.[39] Although it is expected to affect 25% of the US adult population by 2030,[40] the disease process of OA is still poorly understood, especially the early changes. Recent advances in understanding of OA have shown that the disease process involves multiple joint tissues, is influenced by biomechanics, and may have an inflammatory component in some patients.

MR imaging alone is a noninvasive imaging technique that has been used to study OA. The appeal of MR imaging is its ability to produce varying contrasts, which allows for the assessment of soft tissue quality (ie, cartilage, menisci, ligaments), bone changes (ie, bone marrow lesions, cysts, osteophytes), and synovitis presence.[39,41] Even with the high utility of MR imaging in identifying structural changes associated with OA, these changes are typically at a later stage in the OA disease process where tissue loss has occurred, and anatomic MR imaging cannot give insight into the physiologic mechanisms leading to OA.

$^{18}$F-NaF PET can help detect changes in bone remodeling, which can be applied to OA because increased bone remodeling leading to changes in bone and cartilage has been linked to the progression of OA.[42,43] For example, SUV$_{max}$ was significantly elevated in hip joints with abnormal findings in bone on MR imaging, and the severity of hip pain positively correlated with SUV$_{max}$.[44] Similarly, patellofemoral pain coincided with increased metabolic activity in bone at the patellofemoral joint.[45] Furthermore, abnormal findings in bone on MR imaging overlapped with areas of increased $^{18}$F-NaF uptake on PET images, but, notably, increased SUV$_{max}$ on $^{18}$F-NaF PET did not always match to bone or cartilage degeneration found on MR imaging.[46] The associations between symptoms of OA, increased $^{18}$F-NaF uptake, and abnormal findings on MR imaging shows how PET–MR imaging hybrid needs to be studied further, as it presents an opportunity to combine the metabolic information of PET with the structural information of MR imaging to detect OA progression.

Similar to $^{18}$F-NaF, $^{18}$F-FDG has the potential to elucidate OA progression but through its role of characterizing inflammation via increased glucose usage in tissues. Synovitis is inflammation of the synovial membrane in joints and has been recognized as a part of the progression of OA.[47,48] According to studies that assessed patients with clinically diagnosed OA of the shoulder and knee, there was an increase in $^{18}$F-FDG uptake when comparing the patients with healthy volunteers, which was interpreted as presence of synovitis.[49,50] FDG PET–MR imaging could allow for identification of synovitis while visualizing the entire joint for other abnormalities that are present in OA.

Furthermore, bone marrow lesions (BMLs) are hypothesized to have an inflammatory element, and they play a role in the progression of OA.[51] Typically, BMLs are identified through MR imaging, but PET–MR imaging could be a resource to further study the inflammatory mechanism of BMLs. A study on the use of PET–MR imaging for possible OA identification found that BMLs observed on MR imaging correlated with high $^{18}$F-fluoride PET uptake identified as volumes of interest ($VOI_{High}$) 33 (97%) of 34 times (**Fig. 3**).[52] Also, the $SUV_{max}$ in all subchondral bone lesions (BMLs, osteophytes, sclerosis) was significantly elevated compared with the $SUV_{max}$ for normal-appearing bone, as identified on MR imaging. Of note, the uptake of $^{18}$F-FDG in subchondral BMLs was much lower than the uptake of $^{18}$F-fluoride, which suggests that bone remodeling processes might play a larger role in BMLs compared with inflammatory processes. The overlap in information from MR imaging and PET in the study demonstrates the reliability of the 2 modalities in identifying BMLs and other mechanisms thought to play a role in osteoarthritis development. Therefore, PET–MR imaging could be used to detect BMLs and other mechanisms at an earlier time in the progression of OA.

### Rheumatoid Arthritis

Rheumatoid arthritis (RA) is the most common form of inflammatory arthritis and affects 1% of the population.[53] It is a systemic inflammatory autoimmune disorder and affects joints of varying sizes. Although the disease has numerous etiologies, it is predominantly characterized by degenerative synovitis with leukocyte infiltration and proliferation, which leads to cartilage and bone degradation. RA typically progresses more rapidly than OA and most diagnoses for RA occur at a late stage in the disease process. Furthermore, better patient outcomes are dependent on administering aggressive anti-inflammatory drugs early in the disease progression; earlier detection of RA through novel methods has become imperative.

Given that FDG builds up in activated leukocytes and inflammation is a key part of RA pathogenesis, FDG PET is a logical tracer that could be used to reveal the inflammatory process before further changes such as hyperemia and erosion are seen on other radiographic imaging modalities.[54–56] A study that used FDG PET to examine the joints of patients with RA found that the number of PET-positive joints and the cumulative SUV were significantly correlated with RA disease

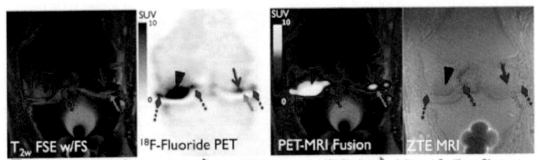

**Fig. 3.** $^{18}$F-Fluoride PET (SUV) and MR imaging images of a male patient with posttraumatic osteoarthritis showing concordance between a BML (*blue arrowhead*) and osteophytes (*red diamond arrows*) on MR imaging with high $^{18}$F-fluoride uptake on PET. Additionally, a focal region of high uptake on PET (*magenta line arrow*) did not exhibit bone abnormalities on MR imaging but was adjacent to a grade 2 cartilage defect (*light blue solid arrow*). (*From* Kogan F, Fan AP, McWalter EJ, et al. PET/MRI of metabolic activity in osteoarthritis: a feasibility study. J Magn Reson Imaging 2017;45(6):1737; with permission.)

activity (**Fig. 4**).[57] Animal models with induced RA have shown that increased FDG uptake correlated with imminent bone destruction and pannus formation.[58]

Alternatively, other PET tracers may be able to elucidate parts of RA processes. One study found that both the uptake of [11]C-choline, a measure of cell proliferation, and the uptake of [18]F-FDG correlated highly with the volume of synovium, which suggests [11]C-Choline could be a promising tracer for quantitative imaging of proliferative arthritis changes.[59] Additionally, the PET tracer, [11]C-(*R*)-PK11195, tags macrophages in the inflammatory response so it could provide a direct measure of the inflammation associated with RA.[60,61]

Similar to OA, RA has been studied with hybrid imaging modalities with further research still ongoing. MR imaging enables synovial inflammation to be delineated as contrast-enhanced lesions with high anatomic resolution, especially for finger lesions in RA.[62] MR imaging also has recently advanced capabilities that could aid in the diagnosis and treatment of RA. For example, early detection of bone erosions can influence the type of treatment,[63] and scoring systems that evaluate RA features based on MR imaging can be used to

monitor responses to treatments.[64] Furthermore, measurement of apparent diffusion coefficient and pharmacokinetic modeling of Gadolinium enhancement and washout are new MR imaging methods that could allow for more understanding of RA pathogenesis.[65] There has been a study that used a hybrid PET–MR imaging system to study early RA in the hand, and it found that FDG uptake overlapped with sites of synovitis and tenosynovitis, which are components of RA progression (**Fig. 5**).[66] It has been demonstrated that PET–MR imaging can be used to image the inflammation associated with RA, but further studies using the hybrid modality are needed. Furthermore, RA is usually not isolated to a single joint and affects joints throughout the body, so the application of PET–MR imaging needs to have the possibility of imaging many joints.

Relative to PET–MR imaging studies on RA, PET-CT has been used for a longer period of time. A study that examined patients with RA found that whole-body FDG PET-CT delineated large joint lesions in patients with RA, and the metabolic activity of inflammation was accurately overlaid on the anatomy of the joints.[67] Furthermore, the investigators

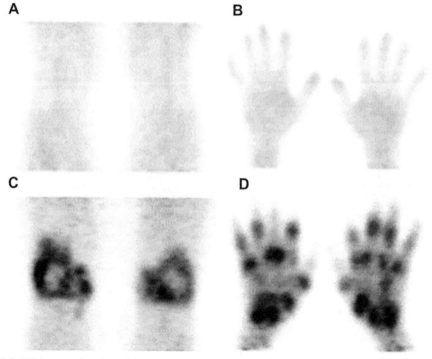

**Fig. 4.** [18]F-FDG PET images. (*A, B*) Healthy control subject. (*C, D*) Patient with RA with active disease. (*A*) Three-dimensional projection image of normal tracer distribution in knee. (*B*) Normal distribution in hand and wrist. (*C*) Rheumatoid knee and (*D*) rheumatoid hand and wrist with elevated FDG uptake. (*From* JNM. Beckers C, Ribbens C, André B, et al. Assessment of disease activity in rheumatoid arthritis with (18)F-FDG PET. J Nucl Med 2004;45:956–64. © Society of Nuclear Medicine and Molecular Imaging.)

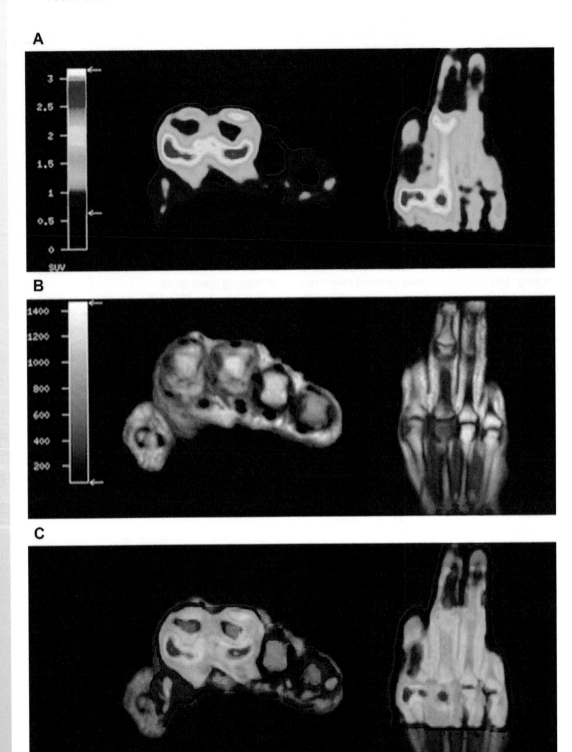

**Fig. 5.** Hybrid [18]F-FDG PET–MR imaging of the hand in early RA. (*A*) Axial and coronal images of PET coregistered with (*B*) axial and coronal T1-weighted MR imaging. (*C*) True hybrid [18]F-FDG PET–MR imaging of the hand. (*Reprinted by permission from* Springer Nature. From Miese F, Scherer A, Ostendorf B, et al. Hybrid [18]F-FDG PET-MRI of the hand in rheumatoid arthritis: initial results. Clin Rheumatol 2011;30:1247–50.)

concluded that the FDG PET-CT findings represented the inflammatory activity in large joints in patients with RA accurately and sensitively and could be helpful for early evaluations of the extent of RA throughout the whole body, including high-risk lesions of the atlantoaxial joint. The PET-CT system also could differentiate increased FDG uptake by enthesopathies from synovitis due to RA.

## Trauma

Musculoskeletal trauma includes injuries to bone, cartilage, tendons, ligaments, and muscle. These injuries are accompanied by the body's inflammation response, so theoretically PET-CT and PET–MR imaging could be used to assess these injuries and manage the recovery process, molecularly and structurally. For example, PET–MR imaging cannot only be used to depict meniscal tears and their exact locations, but also the severity of the tear and the associated synovitis.[1,68,69] This specific information could help to reduce exploratory arthroscopies/surgeries and aid in the surgical repair or meniscectomy.

Similarly, PET–MR imaging and PET-CT could be used to reveal the presence, severity, and recovery of ligament and tendon tears with greater accuracy. Anterior cruciate ligament (ACL) injuries are of particular interest due to their high frequency and the associated postinjury osteoarthritis development.[70] One study investigated the development of posttraumatic OA (PTOA) after ACL transection (ACLT) of the knee in 5 in vivo canine models with Na[18]F PET-CT coregistered with MR imaging scanning (**Fig. 6**).[71] It was found that before ACLT, both knees of all canines did not show Na[18]F uptake above background. The uptake of Na[18]F in the bone of the ACLT knees posttransection increased exponentially, presenting significantly higher uptake at 12 weeks in every region compared with the ACLT knees at baseline. The investigators concluded that Na[18]F PET-CT coregistered with MR imaging is a feasible molecular imaging biomarker to assess knee osseous metabolic changes serially in an in vivo canine model of knee PTOA. Therefore, PET-CT coregistered with MR imaging could be used to track ACL reconstruction healing and associated PTOA development.

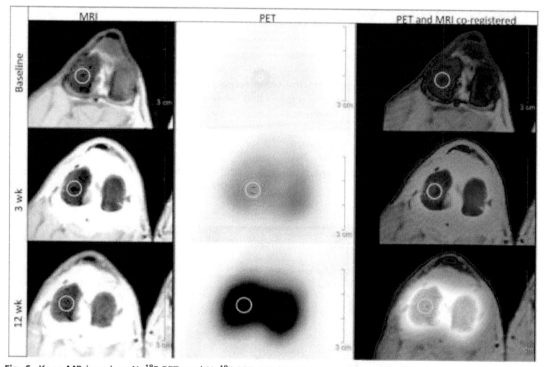

**Fig. 6.** Knee MR imaging, Na[18]F PET, and Na[18]F PET–MR imaging coregistered (*left to right*). Axial views of the knee femoral condyles at baseline, 3 weeks, and 12 weeks after ACLT (*top to bottom*). The images show Na[18]F background uptake at baseline, higher uptake at 3 weeks, and significantly higher uptake at 12 weeks post-ACLT (*bottom row*). The elevated uptake represented increased bone metabolism, caused by the injury-induced trauma. (*From* Menendez MI, Hettlich B, Wei L, et al. Feasibility of Na18F PET/CT and MRI for noninvasive in vivo quantification of knee pathophysiological bone metabolism in a canine model of post-traumatic osteoarthritis. Mol Imaging 2017;16:1536012117714575; with permission.)

A recent study examined ACL grafts after ACL reconstruction surgery in a human population using PET–MR imaging (**Fig. 7**).[72] The study found that metabolic activity was significantly lower in grafts that were imaged more than 2 years after reconstruction relative to those grafts that had been in place for shorter periods of time. The investigators concluded that [18]FDG PET–MR imaging can assess the metabolic activity of ACL grafts in vivo. [18]FDG PET–MR imaging can provide insight into the process of graft ligamentization in patients following ACL reconstruction, which could impact graft selection and recovery timelines for patients.

## METABOLIC BONE DISORDERS

Metabolic bone disorders are often associated with changes in bone turnover and metabolism that can lead to bone fractures, bone deformities, and disability if untreated. Hence, [18]F-NaF and FDG are logical PET tracers to use when tracking these diseases, and MR imaging and CT provide the anatomic detail needed. Studies have shown that maximum SUVs for [18]F-NaF PET correlate well with net uptake of fluoride to bone mineral and osteoblastic activity due to disease.[73] Furthermore, treatments that lead to a decrease in osteoblastic activity correlate with a decrease in SUV, so SUV can be used to assess these metabolic bone disorders.

Paget disease involves increases in the resorption and formation of bone, which leads to fragile and misshapen bones.[74] Treatment for Paget disease relies on reducing the breakdown of bone, typically through the administration of bisphosphonates,[75] so [18]F-NaF PET could be used to assess patients' responses to medication.[76]

A study used [18]F-NaF PET to examine patients with renal osteodystrophy and found that the incorporation of [18]F-NaF into bone correlated closely with serum alkaline phosphatase, a marker of bone turnover and serum parathyroid hormone levels.[77] Additionally, the incorporation of [18]F-NaF into bone correlated well with histomorphometric indices of bone turnover in iliac crest biopsies. The indices were higher in patients with high-turnover renal osteodystrophy and lower in patients with low bone turnover or healthy subjects.

[18]F-NaF PET has been used to study osteoporosis, specifically in postmenopausal women. Compared with premenopausal women, postmenopausal women have been found to experience increased bone turnover.[78,79] A study on postmenopausal women used [18]F-NaF PET and found a significant difference in bone turnover between patients treated with hormone replacement and untreated women,[80] which demonstrates the utility of using [18]F-NaF PET to monitor changes in bone turnover in patients undergoing treatment for osteoporosis.

[18]F-FDG PET has the potential to differentiate between traumatic fractures and fractures due to malignancies. Studies have found that acute osteoporotic or traumatic fractures do not show increases in [18]F-FDG uptake.[81,82] On the contrary, fractures due to malignant or infectious processes do show increases in [18]F-FDG uptake via increased glucose needs of macrophages and other inflammatory cells. Therefore, [18]F-FDG could be used to distinguish fracture types throughout the body.

The metabolic information from PET about bone remodeling/strength could supplement the information from CT or MR imaging for metabolic bone disorders such as osteoporosis,

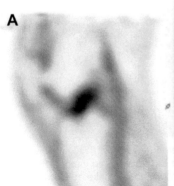
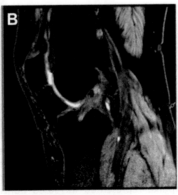
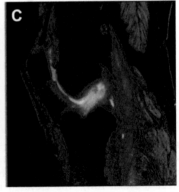

**Fig. 7.** (*A*) PET image, (*B*) MR image, and (*C*) combined PET–MR image of an ACL graft. PET–MR imaging can help to track and manage ACL reconstruction recovery. (*From* Magnussen RA, Binzel K, Zhang J, et al. ACL graft metabolic activity assessed by 18FDG PET-MRI. Arthroscopy 2017;33(10):e79; with permission.)

osteomalacia, Paget disease, parathyroid disorders, and renal osteodystrophy. One of the advantages of using hybrid PET-CT or PET–MR imaging systems for imaging metabolic disorders is that the molecular changes often precede the structural changes (ie, fractures, bone deformities) so hybrid imaging could highlight both of these changes if they are present.

## PAIN (ACUTE AND CHRONIC) AND PERIPHERAL NERVE IMAGING

Acute and chronic pain continues to be a heavily researched topic given patients' varying experiences and the frequency of patients seeking medical assistance for pain. The imaging of pain is challenging and focuses on potential anatomic abnormalities. However, anatomic variation is present throughout patient populations, so a consistent, quantitative imaging modality could help to elucidate potential causes or sites of pain.

FDG PET imaging has shown promise in identifying pain because uptake of FDG is increased when inflamed or overactive neurons have increased metabolic needs for glucose. For example, a study that used rat models found that there was an increase in FDG uptake in injured nerves after the rats had unilateral, induced neuropathic limb pain (**Fig. 8**).[83] Additionally, there was not an increase in FDG uptake in the contralateral, or uninjured, limbs or in the control animals. FDG PET-CT scanning has been done on a human subject who initially presented with progressive difficulty walking, and an increase in FDG uptake was found in his lower spinal cord and sciatic

nerves.[84] A biopsy of the nerves confirmed neuropathy. A study using PET–MR imaging on patients with neuropathic pain of the lower extremities found that FDG uptake could be localized to the affected nerves.[85]

Other PET tracers have the potential to identify pain-related activity, such as [11]C-PK11195 and [18]F-FTC-146. [11]C-PK11195 can image neuroinflammation because it can mark activated microglia and macrophages.[86,87] [18]F-FTC-146, a recently discovered tracer, has the potential to directly assess signaling pathways because it marks sigma 1 receptors, which have been implicated in nociception.[88] It has been recently determined that [18]F-FTC-146 is safe for use in humans, and human studies using PET–MR imaging have been initiated.[89]

According to the Global Burden of Disease 2010 Study, the estimated prevalence of low back pain was 9.4%.[90] PET has the potential to identify low back pain and back pain in general, especially in spondylolysis. Because [18]F-NaF PET characterizes bone remodeling, it may be able to show osseous changes before fractures develop. In a study assessing adolescents with back pain, the investigators concluded that 18F-sodium fluoride PET-CT can detect spinal lesions with high diagnostic accuracy.[91] Another study that included patients who presented with back pain found that [18]F-NaF PET-CT showed abnormal uptake in the spine of 84% of the patients.[92]

Although MR imaging and CT provide high-resolution images of peripheral nerves and general anatomy, they have difficulty specifying sites of nerve inflammation or injury. Hybrid PET–MR

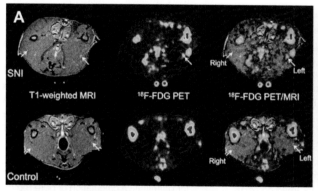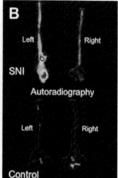

**Fig. 8.** (*A*) Spared-nerve injury (SNI) (*top row*) and control (*bottom row*) rat models showing sciatic nerves (*arrows*) on transaxial MR imaging, PET, and PET–MR imaging. [18]F-FDG PET–MR imaging showed significantly increased [18]F-FDG uptake on the side with SNI (*left*), compared with control side (*right*). Control animals did not show any significant difference between right and left nerves. (*B*) Autoradiography of sciatic nerve specimens from SNI animals showed that normalized radiotracer uptake is higher in injured sciatic nerve (*left*) than in control sciatic nerve (*right*). (*From* Behera D, Jacobs KE, Behera S, et al. (18)F-FDG PET-MRI can be used to identify injured peripheral nerves in a model of neuropathic pain. J Nucl Med 2011;52:1308–12. © Society of Nuclear Medicine and Molecular Imaging.)

imaging and PET-CT imaging modalities can combine the PET information that can potentially localize pain with the MR imaging or CT information that can identify abnormal anatomy. Given the novelty of imaging pain and using hybrid imaging modalities, more research in human subjects is warranted.

## SUMMARY

PET–MR imaging and PET-CT are recently available advanced tools for the diagnosis of musculoskeletal disorders. These methods show considerable promise to improve early detection and characterization of disorders. Currently [18]F-FDG is useful for detection of changes in glucose metabolism, whereas [18]F-NaF is useful to see early areas of bone remodeling. New radiotracers combined with these modalities promise even more specificity for diagnosis of benign musculoskeletal disease.

## REFERENCES

1. Chen K, Blebea J, Laredo JD, et al. Evaluation of musculoskeletal disorders with PET, PET/CT, and PET/MRI. PET Clin 2008;3(3):451–65.
2. Brady Z, Taylor ML, Haynes M, et al. The clinical application of PET/CT: a contemporary review. Australas Phys Eng Sci Med 2008;31:90–109.
3. Griffeth LK. Use of PET/CT scanning in cancer patients: technical and practical considerations. Proc (Bayl Univ Med Cent) 2005;18:321–30.
4. Judenhofer MS, Wehrl HF, Newport DF, et al. Simultaneous PET-MRI: a new approach for functional and morphological imaging. Nat Med 2008; 14:459–65.
5. Chaudhry AA, Gul M, Gould E, et al. Utility of positron emission tomography-magnetic resonance imaging in musculoskeletal imaging. World J Radiol 2016;8:268–74.
6. Hirsch FW, Sattler B, Sorge I, et al. PET/MR in children. Initial clinical experience in paediatric oncology using an integrated PET/MR scanner. Pediatr Radiol 2013;43:860–75.
7. Etchebehere EC, Hobbs BP, Milton DR, et al. Assessing the role of (1)(8)F-FDG PET and (1)(8)F-FDG PET/CT in the diagnosis of soft tissue musculoskeletal malignancies: a systematic review and meta-analysis. Eur J Nucl Med Mol Imaging 2016; 43:860–70.
8. Schelbert HR, Hoh CK, Royal HD, et al. Procedure guideline for tumor imaging using fluorine-18-FDG. Society of nuclear medicine. J Nucl Med 1998;39: 1302–5.
9. Crymes WB Jr, Demos H, Gordon L. Detection of musculoskeletal infection with 18F-FDG PET: review of the current literature. J Nucl Med Technol 2004; 32:12–5.
10. Czernin J, Satyamurthy N, Schiepers C. Molecular mechanisms of bone 18F-NaF deposition. J Nucl Med 2010;51:1826–9.
11. Schiepers C, Nuyts J, Bormans G, et al. Fluoride kinetics of the axial skeleton measured in vivo with fluorine-18-fluoride PET. J Nucl Med 1997;38: 1970–6.
12. Kobayashi N, Inaba Y, Tateishi U, et al. New application of 18F-fluoride PET for the detection of bone remodeling in early-stage osteoarthritis of the hip. Clin Nucl Med 2013;38:e379–83.
13. Blau M, Ganatra R, Bender MA. 18 F-flouride for bone imaging. Semin Nucl Med 1972;2:31–7.
14. Forest M, Coindre JM, Diebold J. Pathology of tumors. In: Forest M, Tomeno B, Vanel D, editors. Orthopedic surgical pathology: diagnosis of tumors and pseudotumoral lesions of bone and joints. Edinburgh (Scotland): Churchill Livingstone; 1997.
15. Resnick D. Tumors and tumor-like lesions of bone: radiographic principles. In: Resnick D, editor. Diagnosis of bone and joint disorders. Philadelphia: Saunders; 1995. p. 3613–27.
16. Resnick D, Kyriakos M, Greenway GD. Tumors and tumor-like lesions of bone: imaging and pathology of specific lesions. In: Resnick D, editor. Diagnosis of bone and joint disorders. Philadelphia: Saunders; 1995. p. 3628–938.
17. Magid D. Two-dimensional and three-dimensional computed tomographic imaging in musculoskeletal tumors. Radiol Clin North Am 1993;31:425–47.
18. Bloem JL, Kroon HM. Imaging of bone and soft tissue tumors: osseous lesions. Radiol Clin North Am 1993;31:261–78.
19. Berquist TH. Magnetic resonance imaging of primary skeletal neoplasms. Radiol Clin North Am 1993;31:411–24.
20. Torigian DA, Zaidi H, Kwee TC, et al. PET/MR imaging: technical aspects and potential clinical applications. Radiology 2013;267:26–44.
21. Torigian DA, Lopez RF, Alapati S, et al. Feasibility and performance of novel software to quantify metabolically active volumes and 3D partial volume corrected SUV and metabolic volumetric products of spinal bone marrow metastases on 18F-FDG-PET/CT. Hell J Nucl Med 2011;14(1):8–14.
22. Basu S, Houseni M, Bural G, et al. Magnetic resonance imaging based bone marrow segmentation for quantitative calculation of pure red marrow metabolism using 2-deoxy-2-[F-18]fluoro-D-glucose-positron emission tomography: a novel application with significant implications for combined structure-function approach. Mol Imaging Biol 2007;9(6): 361–5.
23. Derlin T, Alchalby H, Bannas P, et al. Assessment of bone marrow inflammation in patients with

myelofibrosis: an [18]F-fluorodeoxyglucose PET/CT study. Eur J Nucl Med Mol Imaging 2015;42:696.

24. Stegger L, Juergens KU, Kliesch S, et al. Unexpected finding of elevated glucose uptake in fibrous dysplasia mimicking malignancy: contradicting metabolism and morphology in combined PET/CT. Eur Radiol 2007;17:1784.

25. Langsteger W, Heinisch M, Fogelman I. The role of fluorodeoxyglucose, 18F-dihydroxyphenylalanine, 18F-choline, and 18F-fluoride in bone imaging with emphasis on prostate and breast. Semin Nucl Med 2006;36:73–92.

26. Lipsky BA, Berendt AR, Deery HG, et al. Diagnosis and treatment of diabetic foot infections. Plast Reconstr Surg 2006;117:212S–38S.

27. Basu S, Chyrssikos T, Houseni M, et al. Potential role of FDG PET in the setting of diabetic nueroosteoarthropathy: can it differentiate uncomplicated Charcot's neuroarthropathy from osteomyelitis and soft-tissue infection? Nucl Med Commun 2007; 28(6):465–72.

28. Nawaz A, Torigian DA, Siegelman ES, et al. Diagnostic performance of FDG-PET, MRI, and plain film radiography (PFR) for the diagnosis of osteomyelitis in the diabetic foot. Mol Imaging Biol 2010; 12(3):335–42.

29. Furnes O, Lie SA, Espehaug B, et al. Hip disease and the prognosis of total hip replacements. A review of 53,698 primary total hip replacements reported to the Norwegian Arthroplasty Register 1987-99. J Bone Joint Surg Br 2001;83:579–86.

30. Lu W, Pauly KB, Gold GE, et al. SEMAC: slice encoding for metal artifact correction in MRI. Magn Reson Med 2009;62:66–76.

31. Chryssikos T, Parvizi J, Ghanem E, et al. FDG-PET imaging can diagnose periprosthetic infection of the hip. Clin Orthop Relat Res 2008; 466:1338–42.

32. Zhuang H, Duarte PS, Pourdehnad M, et al. The promising role of 18F-FDG PET in detecting infected lower limb prosthesis implants. J Nucl Med 2001;42: 44–8.

33. Koch KM, Lorbiecki JE, Hinks RS, et al. A multispectral three-dimensional acquisition technique for imaging near metal implants. Magn Reson Med 2009;61:381–90.

34. Ladefoged CN, Andersen FL, Keller SH, et al. PET/MR imaging of the pelvis in the presence of endoprostheses: reducing image artifacts and increasing accuracy through inpainting. Eur J Nucl Med Mol Imaging 2013;40:594–601.

35. Gunzinger JM, Delso G, Boss A, et al. Metal artifact reduction in patients with dental implants using multispectral three-dimensional data acquisition for hybrid PET/MRI. EJNMMI Phys 2014;1:102.

36. Schiepers C, Broos P, Miserez M, et al. Measurement of skeletal flow with positron emission tomography and 18F-fluoride in femoral head osteonecrosis. Arch Orthop Trauma Surg 1998;118: 131–5.

37. Piert M, Winter E, Becker GA, et al. Allogenic bone graft viability after hip revision arthroplasty assessed by dynamic [18F]fluoride ion positron emission tomography. Eur J Nucl Med 1999;26:615–24.

38. Sorensen J, Ullmark G, Langstrom B, et al. Rapid bone and blood flow formation in impacted morselized allografts: positron emission tomography (PET) studies on allografts in 5 femoral component revisions of total hip arthroplasty. Acta Orthop Scand 2003;74:633–43.

39. Braun HJ, Gold GE. Diagnosis of osteoarthritis: imaging. Bone 2012;51(2):278–88.

40. Hootman JM, Helmick CG. Projections of US prevalence of arthritis and associated activity limitations. Arthritis Rheum 2006;54(1):226–9.

41. Guermazi A, Roemer FW, Hayashi D, et al. Assessment of synovitis with contrast-enhanced MRI using a whole-joint semiquantitative scoring system in people with, or at high risk of, knee osteoarthritis: the MOST study. Ann Rheum Dis 2011;70:805–11.

42. Burr DB, Gallant MA. Bone remodeling osteoarthritis. Nat Rev Rheumatol 2012;8:665–73.

43. Hayami T, Pickarski M, Wesolowski GA, et al. The role of subchondral bone remodeling in osteoarthritis: reduction of cartilage degeneration and prevention of osteophyte formation by alendronate in the rat anterior cruciate ligament transection model. Arthritis Rheum 2004;50:1193–206.

44. Kobayashi N, Inaba Y, Tateishi U, et al. Comparison of 18F-fluoride positron emission tomography and magnetic resonance imaging in evaluating earlystage osteoarthritis of the hip. Nucl Med Commun 2015;36:84–9.

45. Draper CE, Fredericson M, Gold GE, et al. Patients with patellofemoral pain exhibit elevated bone metabolic activity at the patellofemoral joint. J Orthop Res 2012;30:209–13.

46. Draper CE, Quon A, Fredericson M, et al. Comparison of MRI and (1)(8)F-NaF PET/CT in patients with patellofemoral pain. J Magn Reson Imaging 2012; 36:928–32.

47. Hayashi D, Roemer FW, Katur A, et al. Imaging of synovitis in osteoarthritis: current status and outlook. Semin Arthritis Rheum 2011;41:116–30.

48. Sellam J, Berenbaum F. The role of synovitis in pathophysiology and clinical symptoms of osteoarthritis. Nat Rev Rheumatol 2010;6:625–35.

49. Nakamura H, Masuko K, Yudoh K, et al. Positron emission tomography with 18F-FDG in osteoarthritic knee. Osteoarthritis Cartilage 2007;15:673–81.

50. Wandler E, Kramer EL, Sherman O, et al. Diffuse FDG shoulder uptake on PET is associated with clinical findings of osteoarthritis. AJR Am J Roentgenol 2005;185:797–803.

51. Felson DT, Chaisson CE, Hill CL, et al. The association of bone marrow lesions with pain in knee osteoarthritis. Ann Intern Med 2001;134:541–9.

52. Kogan F, Fan AP, McWalter EJ, et al. PET/MRI of metabolic activity in osteoarthritis: a feasibility study. J Magn Reson Imaging 2017;45(6):1736–45.

53. Scott DL, Symmons DP, Coulton BL, et al. Long-term outcome of treating rheumatoid arthritis: results after 20 years. Lancet 1987;1:1108–11.

54. Polisson RP, Schoenberg OI, Fischman A, et al. Use of magnetic resonance imaging and positron emission tomography in the assessment of synovial volume and glucose metabolism in patients with rheumatoid arthritis. Arthritis Rheum 1995;38:819–25.

55. Palmer WE, Rosenthal DI, Schoenberg OI, et al. Quantification of inflammation in the wrist with gadolinium-enhanced MR imaging and PET with 2-[F-18]-fluoro-2-deoxy-D-glucose. Radiology 1995;196:647–55.

56. Carey K, Saboury B, Basu S, et al. Evolving role of FDG PET imaging in assessing joint disorders: a systematic review. Eur J Nucl Med Mol Imaging 2011;38:1939–55.

57. Beckers C, Ribbens C, André B, et al. Assessment of disease activity in rheumatoid arthritis with (18) F-FDG PET. J Nucl Med 2004;45:956–64.

58. Matsui T, Nakata N, Nagai S, et al. Inflammatory cytokines and hypoxia contribute to 18F-FDG uptake by cells involved in pannus formation in rheumatoid arthritis. J Nucl Med 2009;50:920–6.

59. Roivainen A, Parkkola R, Yli-Kerttula T, et al. Use of positron emission tomography with methyl-11C-choline and 2-18F-fluoro-2-deoxy-D-glucose in comparison with magnetic resonance imaging for the assessment of inflammatory proliferation of synovium. Arthritis Rheum 2003;48:3077–84.

60. Zeman MN, Scott PJ. Current imaging strategies in rheumatoid arthritis. Am J Nucl Med Mol Imaging 2012;2:174–220.

61. van der Laken CJ, Elzinga EH, Kropholler MA, et al. Noninvasive imaging of macrophages in rheumatoid synovitis using 11C-(R)-PK11195 and positron emission tomography. Arthritis Rheum 2008;58:3350–5.

62. Boutry N, More M, Flipo RM, et al. Early rheumatoid arthritis: a review of MRI and sonographic findings. AJR Am J Roentgenol 2007;189:1502–9.

63. Emery P. Evidence supporting the benefit of early intervention in rheumatoid arthritis. J Rheumatol Suppl 2002;66:3–8.

64. Crowley AR, Dong J, McHaffie A, et al. Measuring bone erosion and edema in rheumatoid arthritis: a comparison of manual segmentation and RAMRIS methods. J Magn Reson Imaging 2011;33:364–71.

65. Hodgson RJ, Connolly S, Barnes T, et al. Pharmacokinetic modeling of dynamic contrast-enhanced MRI of the hand and wrist in rheumatoid arthritis and the response to anti-tumor necrosis factor-alpha therapy. Magn Reson Med 2007;58:482–9.

66. Miese F, Scherer A, Ostendorf B, et al. Hybrid 18F-FDG PET-MRI of the hand in rheumatoid arthritis: initial results. Clin Rheumatol 2011;30:1247–50.

67. Kubota K, Ito K, Morooka M, et al. Whole-body FDG-PET/CT on rheumatoid arthritis of large joints. Ann Nucl Med 2009;23:783–91.

68. Beckers C, Jeukens X, Ribbens C, et al. (18)F-FDG PET imaging of rheumatoid knee synovitis correlates with dynamic magnetic resonance and sonographic assessments as well as with the serum level of metalloproteinase-3. Eur J Nucl Med Mol Imaging 2006;33(3):275–80.

69. El-Haddad G, Kumar R, Pamplona R, et al. PET/MRI depicts the exact location of meniscal tear associated with synovitis. Eur J Nucl Med Mol Imaging 2006;33(4):507–8.

70. Lohmander LS, Ostenberg A, Englund M, et al. High prevalence of knee osteoarthritis, pain, and functional limitations in female soccer players twelve years after anterior cruciate ligament injury. Arthritis Rheum 2004;50(10):3145–52.

71. Menendez MI, Hettlich B, Wei L, et al. Feasibility of Na18F PET/CT and MRI for noninvasive in vivo quantification of knee pathophysiological bone metabolism in a canine model of post-traumatic osteoarthritis. Mol Imaging 2017;16. 1536012117714575.

72. Magnussen RA, Binzel K, Zhang J, et al. ACL graft metabolic activity assessed by 18FDG PET-MRI. Arthroscopy 2017;33(10):e79.

73. Installe J, Nzeusseu A, Bol A, et al. (18)F-fluoride PET for monitoring therapeutic response in Paget's disease of bone. J Nucl Med 2005;46:1650–8.

74. Meunier PJ, Coindre JM, Edouard CM, et al. Bone histomorphometry in Paget's disease. Quantitative and dynamic analysis of pagetic and nonpagetic bone tissue. Arthritis Rheum 1980;23:1095–103.

75. Devogelaer JP. Modern therapy for Paget's disease of bone: focus on bisphosphonates. Treat Endocrinol 2002;1:241–57.

76. Cook GJ, Lodge MA, Blake GM, et al. Differences in skeletal kinetics between vertebral and humeral bone measured by 18F-fluoride positron emission tomography in postmenopausal women. J Bone Miner Res 2000;15:763–9.

77. Messa C, Goodman WG, Hoh CK, et al. Bone metabolic activity measured with positron emission tomography and [18F]fluoride ion in renal osteodystrophy: correlation with bone histomorphometry. J Clin Endocrinol Metab 1993;77:949–55.

78. Fogelman I, Bessent R. Age-related alterations in skeletal metabolism-24-hr whole-body retention of diphosphonate in 250 normal subjects: concise communication. J Nucl Med 1982;23:296–300.

79. Thomsen K, Johansen J, Nilas L, et al. Whole body retention of 99mTc-diphosphonate. Relation to biochemical indices of bone turnover and to total body calcium. Eur J Nucl Med 1987;13:32–5.

80. Blake GM, Park-Holohan SJ, Fogelman I. Quantitative studies of bone in postmenopausal women using (18)F-fluoride and (99m)Tc-methylene diphosphonate. J Nucl Med 2002;43:338–45.

81. Kato K, Aoki J, Endo K. Utility of FDG-PET in differential diagnosis of benign and malignant fractures in acute to subacute phase. Ann Nucl Med 2003; 17:41–6.

82. Schmitz A, Risse JH, Textor J, et al. FDG-PET findings of vertebral compression fractures in osteoporosis: preliminary results. Osteoporos Int 2002;13: 755–61.

83. Behera D, Jacobs KE, Behera S, et al. (18)F-FDG PET/MRI can be used to identify injured peripheral nerves in a model of neuropathic pain. J Nucl Med 2011;52:1308–12.

84. Cheng G, Chamroonrat W, Bing Z, et al. Elevated FDG activity in the spinal cord and the sciatic nerves due to neuropathy. Clin Nucl Med 2009;34:950–1.

85. Biswal S, Behera D, Yoon DH, et al. [18F]FDG PET/MRI of patients with chronic pain alters management: early experience. EJNMMMI Phys 2015; 2:A84.

86. Gerhard A, Neumaier B, Elitok E, et al. In vivo imaging of activated microglia using [11C]PK11195 and positron emission tomography in patients after ischemic stroke. Neuroreport 2000;11:2957–60.

87. Imamoto N, Momosaki S, Fujita M, et al. [11C] PK11195 PET imaging of spinal glial activation after nerve injury in rats. Neuroimage 2013;79:121–8.

88. James ML, Shen B, Nielsen CH, et al. Evaluation of sigma-1 receptor radioligand 18F-FTC-146 in rats and squirrel monkeys using PET. J Nucl Med 2014; 55:147–53.

89. Hjørnevik T, Cipriano PW, Shen B, et al. Biodistribution and radiation Dosimetry of $^{18}$F-FTC-146 in humans. J Nucl Med 2017;58:2004–9.

90. Hoy D, March L, Brooks P, et al. The global burden of low back pain: estimates from the Global Burden of Disease 2010 study. Ann Rheum Dis 2014;73: 968–74.

91. Ovadia D, Metser U, Lievshitz G, et al. Back pain in adolescents: assessment with integrated 18F-fluoride positron-emission tomography-computed tomography. J Pediatr Orthop 2007;27:90–3.

92. Gamie S, El-Maghraby T. The role of PET/CT in evaluation of facet and disc abnormalities in patients with low back pain using (18) F-Fluoride. Nucl Med Rev Cent East Eur 2008;11:17–21.

# Imaging of Osteoarthritis by Conventional Radiography, MR Imaging, PET–Computed Tomography, and PET–MR Imaging

Daichi Hayashi, MD, PhD[a,b,*], Frank W. Roemer, MD[a,c],
Ali Guermazi, MD, PhD[a]

## KEYWORDS

- Osteoarthritis • MR imaging • PET • CT • Radiography

## KEY POINTS

- Conventional radiography remains the first line of imaging in both clinical and research settings, but MR imaging continues to play a large role in OA research endeavors.
- Compositional MR imaging enables evaluation of the biochemical properties of joint tissues, allowing assessment of early premorphologic changes that cannot be depicted on conventional MR imaging.
- Hybrid PET-CT and PET–MR imaging systems allow integration of high-resolution structural information on CT and MR imaging with metabolic information obtained from PET related to OA disease process.

## INTRODUCTION

Imaging of osteoarthritis (OA) can be performed by multiple imaging modalities. Conventional radiography is the most widely available and commonly used modality for evaluation of osteoarthritis.[1] In daily clinical practice, conventional radiography may be the only imaging modality used for initial diagnosis and routine follow-up, despite known limitations.[2] Recently, a series of recommendations regarding the use of imaging in OA clinical trials were published by the Osteoarthritis Research Society International.[3–5] The European League Against Rheumatism (EULAR) task force also published recommendations regarding the use of imaging in the routine clinical management of OA patients.[1] In brief, the EULAR recommendation states that conventional radiography should be the primary imaging modality and use of additional more sophisticated imaging such as MR imaging should be restricted to atypical cases or patients showing rapid progression of symptoms. However, it needs to be emphasized that these EULAR recommendations are not applicable to OA research. MR imaging, hybrid PET–computed tomography (CT), and PET–MR imaging are relatively expensive but enable us to obtain much more information than conventional radiography

Disclosure Statement: D. Hayashi: nothing to disclose. F.W. Roemer: Stockholder of Boston Imaging Core Lab, LLC. A. Guermazi: Stockholder of Boston Imaging Core Lab, LLC. Consultant to MerckSerono, TissueGene, OrthoTrophix, AstraZeneca, Genzyme.
[a] Department of Radiology, Quantitative Imaging Center, Boston University School of Medicine, 820 Harrison Avenue, FGH Building, 3rd Floor, Boston, MA 02118, USA; [b] Department of Radiology, Stony Brook University Hospital, HSC Level 4, Room 120, Stony Brook, NY, 11794, USA; [c] Department of Radiology, University of Erlangen-Nuremberg, Maximilianspl. 1, 91054 Erlangen, Germany
* Corresponding author.
E-mail address: dhayashi@bu.edu

and thus play an important role in clinical trials and epidemiologic observational studies of OA in research. In this review article, in line with the theme of the current issue of *PET Clinics*, we focus on imaging of OA by means of conventional radiography, MR imaging, and hybrid PET-CT and PET–MR imaging.

## CONVENTIONAL RADIOGRAPHY
### Semiquantitative Assessment

Radiography shows characteristic OA features such as osteophytes, subchondral sclerosis and cysts, and joint space narrowing (JSN). Diagnosis of radiographic OA can be made based on Kellgren and Lawrence (KL) grading (grade 0 = normal; grade 1 = presence of equivocal osteophyte; grade 2 = presence of definite osteophyte without JSN; grade 3 = presence of JSN; grade 4 = complete loss of joint space, "bone-on-bone" appearance).[6] Limitations of the KL grading system for semiquantitative assessment of OA have been recognized. For instance, a large proportion of KL grade 0 (radiographically "normal") knees have OA features that can be depicted on MR imaging.[7] Also, KL grade 4 ("end-stage" radiographic OA) cannot progress further based on radiography because it has already reached "bone-on-bone" JSN, but MR imaging can reveal that even KL grade 4 knees can still progress further regarding OA features that cannot be visualized on radiography such as cartilage damage and bone marrow lesions (BMLs).[8] An additional limitation of KL grading is that grade 3 includes any severity of JSN (other than complete loss), and therefore it is insensitive to change over time.[2] Because of these limitations, suggestions for modifications of KL grading have been published.[9]

Semiquantitative radiographic assessment of OA can also be performed using another scoring system developed by Osteoarthritis Research Society International (OARSI), published as an OARSI atlas.[10] In this scoring system, knee osteoarthritis is assessed on a compartmental basis with regard to JSN, which is graded as 0 (none), 1 (mild), 2 (moderate), and 3 (severe), and osteophytes that are graded as 0 (none), 1 (small), 2 (moderate), and 3 (large). Many epidemiologic observational studies such as the Osteoarthritis Initiative (OAI) and the Multicenter Osteoarthritis Study (MOST) use radiographic outcomes to determine incidence and progression of OA based on semiquantitative assessment.[11,12] Recent Osteoarthritis Initiative (OAI)-based studies showed that lower thigh muscle specific strength was a predictor of incident radiographic knee OA in women (odds ratio [OR] 1.47, 95% confidence interval

[CI] 1.10–1.96),[11] and that meniscal surgery was associated with increased risk of radiographic JSN progression in persons without prior history of knee trauma (adjusted hazard ratio 1.27, 95% CI 1.00–1.63).[12] An important methodological issue to note is that radiographic techniques are highly influenced by positioning issues despite standardization and it is of paramount importance in longitudinal studies of OA to acquire identical high-quality radiographic data that are comparable from baseline to future follow-up.[13] Slight variations in knee flexion will result in false-positive or false-negative assessments of progression. An example of how positioning may influence radiographic assessment is given in **Fig. 1**. In multicenter trials, semiquantitative radiographic interpretation should be performed by trained and validated central readers.[14]

### Quantitative Assessment

Joint space width (JSW) can be assessed using quantitative approaches, in which JSW are measured manually or by means of computer software. In the knee, JSW is the distance between the projected femoral and tibial margins. Quantification of JSW using image processing software requires a digital radiographic image. Some investigators advocate the use of minimum JSW, whereas others use location-specific JSW.[15,16] Various degrees of responsiveness have been reported depending on the degree of OA severity, length of the follow-up period, and the knee-positioning protocol.[16,17] More recent studies deploying quantitative JSW measurement have shown findings worth mentioning. In patients without gout with knee OA, high serum urate levels predicted progression of JSN over 24 months (baseline serum uric acid levels distinguished progressors [joint space loss >0.2 mm] from nonprogressors, $P = .03$ by multivariate analysis).[18] Fixed-location JSW measurement was shown to better predict knee replacement surgery (OR 1.57, 95% CI 1.23–2.01) than minimum JSW measurement (OR 1.38, 95% CI 1.11–1.71).[19] Moreover, radiographic JSW measurement could predict future knee replacement surgery with similar accuracy compared with femoral cartilage thickness measurement on MR imaging ($P = .001$ by paired $t$-test and OR 1.38).[20] However, a major limitation of JSW measurement as a surrogate for articular cartilage thickness is that JSW reflects a combination of 3-dimensional (3D) quantitative measures of cartilage and meniscus in the knee.[21] In an attempt to overcome this issue, a new analytical approach to measure JSW using 3D standing CT has been proposed, and seems to have a potential

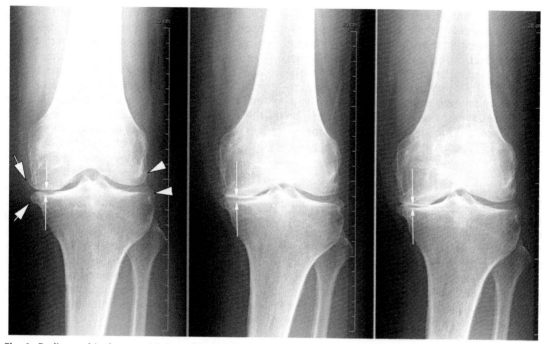

**Fig. 1.** Radiographic characterization of osteoarthritis. Left image in panel shows a posterior-anterior knee radiograph acquired with a positioning frame in standardized knee flexion to optimize visualization of the medial joint space. There are large marginal osteophytes at the medial joint space (*large arrows*) and smaller but also definite osteophytes at the lateral femur and tibia (*arrowheads*). In addition there is definite medial JSN. (*thin, long arrows*). Radiograph was acquired with 15° of beam angulation. Middle image in panel shows another radiograph of the same knee acquired a few minutes later with a slightly different degree of beam angulation (12°). The result is apparent JSN compared with left image (*thin, long arrows* in middle image). Finally, image on the right shows again the same knee now acquired with 10° of beam angulation. In comparison with the other images, joint space seems to be even more narrowed, which is an incorrect assumption and purely based on positioning parameters. For these reasons, reproducible knee positioning is paramount in longitudinal studies of knee OA to ensure correct evaluation of the joint space and potential assessment of progression.

to be used as a tool to stratify participants in clinical trials.[22]

## Clinical Trials of Osteoarthritis Using Radiographic Analysis

Both semiquantitative and quantitative radiographic analyses of OA are widely used to define inclusion/exclusion criteria and outcome measures in OA clinical trials. There have been a multitude of such studies and examples include, but are not limited to, clinical trials of chondroitin sulfate,[23] glucosamine,[24,25] sprifermin,[26] strontium ranelate,[27] meniscal surgery,[10] and gene therapy.[28]

## Advanced Radiographic Technique

Finally, tomosynthesis, which is nowadays commonly used for breast cancer screening, has been shown to be potentially applicable for evaluation of OA joints, with better diagnostic performance than conventional radiography for assessment of JSN[29] and osteophytes and subchondral cysts[30]

in knee OA, as well as OA changes involving small joints of hand,[31] when MR imaging and CT were used as reference. However, to date there are no longitudinal studies looking at tomosynthesis to evaluate progression.

## MR IMAGING
### Analytical Approaches and Technical Considerations

In general, MR imaging analysis in OA research can be classified into semiquantitative and quantitative approaches. Additionally, compositional imaging can be performed using advanced MR imaging techniques, which are mainly restricted to research use at present. Whatever analytical approach is used for a purpose of research, it is critical to use appropriate MR imaging pulse sequences tailored for specific pathologic features to be assessed. For evaluation of focal cartilage defects and BMLs, fluid-sensitive fat-suppressed fast/turbo spin-echo sequences (eg,

T2-weighted, proton density–weighted, or intermediate-weighted [IW]) or short tau inversion recovery sequences should be used so as to be able to detect a small focal defect that may not be visible on gradient recalled echo (GRE)-type sequences.[32–34] Moreover, MR imaging may be affected by artifacts that mimic pathologic findings. For example, susceptibility artifacts can be misinterpreted as focal cartilage defects or meniscal tears. GRE sequences are known to be particularly prone to this type of artifact.[25]

## Semiquantitative Analysis

Detailed description of available MR imaging–based semiquantitative scoring systems can be found in the literature.[35,36] In essence, these scoring systems divide the joint into multiple "subregions" and enable grading of OA features, such as cartilage loss, meniscal lesions, osteophytes, BMLs, effusion, and synovitis, in each subregion and also as a whole joint. Existing semiquantitative scoring systems include, but are not limited to, Whole Organ MRI Score (WORMS),[37] MRI OA Knee Score (MOAKS),[38] Hip OA MRI Score (HOAMS),[39] Outcome Measures in Rheumatology (OMERACT) hand OA MRI scoring system (HOAMRIS).[40] Other newer and more specific scoring systems include Anterior Cruciate Ligament Osteoarthritis Score (ACLOAS), Scoring Hip Osteoarthritis with MRI (SHOMRI), Knee Inflammation MRI Scoring System (KIMRISS), and Thumb Base OA MRI Score (TOMS). ACLOAS allows reliable whole-organ scoring of acute anterior cruciate ligament (ACL) injury and longitudinal changes relevant to knee OA.[41] ACLOAS is the only scoring system that has a specific focus on ACL injury in the context of knee OASHOMRI enables a whole joint semiquantitative evaluation of hip OA with excellent intrareader and interreader reproducibility.[42] KIMRISS was developed to focus on potentially reversible MR imaging biomarkers of active knee OA, namely BMLs, with the use of an online interface.[43] The OMERACT MRI Task Force developed the TOMS, based on the existing HOAMRIS to enable assessment of inflammatory and structural abnormalities in this specific hand OA subset.[44] In this scoring system, interreader reliability was good for all features, with similar intrareader reliability.

OA research studies using semiquantitative MR imaging scoring systems continue to play an important role for OA researchers to further their understanding of OA disease mechanism and to assist in their efforts to develop efficacious therapies for OA. The use of within-grade changes for longitudinal assessment is commonly applied in OA research using semiquantitative MR imaging approaches.[45] Within-grade scoring describes progression or improvement of a lesion that does not meet the criteria for a full-grade change but does represent a definite visual change in comparison with the prior time point. It has been shown that within-grade changes in semiquantitative MR imaging assessment of cartilage and BMLs are valid and their use may increase the sensitivity for detecting longitudinal changes.[45] Using data from the Foundation for the National Institute of Health (FNIH) biomarkers consortium project, studies showed 24-month MOAKS changes in cartilage thickness, cartilage surface area, effusion-synovitis, Hoffa synovitis, and meniscal morphology were independently associated with progression of OA, indicating that these factors can potentially serve as biomarkers in clinical trials of disease-modifying interventions for knee OA.[46,47] An example of the fluctuation of OA features over time in light of semiquantitative assessment is given in **Fig. 2**.

## Semiquantitative Evaluation of Cartilage

Cartilage damage is a central component of OA pathogenesis. Partial-thickness and full-thickness focal cartilage defects seem to be equally important for development of new cartilage damage in knee OA.[48] For patellofemoral OA, sagittal dynamic joint stiffness may be a potentially modifiable risk factor for patellofemoral cartilage damage worsening over 2 years.[49] In contrast, large cross-sectional areas of thigh extensors and vastus medialis muscle are associated with patellofemoral WORMS cartilage damage score increase over 48 months, indicating the importance of maintenance of adequate extensor/flexor muscle balance for prevention of patellofemoral cartilage loss.[50] The presence of mediopatellar plica may also be associated with MR imaging–detected medial patellar cartilage damage.[51]

## Semiquantitative Evaluation of Bone

Osteophytes and BMLs are also important features of OA. Marginal osteophytes were consistently associated with knee pain both cross-sectionally and longitudinally.[52] BMLs are strong predictors of subsequent structural progression in knee OA, including cartilage loss. Serum inflammatory markers were associated with BMLs in men and women with knee OA and predicted increased WORMS BML score in women, suggesting involvement of inflammation in BML pathogenesis in knee OA.[53] Knee malalignment was shown to be associated with increased risk of incident and enlarging BMLs in the more loaded

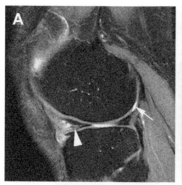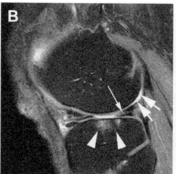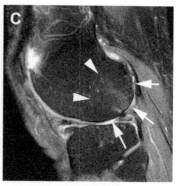

**Fig. 2.** Semiquantitative assessment. (A) Sagittal intermediate-weighted fat-suppressed MR imaging at baseline shows focal full-thickness cartilage defect at the posterior lateral femoral condyle (*arrow*). There is also a horizontal tear of the anterior horn of the lateral meniscus (*arrowhead*). (B) Follow-up MR imaging 1 year later shows progression of posterior femoral cartilage loss (*short arrows*) and incident bone marrow lesion at the tibia (*arrowheads*). In addition there is an incident horizontal meniscal tear at eh medial posterior horn (*long arrow*). (C) At 3-year follow-up, there is further increase in full-thickness femoral cartilage loss (*arrows*). Note incident subchondral convexity of the tibial surface, that is, bone attrition at the tibia, a finding commonly preceded by BMLs in the same joint subregion. In addition, there is a new bone marrow lesion at the lateral femur (*arrowheads*), progressive maceration of the anterior horn of the lateral meniscus, and progression in size of anterior tibial osteophyte.

tibiofemoral compartment in the knee.[54] In hand OA, BMLs are associated with pain, radiographic hand OA progression, and incident joint tenderness.[55–57] All in all, BMLs can be a good target for OA clinical trials.

## Semiquantitative Evaluation of Meniscus

Meniscus is an important structure in the knee, thought to play an important role in OA pathogenesis and serves as a potential target for early detection of persons at risk of developing knee OA. In a study involving 407 subjects, baseline presence of meniscal extrusion was associated with incident radiographic knee OA (OR 2.61, 95% CI 1.11–6.13) and medial JSN (OR 3.19, 95% CI 1.59–6.41) after 30 months.[58] Of note, meniscal root tear is considered a separate entity and is associated with greater pain than meniscal tears or maceration in knee OA.[10] History of meniscal surgery can also affect knee OA incidence. In a study based on OAI data involving 355 knees, 31 knees that had undergone partial meniscectomy demonstrated strong association between prior partial meniscectomy and incident knee OA in 1 year.[59]

## Semiquantitative Evaluation of Synovitis

Synovitis in OA can be assessed using MR imaging without or with intravenous gadolinium. MR imaging signal changes within the Hoffa fat pad ("Hoffa synovitis") and the presence of effusion ("effusion-synovitis") are 2 indirect markers of synovitis in knee OA.[37,38,60] Hoffa synovitis has

been shown to have strong association with knee pain.[61] However, effusion-synovitis may be preferred over Hoffa synovitis as a surrogate marker when contrast-enhanced MR imaging (CEMRI) is not available, based on the finding that effusion-synovitis showing superior correlations compared with Hoffa synovitis, using CEMRI-assessed synovial thickness as the reference.[62] Synovitis in OA should ideally be assessed using CEMRI, which enables direct visualization of inflamed synovium and thus more accurate assessment of synovitis.[63] Studies have shown CEMRI-detected synovitis is strongly associated with tibiofemoral radiographic OA and widespread cartilage damage.[64] Increased severity of CEMRI-detected synovitis was shown to be strongly associated with Western Ontario and McMaster Universities Arthritis Index (WOMAC) pain score increase[65] and increase in synovitis was shown to be associated with worsening cartilage damage.[66] An image example of non-CE versus CEMRI with regard to synovitis visualization is given in **Fig. 3**.

## Quantitative Analysis

Quantitative MR imaging analyses include measurement of the size, thickness, shape, and volume of tissues such as cartilage, meniscus, effusion, synovitis, bone, and BMLs. For quantitative MR imaging analysis of cartilage measures, the use of location-independent analysis has been proposed, given the spatial heterogeneity of cartilage loss in knee OA.[67] A novel Local-

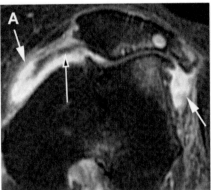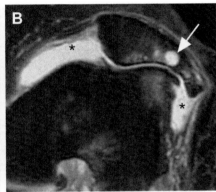

**Fig. 3.** Synovitis assessment on MR imaging. (*A*) Axial T1-weighted contrast-enhanced image shows marked contrast enhancement and synovial thickening (*thick short arrows*), while the true intra-articular amount of joint fluid is only minimal (*thin long arrow*). (*B*) In contrast, axial proton density-weighted MRI of the same knee shows marked distension of the joint capsule due to joint effusion (*asterisks*), but synovial thickening versus intra-articular fluid cannot be differentiated. There is a subchondral cyst at the lateral patella. Pathology of the synovial membrane can be differentiated from intra-articular fluid only by using contrast-enhanced MR imaging.

Area Cartilage Segmentation software method seems to enable fast and responsive cartilage volume measurement on MR imaging.[68]

Studies deploying quantitative analyses have shown baseline lateral femoral cartilage volume is directly associated with medial JSN progression at 48 months follow-up,[69] and bone curvature changes can predict efficacy of OA treatment on cartilage volume reduction in a 2-year clinical trial of chondroitin sulfate.[70] In women only, low serum levels of endogenous estradiol, progesterone, and testosterone were shown to be associated with increased knee effusion-synovitis volume,[71] which might explain observed sex difference in OA. Stronger increase in 3D infrapatellar fat pad (IPFP) MR imaging signal and signal heterogeneity, but not IPFP volume, might be associated with radiographic/symptomatic progression of OA, compared with nonprogressive OA or healthy knee.[72] Quantitative measures of meniscal extrusion were shown to predict incident radiographic knee OA.[73] A pilot study showed longitudinal change in quantitative 3D meniscus measurements, such as meniscal volume, area of tibial plateau coverage, and extent of meniscal extrusion, may provide improved sensitivity to change compared with single slice analysis.[74]

Importance of choice of appropriate MR imaging pulse sequence is also applicable to quantitative BML volume assessment. Changes in Western Ontario and McMaster Universities Osteoarthritis Index (WOMAC) pain score was correlated with BML volume change on IW FS sequence but not GRE sequence.[32] Overall, it was shown that BML quantification on IW FS sequence offered better validity and statistical power than BML quantification using a GRE sequence.

Detailed review and overview of quantitative MR imaging research of OA has been published recently for interested readers.[75] An example of segmentation-based quantitative approaches is shown in **Fig. 4**.

### Compositional (physiologic) MR imaging

Compositional MR imaging enables evaluation of the biochemical properties of joint tissues. Early, premorphologic changes that cannot be depicted on conventional MR imaging may be assessed. Compositional MR imaging has been mostly applied for assessment of cartilage.[76,77] However, the technique can be applied to other tissues, such as meniscus[78] and ligaments.[79] The application of compositional MR imaging techniques including, but not limited to, T2/T2*/T1rho mapping, delayed gadolinium-enhanced MR imaging of cartilage (dGEMRIC), sodium imaging, gagC-EST imaging, and diffusion MR imaging, to cartilage and other articular and periarticular tissues continue to increase in the research setting.[76,77]

T2 mapping is compatible with most MR systems and is a well-validated technique. T2* mapping can be performed with shorter acquisition time than T2 mapping because of 3D acquisition of data. Typically, pulse sequences based on spin-echoes are required for T2 mapping, whereas gradient echoes are required for field mapping. In an attempt to solve this problem, a dual-pathway multi-echo steady state sequence and reconstruction algorithm have been developed to capture T2, T2* and field map information, enabling generation of T2 and field maps from the same acquired data rather than from separately.[80] Another novel approach, Extended Phase Graph modeling, was also developed to allow a simple linear

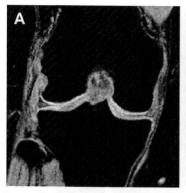 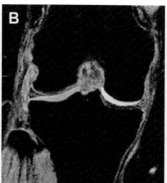 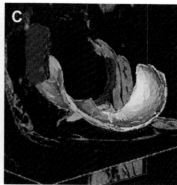

**Fig. 4.** Quantitative assessment. High-resolution knee MR imaging obtained with spoiled gradient-echo sequences with water excitation, in the same person: (*A*) coronal image; (*B*) same coronal image with the medial tibial cartilage marked (ie, segmented) blue, medial femoral cartilage marked yellow, lateral tibial cartilage marked green, and lateral femoral cartilage marked red. The composite 3D reformation is shown in (*C*) Patellar cartilage is shown in purple and trochlear cartilage shown in light blue. (*Courtesy of* Dr Wolfgang Wirth, Chondrometrics GmbH, Ainring, Germany.)

approximation of the relationship between the 2 dual-echo steady-state (DESS) signals, enabling accurate T2 estimation from one DESS scan.[81] However, it should be noted that there can be potential discrepancies in T2 relaxation time quantification between different sequences, and therefore care should be taken when comparison is made among different studies.[82] As stated before, compositional MR imaging techniques have an advantage over conventional "morphologic" MR imaging in that they can be used for imaging of early "premorphologic" stage of OA. For example, T2 map signal variation can potentially predict symptomatic knee OA progression in asymptomatic individuals to serve as a possible early OA imaging marker.[83] Also short-term longitudinal evaluation of T2 map and texture changes may provide early warning of cartilage at risk for progressive degeneration after ACL injury and reconstruction.[84] Moreover, computer-aided diagnosis of early cartilage degeneration in knee OA with T2 mapping has been shown to be technically feasible.[85]

T1rho mapping is sensitive to early cartilage degeneration and may complement T2/T2* mapping, but it is limited due to requirement for special pulse sequences that are only available at select few academic centers and long acquisition time.[86] Sodium imaging correlates directly with GAG content, but is limited by the need for specialized hardware, long examination times, and low spatial resolution. Interestingly, machine learning seems to be a potentially applicable technique for classifying patients with OA and controls using sodium MR imaging.[87] dGEMRIC can help accurately measure cartilage GAG content in vivo in patients with knee OA,[88] but requires

intravenous injection of gadolinium and examination time is prolonged by the need for time gap between injection and imaging. gagCEST is a relatively newer technique and research efforts to optimize image acquisition technique continue.[89,90] However, at present gagCEST is only available for high-field system using 7T MR imaging. Technical feasibility of the diffusion-weighted stimulated echo-based sequence as a tool for early diagnosis and characterization of knee OA at 3T has been shown.[91]

In summary, compositional MR imaging techniques seem to increasingly gain popularity in the OA research community because they can potentially supplement conventional MR imaging sequences to identify degeneration of cartilage or other tissues at an earlier stage than is currently possible. Different techniques are complementary and offer information on different biochemical components of cartilage and other joint tissues. The applicability and responsiveness of these techniques in OA clinical trials need to be validated with future studies. Image examples of compositional assessment over time are presented in **Fig. 5**.

## PET-CT AND PET–MR IMAGING

PET imaging with 18F-fluorodeoxyglucose (FDG) or 18F-fluoride (18F⁻) enable imaging of active metabolism and visualization of bone turnover changes seen in the OA disease process. 18-FDG-PET demonstrates the site of active synovitis and BMLs associated with OA.[92] A pathologic feature of OA that is particularly important to PET imaging is synovitis. Detection of active synovitis in OA is clinically meaningful, because increased

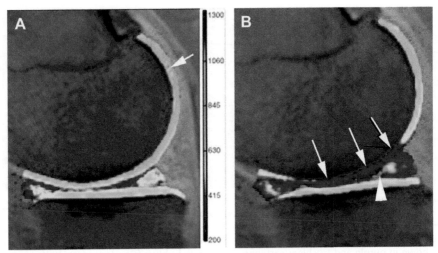

**Fig. 5.** Compositional MR imaging evaluation using the dGEMRIC technique. (*A*) Sagittal T1-weighted fat-suppressed image of the medial tibio-femoral compartment shows normal dGEMRIC indices within the femoral and tibial cartilage (*color-coded in green*). There is a focal spot of T1 prolongation posteriorly, a finding of unknown significance (*arrow*). (*B*) The 2-year follow-up image shows a decrease in dGEMRIC values at the central weight-bearing subregion of the medial femur coded in red consistent with a decrease in GAG content (*arrows*). Note also a decrease in dGEMRIC values in the medial meniscus over time. In addition, there is incident partial maceration of the posterior horn of the medial meniscus (*arrowhead*).

18F-FDG uptake by knee synovium was shown to be associated with knee pain in patients with OA.[93] 18-F⁻ PET can be used for bone imaging because the amount of tracer uptake depends on the regional blood flow and bone remodeling conditions.[94] An in vivo study by Temmerman and colleagues[95] demonstrated a significant increase in bone metabolism in the proximal femur of patients with symptomatic hip OA, showing that 18-F⁻ PET is a potentially useful technique for detection of early OA changes.

To overcome the major limitation of PET imaging, that is, lack of high anatomic resolution, utilization of PET/CT and PET/MR imaging hybrid imaging has been explored and the feasibility was demonstrated for assessment of early metabolic and morphologic markers of knee OA across multiple tissues.[96] Namely, all subchondral bone lesions (BMLs, osteophytes, and sclerosis) show hypermetabolism compared with normal-appearing bone on MR imaging.[96] A study by Moon and coworkers[97] demonstrated PET-CT could detect active inflammation in patients with OA of the shoulder. Preclinical studies using a canine model have been reported exploring the use of NA-18F PET/CT and MR imaging for noninvasive quantification of knee bone metabolism in knee OA.[98,99] A study deploying hybrid Na-18F PET–MR imaging showed increases in cartilage T1rho (which indicates degenerative changes) were associated with increased turnover in the adjoining bone, highlighting the complex biomechanical and biochemical interactions between articular cartilage and adjoining bone in knee OA.[100] Techniques to achieve the optimum registration of PET and MR images have been published.[101] Although originally developed for breast imaging, small-part scanners may be useful for imaging of joints.[102] The small-part PET scanners have the advantages of lower operating costs and lower radiation exposure, while retaining high spatial resolution and sensitivity for detection of lesions.

In addition, increasing research efforts have been made to deploy single-photon emission CT (SPECT)/CT for imaging of OA.[103–105] SUVmax of quantitative bone SPECT/CT was shown to be highly correlated with radiographic and MR imaging parameters for medial compartment knee OA.[104] Also, bone tracer uptake on SPECT/CT imaging demonstrated positive correlation with the degree and size of cartilage lesions depicted by conventional MR imaging.[105] Although the use of hybrid PET-CT/MR imaging or SPECT imaging of OA is essentially limited to studies showing feasibility of these techniques in OA imaging research, ability to combine structural and molecular/metabolic information is promising and further research development in this field is expected. Image examples of FDG-PET CT for the visualization of synovitis are shown in **Fig. 6**.

A                                    B

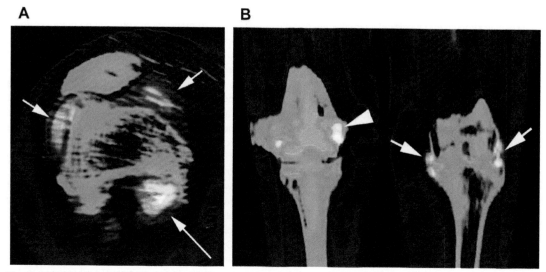

**Fig. 6.** PET-CT. (*A*) Axial fusion image of CT and FDG-PET shows marked intra-articular FDG accumulation in the peripatellar region (*short arrows*) and posterior to the posterior cruciate ligament (PCL) consistent with synovitis (*long arrow*). The region posterior to the PCL is the most common location affected by synovitis in OA. (*B*) Corresponding fusion image in the coronal plane also shows perimeniscal synovitis in the same knee (*arrows*). The contralateral knee has a total knee replacement with an inflammatory focus at the medial femoral condyle (*arrowhead*).

## SUMMARY

In OA imaging, radiography remains the first line of imaging in both clinical and research settings. However, due to known limitations of radiography, MR imaging continues to play a large role in OA research endeavors, whereas compositional MR imaging techniques will increasingly become important due to their ability to assess "premorphologic" biochemical changes of articular cartilage and other tissues. Newer imaging techniques, such as hybrid PET-CT and PET–MR imaging, enable evaluation of the joint as a whole organ with concomitant assessment of structural alterations and metabolic activities. Therefore, these hybrid systems can be a potentially valuable adjunct imaging tool in OA research by allowing integration of high-resolution structural information on CT and MR imaging with metabolic information obtained from PET related to the OA disease process.

## REFERENCES

1. Sakellariou G, Conaghan PG, Zhang W, et al. EU-LAR recommendations for the use of imaging in the clinical management of peripheral joint osteoarthritis. Ann Rheum Dis 2017;76:1484–94.
2. Guermazi A, Roemer FW, Burstein D, et al. Why radiography should no longer be considered a surrogate outcome measure for longitudinal assessment of cartilage in knee osteoarthritis. Arthritis Res Ther 2011;13:247.
3. Hunter DJ, Altman RD, Cicuttini F, et al. OARSI clinical trials recommendations: knee imaging in clinical trials in osteoarthritis. Osteoarthritis Cartilage 2015;23:698–715.
4. Gold GE, Cicuttini F, Crema MD, et al. OARSI clinical trials recommendations: hip imaging in clinical trials in osteoarthritis. Osteoarthritis Cartilage 2015; 23:716–31.
5. Hunter DJ, Arden N, Cicuttini F, et al. OARSI clinical trials recommendations: hand imaging in clinical trials in osteoarthritis. Osteoarthritis Cartilage 2015;23:732–46.
6. Kellgren JH, Lawrence JS. Radiological assessment of osteo-arthrosis. Ann Rheum Dis 1957;16: 494–502.
7. Guermazi A, Niu J, Hayashi D, et al. Prevalence of abnormalities in knees detected by MRI in adults without knee osteoarthritis: population based observational study (Framingham Osteoarthritis Study). BMJ 2012;345:e5339.
8. Guermazi A, Hayashi D, Roemer FW, et al. Severe radiographic knee osteoarthritis—does Kellgren and Lawrence grade 4 represent end stage disease? The MOST study. Osteoarthritis Cartilage 2015;23:1499–505.
9. Felson DT, Niu J, Guermazi A, et al. Defining radiographic incidence and progression of knee osteoarthritis: suggested modifications of the Kellgren and Lawrence scale. Ann Rheum Dis 2011;70:1884–6.
10. Altman RD, Gold GE. Atlas of individual radiographic features in osteoarthritis, revised. Osteoarthritis Cartilage 2007;15(Suppl. A):A1-56.

11. Culvenor AG, Felson DT, Niu J, et al. Thigh muscle specific strength and the risk of incident knee osteoarthritis: the influence of sex and greater body mass index. Arthritis Care Res (Hoboken) 2017; 69:1266–70.

12. Zikria B, Hafezi-Nejad N, Roemer FW, et al. Meniscal surgery: risk of radiographic joint space narrowing progression and subsequent knee replacement: data from the osteoarthritis initiative. Radiology 2017;282:807–16.

13. Kinds MB, Vincken KL, Hoppinga TN, et al. Influence of variation in semiflexed knee positioning during image acquisition on separate quantitative radiographic parameters of osteoarthritis, measured by Knee Images Digital Analysis. Osteoarthritis Cartilage 2012;20:997–1003.

14. Guermazi A, Hunter DJ, Li L, et al. Different thresholds for detecting osteophytes and joint space narrowing exist between the site investigators and the centralized reader in a multicenter knee osteoarthritis study—data from the osteoarthritis initiative. Skeletal Radiol 2012;41:179–86.

15. Duryea J, Zaim S, Genant HK. New radiographic-based surrogate outcome measures for osteoarthritis of the knee. Osteoarthritis Cartilage 2003; 11:102–10.

16. Nevitt MC, Peterfy C, Guermazi A, et al. Longitudinal performance evaluation and validation of fixed-flexion radiography of the knee for detection of joint space loss. Arthritis Rheum 2007;56:1512–20.

17. Duryea J, Neumann G, Niu J, et al. Comparison of radiographic joint space width with magnetic resonance imaging cartilage morphometry: analysis of longitudinal data from the Osteoarthritis Initiative. Arthritis Care Res (Hoboken) 2010;62:932–7.

18. Krasnokutsky S, Oshinsky C, Attur M, et al. Serum urate levels predict joint space narrowing in non-gout patients with medial knee osteoarthritis. Arthritis Rheumatol 2017;69:1213–20.

19. Arden NK, Cro S, Sheard S, et al. The effect of vitamin D supplementation on knee osteoarthritis, the VIDEO study: a randomized controlled trial. Osteoarthritis Cartilage 2016;24:1858–66.

20. Eckstein F, Boudreau R, Wang Z, et al. Comparison of radiographic joint space width and magnetic resonance imaging for prediction of knee replacement: a longitudinal case-control study from the osteoarthritis initiative. Eur Radiol 2016;26: 1942–51.

21. Roth M, Wirth W, Emmanuel K, et al. The contribution of 3D quantitative meniscal and cartilage measures to variation in normal radiographic joint space width. Data from the Osteoarthritis Initiative healthy reference cohort. Eur J Radiol 2017;87: 90–8.

22. Segal NA, Frick E, Duryea J, et al. Correlations of medial joint space width on fixed-flexed standing computed tomography and radiographs with cartilage and meniscal morphology on magnetic resonance imaging. Arthritis Care Res (Hoboken) 2016;68:1410–6.

23. Roman-Blas JA, Castaneda S, Sanchez-Pernaute O, et al. Combined treatment with chondroitin sulfate and glucosamine sulfate shows no superiority over placebo for reduction of joint pain and functional impairment in patients with knee osteoarthritis: a six-month multicenter, randomized, double-blind, placebo-controlled clinical trial. Arthritis Rheumatol 2017;69:77–85.

24. Kwoh CK, Roemer FW, Hannon MJ, et al. Effect of oral glucosamine on joint structure in individuals with chronic knee pain: a randomized placebo-controlled clinical trial. Arthritis Rheumatol 2014; 66:930–9.

25. Jarraya M, Hayashi D, Guermazi A, et al. Susceptibility artifacts detected on 3T MRI of the knee: frequency, change over time and associations with radiographic findings: data from the joints on glucosamine study. Osteoarthritis Cartilage 2014; 22:1499–503.

26. Roemer FW, Aydemir A, Lohmander S, et al. Structural effects of sprifermin in knee osteoarthritis: a post-hoc analysis on cartilage and non-cartilaginous tissue alterations in a randomized controlled trial. BMC Musculoskelet Disord 2016; 17:267.

27. Roubille C, Martel-Pelletier J, Raynauld JP, et al. Meniscal extrusion promotes knee osteoarthritis structural progression: protective effect of strontium ranelate treatment in a phase III clinical trial. Arthritis Res Ther 2015;17:82.

28. Cherian JJ, Parvizi J, Bramlet D, et al. Preliminary results of a phase II randomized study to determine the efficacy and safety of genetically engineered allogeneic human chondrocytes expressing TGF-1 in patients with grade 3 chronic degenerative joint disease of the knee. Osteoarthritis Cartilage 2015;23:2109–18.

29. Kalinosky B, Sabol JM, Piacsek K, et al. Quantifying the tibiofemoral joint space using x-ray tomosynthesis. Med Phys 2011;38:6672–82.

30. Hayashi D, Xu L, Roemer FW, et al. Detection of osteophytes and subchondral cysts in the knee with use of tomosynthesis. Radiology 2012;263: 206–15.

31. Martini K, Becker AS, Guggenberger R, et al. Value of tomosynthesis for lesion evaluation of small joints in osteoarthritic hands using the OARSI score. Osteoarthritis Cartilage 2016;24:1167–71.

32. Zhang M, Driban JB, Price LL, et al. Magnetic resonance imaging sequence influences the relationship between bone marrow lesions volume and pain: data from the osteoarthritis initiative. Biomed Res Int 2015;2015:731903.

33. Roemer FW, Kwoh CK, Hannon MJ, et al. Semi-quantitative assessment of focal cartilage damage at 3T MRI: a comparative study of dual echo at steady state (DESS) and intermediate-weighted (IW) fat suppressed fast spin echo sequences. Eur J Radiol 2011;80:e126–31.

34. Hayashi D, Guermazi A, Kwoh CK, et al. Semiquantitative assessment of subchondral bone marrow edema-like lesions and subchondral cysts of the knee at 3T MRI: a comparison between intermediate-weighted fat-suppressed spin echo and Dual Echo Steady State sequences. BMC Musculoskelet Disord 2011;12:198.

35. Guermazi A, Roemer FW, Haugen IK, et al. MRI-based semiquantitative scoring of joint pathology in osteoarthritis. Nat Rev Rheumatol 2013;9: 236–51.

36. Jarraya M, Hayashi D, Roemer FW, et al. MR imaging-based semi-quantitative methods for knee osteoarthritis. Magn Reson Med Sci 2016; 15:153–64.

37. Peterfy CG, Guermazi A, Zaim S, et al. Whole-organ magnetic resonance imaging score (WORMS) of the knee in osteoarthritis. Osteoarthritis Cartilage 2004;12:177–90.

38. Hunter DJ, Guermazi A, Lo GH, et al. Evolution of semi-quantitative whole joint assessment of knee OA: MOAKS (MRI Osteoarthritis Knee Score). Osteoarthritis Cartilage 2011;19:990–1002.

39. Roemer FW, Hunter DJ, Winterstein A, et al. Hip Osteoarthritis MRI Scoring System (HOAMS): reliability and associations with radiographic and clinical findings. Osteoarthritis Cartilage 2011;19: 946–62.

40. Haugen IK, Ostergaard M, Eshed I, et al. Iterative development and reliability of the OMERACT hand osteoarthritis MRI scoring system. J Rheumatol 2014;41:386–91.

41. Roemer FW, Frobell R, Lohmander LS, et al. Anterior Cruciate Ligament OsteoArthritis Score (ACLOAS): longitudinal MRI-based whole joint assessment of anterior cruciate ligament injury. Osteoarthritis Cartilage 2014;22:668–82.

42. Lee S, Nardo L, Kumar D, et al. Scoring hip osteoarthritis with MRI (SHOMRI): a whole joint osteoarthritis evaluation system. J Magn Reson Imaging 2015;41:1549–57.

43. Jaremko JL, Jeffery D, Buller M, et al. Preliminary validation of the knee inflammation MRI scoring system (KIMRISS) for grading bone marrow lesions in osteoarthritis of the knee: data from the osteoarthritis initiative. RMD Open 2017;3:e000355.

44. Kroon FP, Conaghan PG, Foltz V, et al. Development and reliability of the OMERACT thumb base osteoarthritis magnetic resonance imaging scoring system. J Rheumatol 2017. https://doi.org/10.3899/jrheum.161099.

45. Roemer FW, Nevitt MC, Felson DT, et al. Predictive validity of within-grade scoring of longitudinal changes of MRI-based cartilage morphology and bone marrow lesion assessment in the tibiofemoral joint—the MOST study. Osteoarthritis Cartilage 2012;20:1391–8.

46. Roemer FW, Guermazi A, Collins JE, et al. Semiquantitative MRI biomarkers of knee osteoarthritis progression in the FNIH biomarkers consortium cohort–Methodologic aspects and definition of change. BMC Musculoskelet Disord 2016;17:466.

47. Collins JE, Losina E, Nevitt MC, et al. Semiquantitative imaging biomarkers of knee osteoarthritis progression: data from the Foundation for the National Institute of Health osteoarthritis biomarker consortium. Arthritis Rheumatol 2016;68:2422–31.

48. Guermazi A, Hayashi D, Roemer FW, et al. Partial- and full-thickness focal cartilage defects contribute equally to development of new cartilage damage in knee osteoarthritis: the Multicenter Osteoarthritis Study. Arthritis Rheumatol 2017;69:560–4.

49. Chang AH, Chmiel JS, Almagor O, et al. Association of baseline knee sagittal dynamic joint stiffness during gait and 2-year patellofemoral cartilage damage worsening in knee osteoarthritis. Osteoarthritis Cartilage 2017;25:242–8.

50. Goldman LH, Tang K, Facchetti L, et al. Role of thigh muscle cross-sectional area and strength in progression of knee cartilage degeneration over 48 months–data from the Osteoarthritis Initiative. Osteoarthritis Cartilage 2016;24:2082–91.

51. Hayashi D, Xu L, Guermazi A, et al. Prevalence of MRI-detected mediopatellar plica in subjects with knee pain and the association with MRI-detected patellofemoral cartilage damage and bone marrow lesions: data from the Joints on Glucosamine study. BMC Musculoskelet Disord 2013;14:292.

52. Sayre E, Guermazi A, Esdaile JM, et al. Associations between MRI features versus knee pain severity and progression: data from the Vancouver longitudinal study of early knee osteoarthritis. PLoS One 2017;12:e0176833.

53. Zhu Z, Otahal P, Wang B, et al. Cross-sectional and longitudinal associations between serum inflammatory cytokines and knee bone marrow lesions in patients with knee osteoarthritis. Osteoarthritis Cartilage 2017;25:499–505.

54. Hayashi D, Englund M, Roemer FW, et al. Knee malalignment is associated with increased risk for incident and enlarging bone marrow lesions in the more loaded compartments: the MOST study. Osteoarthritis Cartilage 2012;20:1227–33.

55. Haugen IK, Slatkowsky-Christensen B, Boyesen P, et al. Increasing synovitis and bone marrow lesions are associated with incident joint tenderness in hand osteoarthritis. Ann Rheum Dis 2016;75: 702–8.

56. Ramonda R, Favero M, Vio S, et al. A recently developed MRI scoring system for hand osteoarthritis: its application in a clinical setting. Clin Rheumatol 2016;35:2079–86.

57. Damman W, Liu R, Bloem JL, et al. Bone marrow lesions and synovitis on MRI associate with radiographic progression after 2 years in hand osteoarthritis. Ann Rheum Dis 2017;76:214–7.

58. van der Voet JA, Runhaar J, van der Plas P, et al. Baseline meniscal extrusion associated with incident knee osteoarthritis after 30 months in overweight and obese women. Osteoarthritis Cartilage 2017;25:1299–303.

59. Roemer FW, Kwoh CK, Hannon MJ, et al. Partial meniscectomy is associated with increased risk of incident radiographic osteoarthritis and worsening cartilage damage in the following year. Eur Radiol 2017;27:404–13.

60. Roemer FW, Jarraya M, Felson DT, et al. Magnetic resonance imaging of Hoffa's fat pad and relevance for osteoarthritis research: a narrative review. Osteoarthritis Cartilage 2016;24:383–97.

61. Kaukinen P, Podlipska J, Guermazi A, et al. Associations between MRI-defined structural pathology and generalized and localized knee pain–the Oulu knee osteoarthritis study. Osteoarthritis Cartilage 2016;24:1565–76.

62. Crema MD, Roemer FW, Li L, et al. Comparison between semiquantitative and quantitative methods for the assessment of knee synovitis in osteoarthritis using non-enhanced and gadolinium-enhanced MRI. Osteoarthritis Cartilage 2017;25:267–71.

63. Hayashi D, Roemer FW, Katur A, et al. Imaging of synovitis in osteoarthritis: current status and outlook. Semin Arthritis Rheum 2011;41:116–30.

64. Guermazi A, Hayashi D, Roemer FW, et al. Synovitis in knee osteoarthritis assessed by contrast-enhanced magnetic resonance imaging (MRI) is associated with radiographic tibiofemoral osteoarthritis and MRI-detected widespread cartilage damage: the MOST study. J Rheumatol 2014;41:501–8.

65. Wallace G, Cro S, Dore C, et al. Associations between clinical evidence of inflammation and synovitis in symptomatic knee osteoarthritis: a substudy of the VIDEO trial. Arthritis Care Res (Hoboken) 2017;69:1340–8.

66. deLange-Brokaar BJ, Ioan-Facsinay A, Yusuf E, et al. Evolution of synovitis in osteoarthritic knees and its association with clinical features. Osteoarthritis Cartilage 2016;24:1867–74.

67. Eckstein F, Buck R, Wirth W. Location-independent analysis of structural progression of osteoarthritis: taking it all apart, and putting the puzzle back together makes the difference. Semin Arthritis Rheum 2017;46:404–10.

68. Shaefer LF, Sury M, Yin M, et al. Quantitative measurement of medial femoral knee cartilage volume–analysis of the OA biomarkers consortium FNIH study cohort. Osteoarthritis Cartilage 2017;25:1107–13.

69. Hafezi-Nejad N, Guermazi A, Roemer FW, et al. Prediction of medial tibiofemoral compartment joint space loss progression using volumetric cartilage measurements: data from the FNIH OA biomarkers consortium. Eur Radiol 2017;27:464–73.

70. Raynauld JP, Pelletier JP, Delorme P, et al. Bone curvature changes can predict the impact of treatment on cartilage volume loss in knee osteoarthritis: data from a 2-year clinical trial. Rheumatology (Oxford) 2017;56:989–98.

71. Jin X, Wang BH, Wang X, et al. Associations between endogenous sex hormones and MRI structural changes in patients with symptomatic knee osteoarthritis. Osteoarthritis Cartilage 2017;25:1100–6.

72. Ruhdorfer A, Haniel F, Petersohn T, et al. Between-group differences in infra-patellar fat pad size and signal in symptomatic and radiographic progression of knee osteoarthritis vs non-progressive controls and healthy knees–data from the FNIH biomarkers consortium study and the osteoarthritis initiative. Osteoarthritis Cartilage 2017;25:1114–21.

73. Emmanuel K, Quinn E, Niu J, et al. Quantitative measures of meniscus extrusion predict incident radiographic knee osteoarthritis—data from the Osteoarthritis Initiative. Osteoarthritis Cartilage 2016;24:262–9.

74. Bloecker K, Wirth W, Guermazi A, et al. Longitudinal change in quantitative meniscus measurements in knee osteoarthritis—data from the Osteoarthritis Initiative. Eur Radiol 2015;25:2960–8.

75. Eckstein F, Peterfy C. A 20 years of progress and future of quantitative magnetic resonance imaging (qMRI) of cartilage and articular tissues-personal perspective. Semin Arthritis Rheum 2016;45:639–47.

76. Guermazi A, Alizai H, Crema MD, et al. Compositional MRI techniques for evaluation of cartilage degeneration in osteoarthritis. Osteoarthritis Cartilage 2015;23:1639–53.

77. Link TM, Neumann J, Li X. Prestructural cartilage assessment using MRI. J Magn Reson Imaging 2017;45:949–65.

78. Wang L, Chang G, Bencardino J, et al. T1rho MRI of menisci in patients with osteoarthritis at 3 Tesla: a preliminary study. J Magn Reson Imaging 2014;40:588–95.

79. Wilson KJ, Surowiec RK, Ho CP, et al. Quantifiable imaging biomarkers for evaluation of the posterior cruciate ligament using 3-T magnetic resonance imaging: a feasibility study. Orthop J Sports Med 2016;4. 2325967116639044.

80. Cheng CC, Mei CS, Duryea J, et al. Dual-pathway multi-echo sequence for simultaneous frequency and T2 mapping. J Magn Reson 2016;265:177–87.

81. Sveinsson B, Chaudhari AS, Gold GE, et al. A simple analytic method for estimating T2 in the knee from DESS. Magn Reson Imaging 2017;38:63–70.

82. Matzat SJ, McWalter EJ, Kogan F, et al. T2 relaxation time quantitation differs between pulse sequences in articular cartilage. J Magn Reson Imaging 2015;42:105–13.

83. Zhong H, Miller DJ, Urish KL. T2 map signal variation predicts symptomatic osteoarthritis progression: data from the Osteoarthritis Initiative. Skeletal Radiol 2016;45:909–13.

84. Williams A, Winalski CS, Chu CR. Early articular cartilage MRI T2 changes after anterior cruciate ligament reconstruction correlate with later changes in T2 and cartilage thickness. J Orthop Res 2017;35:699–706.

85. Wu Y, Yang R, Jia S, et al. Computer-aided diagnosis of early knee osteoarthritis based on MRI T2 mapping. Biomed Mater Eng 2014;24:3379–88.

86. Wang L, Regatte RR. T1rho MRI of human musculoskeletal system. J Magn Reson Imaging 2015;41:586–600.

87. Madelin G, Poidevin F, Makrymallis A, et al. Classification of sodium MRI data of cartilage using machine learning. Magn Reson Med 2015;74:1435–58.

88. van Tiel J, Kotek G, Reijman M, et al. Is T1rho mapping an alternative to delayed gadolinium-enhanced MR imaging of cartilage in the assessment of sulphated glycosaminoglycan content in human osteoarthritic knees? An in vivo validation study. Radiology 2016;279:523–31.

89. Kogan F, Hargreaves BA, Gold GE. Volumetric multislice gagCEST imaging of articular cartilage: optimization and comparison with T1rho. Magn Reson Med 2017;77:1134–41.

90. Krishnamoorthy G, Nanga RPR, Bagga P, et al. High quality three-dimensional gagCEST imaging of in vivo human knee cartilage at 7 Tesla. Magn Reson Med 2017;77:1866–73.

91. Guha A, Wyatt C, Karampinos DC, et al. Spatial variations in magnetic resonance-based diffusion of articular cartilage in knee osteoarthritis. Magn Reson Imaging 2015;33:1051–8.

92. Nakamura H, Masuko K, Yudoh K, et al. Positron emission tomography with 18F-FDG in osteoarthritic knee. Osteoarthritis Cartilage 2007;15:673–81.

93. Parsons MA, Moghbel M, Saboury B, et al. Increased FDG uptake suggests synovial inflammatory reaction with osteoarthritis: preliminary in vivo results in humans. Nucl Med Commun 2015;36:1215–9.

94. Umemoto Y, Oka T, Inoue T&Saito T. Imaging of a rat osteoarthritis model using (18)F-fluoride positron emission tomography. Ann Nucl Med 2010;24:663–9.

95. Temmerman OP, Raijmakers PG, Kloet R, et al. In vivo measurements of blood flow and bone metabolism in osteoarthritis. Rheumatol Int 2013;33:959–63.

96. Kogan F, Fan AP, McWalter EJ, et al. PET/MRI of metabolic activity in osteoarthritis: a feasibility study. J Magn Reson Imaging 2017;45:1736–45.

97. Moon YL, Lee SH, Park SY, et al. Evaluation of shoulder disorders by 2-[F-18]-fluoro-2-deoxy-D-glucose positron emission tomography and computed tomography. Clin Orthop Surg 2010;2:167–72.

98. Menendez MI, Hettlich B, Wei L, et al. Preclinical multimodal molecular imaging using 18F-FDG PET/CT and MRI in a phase I study of a knee osteoarthritis in in vivo canine model. Mol Imaging 2017;16. 1536012117697443.

99. Menendez MI, Hettlich B, Wei L, et al. Feasibility of Na18F PET/CT and MRI for noninvasive in vivo quantification of knee pathophysiological bone metabolism in a canine model of post-traumatic osteoarthritis. Mol Imaging 2017;16. 1536012117714575.

100. Savic D, Pedoia V, Seo Y, et al. Imaging bone-cartilage interactions in osteoarthritis using [18F]-NaF PET-MRI. Mol Imaging 2016;15:1–12.

101. Magee D, Tanner SF, Waller M, et al. Combining variational and model-based techniques to register PET and MR images in hand osteoarthritis. Phys Med Biol 2010;55:4755–69.

102. Omoumi P, Mercier GA, Lecouvet F, et al. CT arthrography, MR arthrography, PET, and scintigraphy in osteoarthritis. Radiol Clin North Am 2009;47:595–615.

103. Maas O, Joseph GB, Sommer G, et al. Association between cartilage degeneration and subchondral bone remodeling in patients with knee osteoarthritis comparing MRI and (99 m)Tc-DPD-SPECT/CT. Osteoarthritis Cartilage 2015;23:1713–20.

104. Kim J, Lee HH, Kang Y, et al. Maximum standardized uptake value of quantitative bone SPECT/CT in patients with medial compartment osteoarthritis of the knee. Clin Radiol 2017;72:580–9.

105. Dordevic M, Hirschmann MT, Rechsteiner J, et al. Do chondral lesions of the knee correlate with bone tracer uptake by using SPECT/CT? Radiology 2016;278:223–31.

# Evolving Role of MR Imaging and PET in Assessing Osteoporosis

Alecxih G. Austin, BS, William Y. Raynor, BS,
Catherine C. Reilly, BS, Mahdi Zirakchian Zadeh, MD, MHM,
Thomas J. Werner, MSE, Hongming Zhuang, MD, PhD,
Abass Alavi, MD, MD (Hon), PhD (Hon), DSc (Hon),
Chamith S. Rajapakse, PhD*

## KEYWORDS

• Bone • MRI • NaF • Osteoporosis

## KEY POINTS

• Molecular imaging with fluorine-18 sodium fluoride (NaF)-PET and technetium-99m methylene diphosphonate ([99m]Tc-MDP) represents a novel approach to measuring bone turnover.
• [99m]Tc-MDP studies and NaF-PET quantification studies that use standardized uptake values are relatively noninvasive and can provide a regional analysis of different skeletal sites.
• The differential effects of treatments on various skeletal sites can be measured and are consistent with their known effects on osteoblast metabolism.
• Additional studies are necessary to assess regional effects of new drugs on bone formation as well as the ability to enhance properties of fracture healing in patients with osteoporosis.

## INTRODUCTION

Bone is a rigid, mineralized tissue that comprises the skeleton of all vertebrates and serves to provide structure and support to the body as well as protection of other organs and the mechanical ability of locomotion.[1] As a living tissue, bone is subject to constant remodeling, a term that implies a chemical balance between the presence of bone-forming osteoblast cells and bone-resorbing osteoclasts. Conditions that interrupt the dynamic equilibrium between new bone formation and damaged bone degradation are classified under a category known as metabolic bone diseases.[2] The most prominent condition within this overarching umbrella term of metabolic bone disease is osteopenia. Upon progression to pathologic clinical symptoms, osteopenia is identified as osteoporosis, a disease of microstructural deterioration resulting in low bone mass, increased osseous fragility, and ultimately an increased risk of fracture incidence.[3] The International Osteoporosis Foundation estimates that this condition accounts for 8.9 million annual fractures globally, which constitutes a staggering rate of an osteoporotic fracture occurrence every 3 seconds.[4] In the United States alone, the incidence of insufficiency fracture is estimated to be approximately 2 million cases annually, which equates to a staggering $17 billion in associated fracture care costs.[5]

## BONE MICROARCHITECTURE

The unique mechanical properties of bone are derived from its chemical composition. Approximately 65% of osseous tissue is composed of calcium hydroxyapatite and other minerals that form an inorganic matrix and provide both stiffness and structural rigidity. The remaining 35% of bone is

Department of Radiology, University of Pennsylvania, 3400 Spruce Street, MRI Education Center, 1 Founders Building, 253 South 45th Street, Philadelphia, PA 19104, USA
* Corresponding author.
E-mail address: chamith@pennmedicine.upenn.edu

PET Clin 14 (2019) 31–41
https://doi.org/10.1016/j.cpet.2018.08.007

composed of an organic matrix, largely type I collagen, which confers the tissues tensile strength.[6] A key distinction in understanding the structure of bone is the division between trabecular or cancellous bone, which forms the internal aspect of osseous structures, and cortical bone, which forms a dense external "cortex." The porosity of cortical bone has been shown to be an important metric in the classification osseous competence and must be accounted for in the setting of osteoporotic degeneration.[7] In regard to bone microarchitecture, the more porous, cancellous bone is composed of a network of interwoven trabeculae or individual osseous building blocks. Trabeculae vary in their 3–dimensional (3D) shape, geometry, and spatial distribution and are a primary contributor to bones' mechanical integrity. In the setting of osteoporosis, trabecular degeneration is a key contributor to skeletal fragility.[8,9]

## Diagnosis of Osteoporosis

The current standard in the diagnosis of osteoporosis, provided that the patient has not already sustained an insufficiency fracture, which carries an inherent diagnosis, is an imaging modality known as dual-energy X-ray absorptiometry (DXA).[2] DXA provides an assessment of mineralized bone mass per a given bone volume referred to as areal bone mineral density (BMD). Patients who have a BMD that falls 2.5 standard deviations below the mean BMD for a population of 30-year-old individuals of the same gender and race (T-score $<-2.5$) are identified as having a positive diagnosis of osteoporosis. Despite the supported correlation between low BMD and increased incidence of insufficiency fracture, DXA technology does not represent an entirely exhaustive means of identifying patients at risk for fragility fractures at various anatomic regions. Although DXA can accurately derive BMD, this metric is limited in scope and is not a comprehensive assessment of bone integrity and mechanical competence. Subsequently there exists a disparity between quantitative BMD values and fracture incidence, especially at anatomic sites where there is a high ratio of trabecular to cortical bone. DXA is a low-resolution, 2D projection that fails to account for the geometry and distribution of the trabecular components of bone microarchitecture that contribute significantly to the mechanical properties of bone.[10]

## HIGH-RESOLUTION MR IMAGING IN ASSESSMENT OF OSTEOPOROSIS

The role of high-resolution MR imaging in the assessment of osseous structures has progressed and expanded extensively from the point when it was first introduced for imaging bones of the distal skeleton over 20 years ago.[11,12] MR imaging is used as a noninvasive means to gain a detailed perspective of bone microarchitecture and structural determinants of mechanical insufficiency.[13] MR imaging is able to capitalize on the variability between fat and water content contained in the bone marrow at differing skeletal sites in vivo, as well as the evident difference in magnetic susceptibility between bone marrow and trabecular bone, which gives rise to magnetic inhomogeneity.[14] MR imaging techniques have succeeded in quantifying these inhomogeneities, thereby characterizing bones complex trabecular network into a concise image portrayal.[15] By exploiting this remarkable functionality, a detailed assessment of fracture risk can now be attained through MR imaging at skeletal sites that include the distal radius, distal tibia, and calcaneus, as well as, with the progression of multichannel radio frequency coils, more proximal sites such as the distal tibia, distal femur, and the proximal femur or hip region.[16,17]

## Distal Radius

There are to date, multiple studies that have been conducted pertaining to MR-based assessment of osteoporosis at the anatomic site of the distal radius. This is, to some extent, a consequence of fact that this osseous region is not subject to signal-to-noise ratio (SNR) limitations by virtue of its superficial position within the skeleton. That is to say, that the distal radius is positioned no more than 2 cm from the skin surface and is thereby in very close proximity to the radiofrequency coil when an MR image is obtained allowing for an inherently higher SNR and image resolution quality within a reasonable scan time. Before the advent of multichannel coils and SNR-efficient pulse sequences, sufficiently resolved MR imaging–based assessment of osteoporotic changes could not be effectively performed at deep skeletal sites.[17] This, in conjunction with the fact that the distal radius is a common anatomic site of osteoporotic degradation, has led to a small collection of MR-related research centered specifically around this bone.

In a study conducted in 2011, Lam and colleagues[18] sought to elucidate the reproducibility of MR-based assessment of the microstructural and mechanical parameters in the distal radius of 20 female subjects ranging in age from 50 to 75 years. Seventeen of these subjects were postmenopausal women, a cohort that commonly undergoes osteoporotic changes due to a rapid decline in estrogen levels. Subjects underwent

MR imaging scanning at 1.5 Tesla (T) strength at 3 separate points with an average time interval of 20.2 days between scans (Standard Deviation was 14.5 days). Volume-derived, sectional regions of interest for trabecular bone were reported to have an aggregate mean coefficient of variation (CV) of 4.4% (1.8%–7.7%) and an aggregate intra-class correlation coefficient (ICC) of 0.946 for microstructural parameters and a CV/ICC of 4.0%/0.974 for assessment of axial stiffness. In regard to subregional trabecular regions of interest, CV/ICC was reported at 5.5%/0.974 for mechanical parameters and 6.5%/0.946 for microstructural parameters[18] (Fig. 1).

A study conducted by Kijowski and colleagues[19] performed an MR-based assessment (1.5 T 3D FLASE, 0.137 x 0.137 × 0.400 mm) of the distal radius of 36 postmenopausal female patients, all of whom who did not carry a clinical diagnosis of osteoporosis by virtue of their BMD attained through DXA (T-score >−2.5 at the sites of the proximal femur, lumbar spine, and radius). Eighteen of the subjects had a history of insufficiency fracture forming a "patient" cohort and 18 had no history of fracture serving as a "control" cohort. The results of this study showed that the patients with a history of fracture had a significantly lower trabecular bone volume fraction (9%, P<0.001) as well as a significantly lower surface-to-curve ratio (14%, P = .04) consistent with trabecular plate breakdown into trabecular rods. Furthermore, fracture patients were found to possess significantly higher erosion index (17%, P = .03) than the nonfracture control cohort. These results were reported in spite of the fact that densitometric criterion (ie, DXA-based T-score) failed to distinguish fracture from nonfracture subjects. These findings support the assertion that MR imaging provides improved insight into mechanical strength of bone and associated fracture risk that is not provided by DXA.

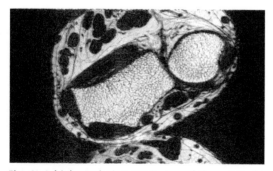

Fig. 1. A high-resolution MR image of the wrist of a human subject showing the trabecular and cortical bone microstructure of the distal radius and ulna.

## Calcaneus

The calcaneus is another osseous structure that lies superficially without a large degree of overlying soft tissue, again making MR imaging of this bone less subject to SNR limitations. Link and colleagues[11] sought to analyze and quantify trabecular structure of the calcaneus in a study that involved MR imaging of 50 postmenopausal female subjects. Twenty-three of these subjects had a history of low-energy hip fracture; the trabecular parameters of these patients were compared with 27 age-matched controls with no prior history of insufficiency fracture. The analysis of microstructural, morphologic parameters obtained through MR imaging (1.5 T) of these patients revealed that the bone volume to total volume ratio and trabecular number were both significantly higher in the control cohort (P = .0001 axial and P = .0019 axial, respectively). Trabecular spacing in the calcaneus was significantly higher for the fracture cohort than that observed in the control cohort (P = .0018 axial).

Rebuzzi and colleagues[20] conducted a study that sought to differentiate between healthy, osteopenic, and osteoporotic bone, as classified by DXA, through application of the MR parameter of internal magnetic field gradient (IMFG) on images (3T) of the calcaneus of 55 women (mean age 62.9 ± 6.6 years). By virtue of increased intertrabecular spacing consistent with osteopenia and to a greater extent with osteoporosis, the IMFG parameter was able to differentiate between the subjects contained in each of the 3 categories. IMFG was found to be significantly different (P<.01) in the subtalar region of the calcaneus between each of the groups, with the greatest value corresponding to the healthy cohort (n = 8), the intermediate value corresponding to the osteopenic cohort (n = 25), and the lowest value corresponding to the cohort with a diagnosis of osteoporosis (n = 22).

## Distal Tibia

A study conducted by Wald and colleagues[21] aimed to assess the sensitivity, reliability, and reproducibility of MR imaging as a means to examine microstructural and mechanical parameters of the trabecular bone that comprises the distal tibia. Seven subjects (5 men, 2 women aged 24–42 years) with no known history of bone mineral degradation were scanned 3 separate times (3T) over a 6-month period at both anisotropic and isotropic resolution qualities (3D FLASE, 0.137 x 0.137 × 0.410 mm and 0.160 x 0.160 × 0.160 mm). Images obtained at anisotropic resolution generally demonstrated better reproducibility with regard to microarchitectural and mechanical parameters. CVs for anisotropic images ranged from 1.0% to 5.2% and ICCs at this resolution category were found to range from 0.75 to 0.99. Data collected from images obtained at isotropic resolution displayed CVs that ranged from 0.87% to 8.1% and ICCs that ranged from 0.62 to 0.99 with respect to both structural and mechanical parameters of distal tibia trabecular bone.

Wehrli and colleagues[22] conducted a longitudinal study that incorporated MR imaging as a means to assess the osseous implications of estradiol therapy for 32 early menopausal female subjects, compared with 33 age-matched female controls that were not on estrogen. Analysis was performed over a 24-month period using both DXA and 1.5 T MR imaging of both the distal tibia and the distal radius to examine temporal changes in architecture and density of trabecular and cortical bone. At 12-month follow-up, the treatment cohort displayed no significant microstructural alterations at either anatomic site; the control group demonstrated a 5.6% decrease in surface-to-curve ratio (P<.0005) in the trabecular bone of the distal tibia as compared with baseline findings consistent with degradative changes of trabecular plates.

The nontreatment group also demonstrated a 7.1% higher erosion index (P<.0005), a metric that assesses the extent of bone network resorption as a consequence of osteoclast deposition.[1] Final assessment at 24 months revealed that microstructural parameters had changed by up to 10.81% relative to baseline values in the treatment group (P = .03) despite the fact that the examination through DXA displayed no significant changes in BMD (P = .52) when compared with baseline values. Average surface-to-curve ratio values between therapy and control groups had deviated 13% (P = .005) at 24 months when compared with baseline values, whereas areal BMD differences between the 2 cohorts had changed less than 5.0% (P<.005). These findings support the utility of MR imaging as a sensitive and comprehensive means to assess bone microarchitectural contributors to mechanical insufficiency (**Figs. 2 and 3**).

## Distal Femur

Chang and colleagues[23] used 7T MR imaging (3D FLASH, 0.234 x 0.234 × 1 mm) to quantify the microarchitectural parameters of the distal femur to determine whether these criterion could effectively differentiate female patients with a history of insufficiency fracture (n = 31) from controls

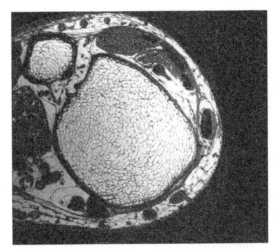

**Fig. 2.** A high-resolution MR image of the ankle of a human subject showing the trabecular and cortical bone microstructure of the distal tibia and fibula.

(n = 25) with healthy bone. Results of the study concluded that 7T MR imaging was able to detect significant degenerative changes in bone microstructural parameters between cohorts, with fracture patients displaying an increased prevalence of trabecular rod–like structure of up to 341% (P<.03) and an increased trabecular isolation of up to 450% (P<.03) than controls with no history of fracture. T-scores generated by DXA were not found to be significant between the 2 cohorts (P>.05), and in a receiver operator characteristic (ROC) analysis, DXA failed to distinguish a significant difference between fracture cases and

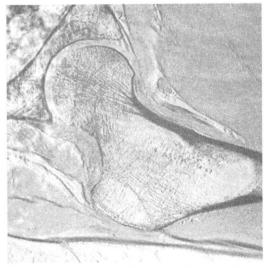

**Fig. 3.** A high-resolution MR image of the hip of a human subject showing the trabecular and cortical bone microstructure of the proximal femur.

controls ($P>.07$). ROC analysis that incorporated microstructural parameters effectively differentiated a significant difference between fracture patients and control subjects ($P<.05$).

In a smaller scale study, Zuo and colleagues[24] again supported the reproducibility of MR imaging in assessment of bone microarchitecture and associated mechanical parameters through conducting 2 separate scans (7T 3D SSFP, 10 cm FOV, 512 x 384 matrix 1 mm slice thickness) on the distal femur of 6 different subjects, each of which were repositioned between scans. CVs of microstructural parameters were demonstrated to be 1.07% to 3.03%.

Modlesky and colleagues[25] designed a study to evaluate disuse osteoporosis in the distal femur of 10 pediatric subjects with cerebral palsy, whose trabecular parameters were compared with 10 healthy age- and gender-matched controls. Analysis of 1.5 T (3D GRE, $0.175 \times 0.175 \times 0.700$ mm) MR images revealed that the pediatric patients who could not ambulate independently displayed significantly lower trabecular thickness (212%, $P<.05$), lower apparent bone volume (230%, $P<.05$), and a higher degree of trabecular separation (148%, $P<.05$) than the healthy control children. Analysis of BMD through DXA also revealed that patients with cerebral palsy possessed a significantly lower bone mineral mass per bone volume (237%, $P<.05$) than the controls.

### Proximal Femur

As discussed before, developments in multichannel radiofrequency coils and effective SNR-efficient pulse sequences as well as the implementation of high-field strength scanning have allowed for MR-based assessment of deep osseous structures like the proximal femur, which typically lie between 6 and 10 cm from the skin surface (see **Fig. 3**).[17,26] The importance of the ability to analyze the microarchitectural parameters and mechanical integrity of the hip cannot be overstated. Low-energy, fragility fracture of the hip is known to be highly prevalent, and the associated implications of proximal femur fracture have been shown to be exceedingly impactful with evidence suggesting a 1-year mortality rate as high as 24%.[27]

Several recent studies focusing on the microarchitectural properties of the proximal femur have applied nonlinear finite element analysis (FEA) to high-resolution MR images. FEA has been shown to be an accurate, reproducible, and sensitive means of identifying structural properties such as trabecular shape, alignment, and

geometry; it has the ability to quantify the impact of those parameters on bones' mechanical sufficiency and associated resistance or susceptibility to fracture.[10,27]

A 2014 study conducted by Chang and colleagues[10] involved 44 postmenopausal women who were largely nondifferentiated on the basis of DXA-generated T-scores ($P>.25$). Twenty-two study subjects sustained some manner of prior low-energy fracture and 22 subjects with no history of fracture incidence or bisphosphonate use served as age, height, weight, and BMI-matched controls. Through the application of finite element analysis to 5 selected volumes of interest (VOIs) (femoral head, femoral neck, ward triangle, intertrochanteric region, greater trochanter) on each patient's high-resolution MR images, it was determined that the cohort who had sustained a prior fracture displayed significantly lower elastic moduli in all 5 of the VOIs as compared with the controls (8.7%–66.8% lower for fracture patients, $P\leq.05$). Elastic modulus is a metric directly correlated to mechanical competence of bone and is negatively correlated with fracture risk.

Finally, Rajapakse and colleagues[27] supported the reproducibility of nonlinear FEA in the assessment of MR-based microarchitectural parameters and mechanical competence of the entire proximal femur. Parameters assessed under 2 different simulated, realistic loading conditions resulted in CVs for yield strain, yield load, ultimate strain, ultimate load, and toughness that were less than 8% and all of which had ICCs of 0.99. As such, the techniques used in this study were shown to support the reproducibility of MR-based FEA in evaluation of femoral microstructure and mechanical strength.

All aforementioned studies denote the progression of the role of MR imaging as a sensitive and comprehensive means to assess bone quality and osteoporotic degradation as it pertains to bone microarchitecture, skeletal fragility, and fracture risk. There is an undeniable requirement to invest resources toward the continued progression of MR imaging as a means to assess the osseous structures of the body. The current utility of this imaging modality and potential for future development and expansion of skeletal applications undoubtedly warrants continued research.

## PET/COMPUTED TOMOGRAPHY IN ASSESSMENT OF OSTEOPOROSIS

MR imaging has been shown to be an incredibly promising tool for detecting the microstructural changes associated with osteoporosis. In spite of this, there still exists a need for development of an imaging modality that can effectively detect early stage skeletal changes before observed microarchitectural deterioration. PET/computed tomography is an imaging tool that provides the unique ability to assess osseous changes at the molecular level through the evaluation of bone turnover providing a critical supplement to information provided by structural imaging techniques. The importance of bone turnover is evident from its independent association with fracture risk,[28,29] which has been observed to change with antiresorptive treatments.[30,31]

Although bone turnover measurements have great potential clinical utility, they are more difficult to obtain compared with bone density measurements. The current gold standard involves double tetracycline labeling followed by bone biopsy, which is invasive, subject to error, costly, and limited to the iliac crest.[32,33] Because of these limitations, enzymes and products of biochemical reactions related to bone turnover, called bone turnover markers (BTM), are commonly measured in urine or serum samples to estimate osteoblast and osteoclast activity in the whole body.[30,31] BTM may be valuable for measuring overall osseous activity but can differentiate neither between skeletal sites nor between cortical and trabecular bones.[34] Instead, a noninvasive and regional approach that examines bone turnover in clinically relevant sites is possible with techniques in molecular imaging using bone tracers such as fluorine-18 sodium fluoride (NaF) and technetium-99m methylene diphosphonate ($^{99m}$Tc-MDP).[35–39] Both bone tracers have affinity for sites of new bone formation and contain radionuclides, allowing for their localization by a detector and the construction of an image portraying levels of bone turnover throughout the skeleton. Determined by their pattern of radioactive decay, NaF studies are suitable to be imaged using PET, and $^{99m}$Tc-MDP studies are suitable to be imaged using either planar scintigraphy or single photon emission computed tomography (SPECT).[40]

## IMAGING WITH FLUORINE-18 SODIUM FLUORIDE-PET AND TECHNETIUM-99M METHYLENE DIPHOSPHONATE

NaF as a radiotracer in molecular imaging predates modern PET technology and was originally used for skeletal scintigraphy.[41] High-quality images with NaF are possible due to high uptake and rapid plasma clearance, ensuring proper contrast in tracer presence between bone and background less than 1 hour after intravenous tracer administration.[42] Sodium and fluoride ions dissociate in the plasma, and $^{18}$F retention begins when fluoride ions exchange with hydroxyl groups on the hydroxyapatite matrix, forming fluoroapatite.[35,43] The fluoride ion is retained in the crystalline matrix of the bone until remodeling occurs. Plasma clearance occurs biexponentially,[44] with first-pass extraction of fluoride ions from blood by bone being near 100%.[45] Once the tracer has reached its target, the location of newly mineralizing bone can be determined from the consequences of radioactive decay of $^{18}$F, by which a proton in the nucleus becomes a neutron and a positron is released. When the positron contacts an electron in the surrounding tissue, the particles are annihilated, and 2 511-keV gamma rays traveling in opposite directions are emitted. These coincident gamma rays are detected by the PET scanner and back-projected to produce a tomographic image.

The structural similarity of $^{99m}$Tc-MDP to bisphosphonates indicates that it is bone-seeking, yet the simple side chain of $^{99m}$Tc-MDP allows for high plasma clearance and high urinary excretion, increasing contrast of bone to background uptake.[46] However, unlike NaF tracer properties, $^{99m}$Tc-MDP is subject to protein binding, which varies between 25% and 50% and limits tracer from being deposited on bone.[47,48] The radioactive decay of $^{99m}$Tc involves the emission of a single 140-keV gamma ray, which must pass through a collimator ensuring only gamma rays traveling in a particular direction are detected in order to localize the tracer in 2 dimensions. Anterior and posterior planar images can be obtained simultaneously, and rotation of the gamma camera around the subject can be used for 3D SPECT.[40]

## QUANTITATIVE PARAMETERS

Studies using NaF and $^{99m}$Tc-MDP can quantify bone formation by measuring either bone uptake or bone plasma clearance. Bone uptake is the parameter measured in the 24-hour $^{99m}$Tc-MDP whole-body retention (24-h WBR) test developed by Fogelman and colleagues,[49] with applications in osteoporosis. In the 24-h WBR test, a whole-body counter measures $^{99m}$Tc-MDP that remains in the bone after most $^{99m}$Tc-MDP in the plasma has been excreted 24 hours after tracer administration, yielding a measure of systemic osteoblast activity. In NaF-PET studies, bone uptake is commonly expressed using standardized uptake values (SUV), which is the activity concentration within a region of interest (ROI) normalized to injected dose and subject body weight.[50] Activity concentration is measured in kilobecquerels per milliliter (kBq/mL), injected dose in megabecquerels (MBq), and body weight in kilograms (kg). The calculation of SUV is given thus:

$$SUV = \frac{activity \left(\frac{kBq}{mL}\right) \times body\ weight(kg)}{injected\ dose\ (MBq)}.$$

Therefore, SUV can be said to be in the units of g/mL. A hypothetical uniform distribution of tracer (assuming mass density of 1.0 g/mL in the ROI) will result in a SUV of 1.0, meaning SUV can also be thought of as a ratio of actual tracer uptake compared with a hypothetical uniform distribution.[40] A limitation of measuring bone uptake is that additional sites of high bone formation or a high renal excretion rate can compete for tracer and decrease the uptake observed at a particular site, resulting in an underestimation of bone formation at that site.

Alternatively, bone plasma clearance is independent of competition for tracers at other sites and indicates the amount of tracer cleared to bone tissue compared with the tracer concentration in the plasma. The unit of bone plasma clearance is mL/min/mL, indicating the amount of tracer present in a volume of plasma cleared in 1.0 minute to 1.0 mL of bone. This parameter therefore accounts for the fact that clearance of tracer to bone tissue is proportional to the concentration of tracer in the plasma.[50] Bone plasma clearance was first measured in NaF-PET by Hawkins and colleagues,[51] whose method of calculation using dynamic scans has become widely adopted.[52–58] The Hawkins method requires that a 60-minute dynamic scan be taken of a 15-cm section within the field of view of the PET scanner. In addition, the arterial input function must be determined, which can be done with an arterial blood line or with venous blood sampling.[51,55,57,59] Next, the changes in concentration of NaF in the bone and in the arterial blood with time are determined with a 3-compartment model, which accounts for NaF in the plasma, in the bone extracellular fluid (ECF), and in the bone mineral. Rate constants are used to describe movement of NaF from one compartment to another, including forward and reverse transport. Specifically, $K_1$ describes movement of NaF from plasma to bone ECF; $k_2$, from bone ECF to plasma; $k_3$, from bone ECF to bone mineral; and $k_4$, from bone mineral to bone ECF. $K_i$ represents overall clearance of NaF from plasma to bone mineral, given by the following equation:

$$K_i = \frac{K_1 \times k_3}{(k_2 + k_3)}\ mL/min/mL$$

$K_i$ is highly correlated with histomorphometric indications of bone formation and mineral apposition rate.[60,61] The Patlak plot method assumes a negligible rate constant $k_4$ and allows for the estimation of $K_i$ using bone uptake as measured in a dynamic scan.[62,63] Although this method avoids the need for arterial sampling, because reverse transport of tracer from bone mineral to bone ECF is not considered, bone plasma clearance is typically underestimated.

Several methods for measuring bone plasma clearance in $^{99m}$Tc-MDP studies have been investigated by Moore and colleagues.[64] In one method, bone clearance is calculated by subtracting renal clearance (estimated from the glomerular filtration rate) from total plasma clearance of NaF. Alternatively, the Patlak plot method with sequential blood samples can be used to determine regional values of bone plasma clearance of $^{99m}$Tc-MDP.[38,64,65]

## EVALUATION OF THE PATHOPHYSIOLOGY OF OSTEOPOROSIS

In a study of 72 subjects by Frost and colleagues,[66] regional NaF $K_i$ measured in the lumbar spine was observed to be lower in postmenopausal women diagnosed with osteoporosis with the BMD T-score compared with those classified as normal or osteopenic. In the same study, bone-specific alkaline phosphatase, which indicates global skeletal bone turnover, was observed to be significantly increased in osteoporotic women, demonstrating the utility of regional measurements. These results were corroborated in a study by Uchida and colleagues,[67] which reported a decrease in SUV of the lumbar spine in osteoporotic patients compared with a healthy and an osteopenic group. Additional studies using quantitative SPECT found that uptake in the lumbar spine, iliac wing, and femoral neck decrease after the onset of menopause[68] and that bone turnover is increased in cortical bone of postmenopausal osteoporotic women.[69] These results indicating lower trabecular bone turnover are consistent with histomorphometric studies that report reduced osteoblast activity with postmenopausal osteoporosis.[33,70–72] Osteoporosis as a result of long-term glucocorticoid treatment was assessed by NaF-PET in a 61-year-old woman with multiple fractures, and reduced activity was observed in nonfractured vertebrae,[73] a finding consistent with suppressed bone formation found in glucocorticoid-induced osteoporosis.[74]

Differences in bone turnover at different skeletal sites and between cortical and trabecular bones have been observed in bone biopsy studies.[75–77] Findings from bone turnover measurements at specific skeletal sites using PET also reflect skeletal heterogeneity. A sample of postmenopausal women with osteoporosis or significant osteopenia found that bone plasma clearance was significantly greater at the lumbar spine than at the humerus, regardless of whether the subject was on antiresorptive therapy.[39] In addition, studies have investigated bone turnover at the clinically relevant sites of the lumbar spine and hip. Puri and colleagues[78] reported greater SUV at the lumbar spine compared with that of the femoral neck and femoral shaft. A study by Uchida and colleagues[67] measured the SUV at the femoral neck and lumbar spine in women treated with corticosteroids, similarly finding that bone turnover is significantly lower at the femoral neck compared with that at the lumbar spine.

## EVALUATION OF RESPONSE TO THERAPY

At the initiation of therapy with bisphosphonates, biochemical markers of bone resorption decrease promptly, followed by a reduction in bone formation markers several weeks later.[79] This decrease in bone turnover was investigated in a study by Frost and colleagues,[58] which reported an 18% decrease in lumbar spine plasma clearance compared with a 23% decrease in markers of bone formation in 18 postmenopausal women undergoing treatment with risedronate. The effects of alendronate were investigated in 24 postmenopausal women, in whom a 14% decrease in SUV at the lumbar spine and 24% decrease at the femoral neck were observed after 12 months of treatment.[67]

Teriparatide is given to prevent osteoporotic fractures by promoting both bone formation and resorption.[80] A study by Frost and colleagues[55] assessed the effect of teriparatide therapy on 18 postmenopausal women. $K_i$ at the spine and SUV at the spine, hip, pelvis, and femoral shaft were assessed with NaF-PET at baseline and after 6 months, with significant increases in bone turnover observed at the spine, femoral shaft, and hip. The investigators concluded that changes in bone turnover as assessed by PET, depend on the skeletal site, with greater changes observed at predominantly cortical sites rather than trabecular sites. In another study, $K_i$ was observed to increase at the total hip, femoral neck, trabecular bone of the hip, and cortical bone of the hip in 13 subjects given teriparatide, calcium, and vitamin D for 12 weeks, compared with no significant increases in a control group that only received calcium and vitamin D.[81] [99m]Tc-MDP scintigraphy was used by Moore and colleagues[38] to further investigate regional effects of teriparatide treatment. Plasma clearance in the whole skeleton

increased by 34% after 18 months, after the start of therapy, with 34% increase in the spine and 128% increase in the calvarium.

In conclusion, molecular imaging with NaF-PET and [99m]Tc-MDP represents a novel approach to measuring bone turnover. [99m]Tc-MDP studies and NaF-PET quantification studies that use SUV are relatively noninvasive and can provide a regional analysis of different skeletal sites. Furthermore, the differential effects of treatments on various skeletal sites can be measured and are consistent with their known effects on osteoblast metabolism. Additional studies are necessary to assess regional effects of new drugs on bone formation as well as the ability to enhance properties of fracture healing in patients with osteoporosis.

## REFERENCES

1. Wehrli FW. Structural and functional assessment of trabecular and cortical bone by micro magnetic resonance imaging. J Magn Reson Imaging 2007; 25(2):390–409.
2. Kanis JA. Diagnosis of osteoporosis and assessment of fracture risk. Lancet 2002;359(9321): 1929–36.
3. Consensus development conference: diagnosis, prophylaxis, and treatment of osteoporosis. Am J Med 1993;94(6):646–50.
4. Johnell O, Kanis JA. An estimate of the worldwide prevalence and disability associated with osteoporotic fractures. Osteoporos Int 2006;17(12):1726–33.
5. Burge R, Dawson-Hughes B, Solomon DH, et al. Incidence and economic burden of osteoporosis-related fractures in the United States, 2005-2025. J Bone Miner Res 2007;22(3):465–75.
6. Linde F. Elastic and viscoelastic properties of trabecular bone by a compression testing approach. Dan Med Bull 1994;41(2):119–38.
7. Bala Y, Zebaze R, Seeman E. Role of cortical bone in bone fragility. Curr Opin Rheumatol 2015;27(4): 406–13.
8. Dempster DW. Bone microarchitecture and strength. Osteoporos Int 2003;14(Suppl 5):S54–6.
9. Kleerekoper M, Villanueva AR, Stanciu J, et al. The role of three-dimensional trabecular microstructure in the pathogenesis of vertebral compression fractures. Calcif Tissue Int 1985;37(6):594–7.
10. Chang G, Honig S, Brown R, et al. Finite element analysis applied to 3-T MR imaging of proximal femur microarchitecture: lower bone strength in patients with fragility fractures compared with control subjects. Radiology 2014;272(2):464–74.
11. Link TM, Majumdar S, Augat P, et al. In vivo high resolution MRI of the calcaneus: differences in trabecular structure in osteoporosis patients. J Bone Miner Res 1998;13(7):1175–82.

12. Wehrli FW, Hwang SN, Ma J, et al. Cancellous bone volume and structure in the forearm: noninvasive assessment with MR microimaging and image processing. Radiology 1998;206(2):347–57.

13. Majumdar S. Magnetic resonance imaging of trabecular bone structure. Top Magn Reson Imaging 2002;13(5):323–34.

14. Majumdar S. Magnetic resonance imaging for osteoporosis. Skeletal Radiol 2008;37(2):95–7.

15. Majumdar S, Bay BK. Noninvasive assessment of trabecular bone architecture and the competence of bone. Advances in experimental medicine and biology. New York: Kluwer/Plenum; 2001. p. xi, 227.

16. Krug R, Banerjee S, Han ET, et al. Feasibility of in vivo structural analysis of high-resolution magnetic resonance images of the proximal femur. Osteoporos Int 2005;16(11):1307–14.

17. Wright SM, Wald LL. Theory and application of array coils in MR spectroscopy. NMR Biomed 1997;10(8):394–410.

18. Lam SC, Wald MJ, Rajapakse CS, et al. Performance of the MRI-based virtual bone biopsy in the distal radius: serial reproducibility and reliability of structural and mechanical parameters in women representative of osteoporosis study populations. Bone 2011;49(4):895–903.

19. Kijowski R, Tuite M, Kruger D, et al. Evaluation of trabecular microarchitecture in nonosteoporotic postmenopausal women with and without fracture. J Bone Miner Res 2012;27(7):1494–500.

20. Rebuzzi M, Vinicola V, Taggi F, et al. Potential diagnostic role of the MRI-derived internal magnetic field gradient in calcaneus cancellous bone for evaluating postmenopausal osteoporosis at 3T. Bone 2013;57(1):155–63.

21. Wald MJ, Magland JF, Rajapakse CS, et al. Structural and mechanical parameters of trabecular bone estimated from in vivo high-resolution magnetic resonance images at 3 tesla field strength. J Magn Reson Imaging 2010;31(5):1157–68.

22. Wehrli FW, Ladinsky GA, Jones C, et al. In vivo magnetic resonance detects rapid remodeling changes in the topology of the trabecular bone network after menopause and the protective effect of estradiol. J Bone Miner Res 2008;23(5):730–40.

23. Chang G, Honig S, Liu Y, et al. 7 tesla MRI of bone microarchitecture discriminates between women without and with fragility fractures who do not differ by bone mineral density. J Bone Miner Metab 2015;33(3):285–93.

24. Zuo J, Bolbos R, Hammond K, et al. Reproducibility of the quantitative assessment of cartilage morphology and trabecular bone structure with magnetic resonance imaging at 7 T. Magn Reson Imaging 2008;26(4):560–6.

25. Modlesky CM, Subramanian P, Miller F. Underdeveloped trabecular bone microarchitecture is detected in children with cerebral palsy using high-resolution magnetic resonance imaging. Osteoporos Int 2008; 19(2):169–76.

26. Techawiboonwong A, Song HK, Magland JF, et al. Implications of pulse sequence in structural imaging of trabecular bone. J Magn Reson Imaging 2005; 22(5):647–55.

27. Rajapakse CS, Hotca A, Newman BT, et al. Patient-specific hip fracture strength assessment with microstructural MR imaging-based finite element modeling. Radiology 2017;283(3):854–61.

28. Johnell O, Odén A, De Laet C, et al. Biochemical indices of bone turnover and the assessment of fracture probability. Osteoporos Int 2002;13(7):523–6.

29. Garnero P, Sornay-Rendu E, Duboeuf F, et al. Markers of bone turnover predict postmenopausal forearm bone loss over 4 years: the OFELY study. J Bone Miner Res 1999;14(9):1614–21.

30. Hochberg MC, Greenspan S, Wasnich RD, et al. Changes in bone density and turnover explain the reductions in incidence of nonvertebral fractures that occur during treatment with antiresorptive agents. J Clin Endocrinol Metab 2002;87(4):1586–92.

31. Eastell R, Barton I, Hannon RA, et al. Relationship of early changes in bone resorption to the reduction in fracture risk with risedronate. J Bone Miner Res 2003;18(6):1051–6.

32. Martin KJ, Olgaard K, Coburn JW, et al. Diagnosis, assessment, and treatment of bone turnover abnormalities in renal osteodystrophy. Am J Kidney Dis 2004;43(3):558–65.

33. Compston JE, Croucher PI. Histomorphometric assessment of trabecular bone remodelling in osteoporosis. Bone Miner 1991;14(2):91–102.

34. Heaney RP. Is the paradigm shifting? Bone 2003; 33(4):457–65.

35. Raynor W, Houshmand S, Gholami S, et al. Evolving role of molecular imaging with (18)F-Sodium Fluoride PET as a biomarker for calcium metabolism. Curr Osteoporos Rep 2016;14(4):115–25.

36. Moore AE, Blake GM, Taylor KA, et al. Changes observed in radionuclide bone scans during and after teriparatide treatment for osteoporosis. Eur J Nucl Med Mol Imaging 2012;39(2):326–36.

37. Lou J, Wen G, Dong K, et al. Early monitoring of osteoporosis treatment response by technetium-99m-methylene diphosphonate bone scan. Nucl Med Commun 2017;38(10):854–7.

38. Moore AE, Blake GM, Taylor KA, et al. Assessment of regional changes in skeletal metabolism following 3 and 18 months of teriparatide treatment. J Bone Miner Res 2010;25(5):960–7.

39. Frost ML, Blake GM, Cook GJ, et al. Differences in regional bone perfusion and turnover between lumbar spine and distal humerus: (18)F-fluoride PET

study of treatment-naive and treated postmenopausal women. Bone 2009;45(5):942–8.

40. Blake GM, Frost ML, Moore AE, et al. The assessment of regional skeletal metabolism: studies of osteoporosis treatments using quantitative radionuclide imaging. J Clin Densitom 2011;14(3):263–71.

41. Grant FD, Fahey FH, Packard AB, et al. Skeletal PET with 18F-fluoride: applying new technology to an old tracer. J Nucl Med 2008;49(1):68–78.

42. Blau M, Ganatra R, Bender MA. 18 F-fluoride for bone imaging. Semin Nucl Med 1972;2(1):31–7.

43. Costeas A, Woodard HQ, Laughlin JS. Depletion of 18F from blood flowing through bone. J Nucl Med 1970;11(1):43–5.

44. Weber DA, Greenberg EJ, Dimich A, et al. Kinetics of radionuclides used for bone studies. J Nucl Med 1969;10(1):8–17.

45. Wootton R, Dore C. The single-passage extraction of 18F in rabbit bone. Clin Phys Physiol Meas 1986; 7(4):333–43.

46. Subramanian G, McAfee JG, Blair RJ, et al. Technetium-99m-methylene diphosphonate–a superior agent for skeletal imaging: comparison with other technetium complexes. J Nucl Med 1975;16(8): 744–55.

47. Moore AE, Hain SF, Blake GM, et al. Validation of ultrafiltration as a method of measuring free 99mTc-MDP. J Nucl Med 2003;44(6):891–7.

48. Blake GM, Moore AE, Park-Holohan SJ, et al. A direct in vivo measurement of 99mTc-methylene diphosphonate protein binding. Nucl Med Commun 2003;24(7):829–35.

49. Fogelman I, Bessent RG, Turner JG, et al. The use of whole-body retention of Tc-99m diphosphonate in the diagnosis of metabolic bone disease. J Nucl Med 1978;19(3):270–5.

50. Blake GM, Siddique M, Frost ML, et al. Imaging of site specific bone turnover in osteoporosis using positron emission tomography. Curr Osteoporos Rep 2014;12(4):475–85.

51. Hawkins RA, Choi Y, Huang SC, et al. Evaluation of the skeletal kinetics of fluorine-18-fluoride ion with PET. J Nucl Med 1992;33(5):633–42.

52. Siddique M, Frost ML, Blake GM, et al. The precision and sensitivity of (18)F-fluoride PET for measuring regional bone metabolism: a comparison of quantification methods. J Nucl Med 2011;52(11):1748–55.

53. Al-Beyatti Y, Siddique M, Frost ML, et al. Precision of (1)(8)F-fluoride PET skeletal kinetic studies in the assessment of bone metabolism. Osteoporos Int 2012;23(10):2535–41.

54. Blake GM, Siddique M, Puri T, et al. A semipopulation input function for quantifying static and dynamic 18F-fluoride PET scans. Nucl Med Commun 2012;33(8):881–8.

55. Frost ML, Siddique M, Blake GM, et al. Differential effects of teriparatide on regional bone formation using (18)F-fluoride positron emission tomography. J Bone Miner Res 2011;26(5):1002–11.

56. Frost ML, Blake GM, Park-Holohan SJ, et al. Long-term precision of 18F-fluoride PET skeletal kinetic studies in the assessment of bone metabolism. J Nucl Med 2008;49(5):700–7.

57. Installe J, Nzeusseu A, Bol A, et al. (18)F-fluoride PET for monitoring therapeutic response in Paget's disease of bone. J Nucl Med 2005;46(10):1650–8.

58. Frost ML, Cook GJ, Blake GM, et al. A prospective study of risedronate on regional bone metabolism and blood flow at the lumbar spine measured by 18F-fluoride positron emission tomography. J Bone Miner Res 2003;18(12):2215–22.

59. Schiepers C, Nuyts J, Bormans G, et al. Fluoride kinetics of the axial skeleton measured in vivo with fluorine-18-fluoride PET. J Nucl Med 1997;38(12): 1970–6.

60. Piert M, Zittel TT, Becker GA, et al. Assessment of porcine bone metabolism by dynamic. J Nucl Med 2001;42(7):1091–100.

61. Messa C, Goodman WG, Hoh CK, et al. Bone metabolic activity measured with positron emission tomography and [18F]fluoride ion in renal osteodystrophy: correlation with bone histomorphometry. J Clin Endocrinol Metab 1993;77(4):949–55.

62. Patlak CS, Blasberg RG, Fenstermacher JD. Graphical evaluation of blood-to-brain transfer constants from multiple-time uptake data. J Cereb Blood Flow Metab 1983;3(1):1–7.

63. Raijmakers P, Temmerman OP, Saridin CP, et al. Quantification of 18F-fluoride kinetics: evaluation of simplified methods. J Nucl Med 2014;55(7):1122–7.

64. Moore AE, Blake GM, Fogelman I. Quantitative measurements of bone remodeling using 99mTc-methylene diphosphonate bone scans and blood sampling. J Nucl Med 2008;49(3):375–82.

65. Moore AE, Blake GM, Fogelman I. Validation of a blood-sampling method for the measurement of 99mTc-methylene diphosphonate skeletal plasma clearance. J Nucl Med 2006;47(4):581–6.

66. Frost ML, Fogelman I, Blake GM, et al. Dissociation between global markers of bone formation and direct measurement of spinal bone formation in osteoporosis. J Bone Miner Res 2004;19(11):1797–804.

67. Uchida K, Nakajima H, Miyazaki T, et al. Effects of alendronate on bone metabolism in glucocorticoid-induced osteoporosis measured by 18F-fluoride PET: a prospective study. J Nucl Med 2009;50(11): 1808–14.

68. Carnevale V, Dicembrino F, Frusciante V, et al. Different patterns of global and regional skeletal uptake of 99mTc-methylene diphosphonate with age: relevance to the pathogenesis of bone loss. J Nucl Med 2000;41(9):1478–83.

69. Israel O, Lubushitzky R, Frenkel A, et al. Bone turnover in cortical and trabecular bone in normal

women and in women with osteoporosis. J Nucl Med 1994;35(7):1155–8.

70. Kimmel DB, Recker RR, Gallagher JC, et al. A comparison of iliac bone histomorphometric data in post-menopausal osteoporotic and normal subjects. Bone Miner 1990;11(2):217–35.

71. Eriksen EF, Hodgson SF, Eastell R, et al. Cancellous bone remodeling in type I (postmenopausal) osteoporosis: quantitative assessment of rates of formation, resorption, and bone loss at tissue and cellular levels. J Bone Miner Res 1990;5(4):311–9.

72. Arlot ME, Delmas PD, Chappard D, et al. Trabecular and endocortical bone remodeling in postmenopausal osteoporosis: comparison with normal postmenopausal women. Osteoporos Int 1990;1(1):41–9.

73. Berding G, Kirchhoff TD, Burchert W, et al. [18F]fluoride PET indicates reduced bone formation in severe glucocorticoid-induced osteoporosis. Nuklearmedizin 1998;37(2):76–9.

74. Canalis E, Delany AM. Mechanisms of glucocorticoid action in bone. Ann N Y Acad Sci 2002;966:73–81.

75. Podenphant J, Engel U. Regional variations in histomorphometric bone dynamics from the skeleton of an osteoporotic woman. Calcif Tissue Int 1987;40(4):184–8.

76. Eventov I, Frisch B, Cohen Z, et al. Osteopenia, hematopoiesis, and bone remodelling in iliac crest and femoral biopsies: a prospective study of 102 cases of femoral neck fractures. Bone 1991;12(1):1–6.

77. Byers RJ, Denton J, Hoyland JA, et al. Differential patterns of altered bone formation in different bone compartments in established osteoporosis. J Clin Pathol 1999;52(1):23–8.

78. Puri T, Frost ML, Curran KM, et al. Differences in regional bone metabolism at the spine and hip: a quantitative study using (18)F-fluoride positron emission tomography. Osteoporos Int 2013;24(2):633–9.

79. Garnero P, Shih WJ, Gineyts E, et al. Comparison of new biochemical markers of bone turnover in late postmenopausal osteoporotic women in response to alendronate treatment. J Clin Endocrinol Metab 1994;79(6):1693–700.

80. McClung MR, San Martin J, Miller PD, et al. Opposite bone remodeling effects of teriparatide and alendronate in increasing bone mass. Arch Intern Med 2005;165(15):1762–8.

81. Frost ML, Moore AE, Siddique M, et al. [18]F-fluoride PET as a noninvasive imaging biomarker for determining treatment efficacy of bone active agents at the hip: a prospective, randomized, controlled clinical study. J Bone Miner Res 2013;28(6):1337–47.

# In Vivo Molecular Imaging of Musculoskeletal Inflammation and Infection

Alok Pawaskar, MBBS, DRM, DNB[a,b], Sandip Basu, MBBS (Hons), DRM, DNB, MNAMS[b,c,*],
Pegah Jahangiri, MD[d], Abass Alavi, MD, MD (Hon), PhD (Hon), DSc (Hon)[d]

## KEYWORDS

- PET/CT • PET/MR Imaging • Musculoskeletal • Infection • Inflammation

## KEY POINTS

- FDG-PET/CT seems to be a promising tool in imaging various infective and inflammatory processes in the musculoskeletal system.
- The procedure is simple, less time consuming, non-invasive and is well tolerated by the patient.
- Apart from FDG, 18F-NaF, FDG-labelled leukocytes, and Ga-68 citrate may be used for infection/inflammation imaging. Newer tracers, such as I-124-fialuridine, are being explored for the same.
- FDG-PET/CT seems to be useful not only in imaging of various skeletal and joint infections, but also for various inflammatory diseases affecting muscles and nerves.
- PET/MR imaging fusion has added strength of metabolic imaging to MR imaging, which is already an established modality for imaging finer details of cartilage, muscles, and nerves. As more data become available, PET/MR seems to be the front runner in imaging of musculoskeletal infection and inflammation.

## INTRODUCTION

Musculoskeletal molecular imaging refers to the noninvasive visualization and measurement of molecular and cell biology of the hard and soft tissues of the musculoskeletal system.[1] The target organs imaged in the musculoskeletal imaging includes bones, joints, muscles, and nerves. Both infection and inflammation are of common occurrence in musculoskeletal system. Conventional imaging modalities, such as radiography, Ultrasonography (USG), computed tomography (CT) scan, and MR imaging, are commonly used for the diagnosis of same. These modalities show anatomic changes happening in later phase of the infective/inflammatory process. However, molecular imaging shows early physiologic/pathophysiologic changes. Molecular imaging offers two key advantages: it detects biologic processes at the underlying molecular level, rather than simply at the tissue level; and compared with conventional anatomic imaging, it provides diagnostic information at an earlier time point during a disease onset or repair process. Together, these advantages are expected to add to an increased precision and prognostic value in diagnostic musculoskeletal imaging.[2]

The molecular imaging of musculoskeletal system today includes (1) optical imaging, (2) contrast ultrasound, and (3) radionuclide imaging.

[a] Oncolife Cancer Centre, Satara, Maharashtra 415519, India; [b] Radiation Medicine Centre, Bhabha Atomic Research Centre, Tata Memorial Centre Annexe, Parel, Mumbai, Maharashtra 400012, India; [c] Homi Bhabha National Institute, Mumbai, Maharashtra, India; [d] Division of Nuclear Medicine, Hospital of University of Pennsylvania, Philadelphia, PA, USA
* Corresponding author. Radiation Medicine Centre, Bhabha Atomic Research Centre, Tata Memorial Centre Annexe, Parel, Mumbai, Maharashtra 400012, India.
E-mail address: drsanb@yahoo.com

PET Clin 14 (2019) 43–59
https://doi.org/10.1016/j.cpet.2018.08.009
1556-8598/19/© 2018 Elsevier Inc. All rights reserved.

Optical imaging consists of bioluminescence imaging and fluorescence reflectance imaging. These optical modalities have been primarily beneficial in small animal models. In humans, issues associated with absorption and scatter of incident photons by biologic materials limit their use. However, the development of tomographic approaches using fluorescence-based optical techniques may enable sufficient tissue penetration to image superficial regions, including joints, in patients.[3] Although ultrasound is primarily used in anatomic imaging of soft tissue and joints, advancements in microbubble contrast agents is expected to make molecular imaging with ultrasound a possibility.

Radionuclide imaging is the only in vivo molecular imaging technique that is widely used in clinical practice for imaging of infection and inflammation. Bone scan, especially three-phase bone scan, is the most commonly performed radionuclide procedure for detection of infection in intact bones. Ga-67 scintigraphy is another imaging that is particularly effective in spondylodiskitis. In-111 or Tc-99m labeled white blood cell (WBC) imaging has high specificity for infection imaging. It has been successfully used in combination with bone marrow imaging for diagnosis of osteomyelitis (OM). Radiolabeled biotin, peptides, and antibiotics have been used with varying degrees of success, but none of these has shown consistent results. PET/CT with powerful and optimal combination of functional and anatomic imaging has opened new frontiers in clinical molecular imaging. Its role is well established in oncologic imaging and it is being explored for infection and inflammation imaging with remarkable success.

## PET/COMPUTED TOMOGRAPHY IMAGING OF INFECTION/INFLAMMATION
### Fluorodeoxyglucose PET/Computed Tomography Imaging

Fluorodeoxyglucose (FDG) is a glucose analogue transported into cells via glucose transporters and is phosphorylated by hexokinase to FDG-6 phosphate. However, unlike glucose, it is not metabolized further. FDG accumulates in neutrophils, macrophages, and activated lymphocytes indicating increased glucose use by these cells at the site and time of infection. Increased FDG uptake in inflammation is probably caused by several factors. There is an increased number of glucose transporters on activated inflammatory cells. In addition, there is an increased affinity of the glucose transporters for FDG in inflammation, probably secondary to the effects of circulating cytokines and growth factors. Hence although FDG accumulates in infection, it is a nonspecific tracer that also accumulates in aseptic inflammation and malignant lesions.[4]

Imaging with FDG-PET/CT has some distinct advantages over other imaging modalities. FDG is a small molecule and penetrates easily even in poorly perfused areas. It accumulates in acute and chronic inflammation/infection. It produces high-resolution tomographic images with accurate localization of the abnormality. Entire PET/CT scan is undertaken within 1 to 2 hours' time with quantitative/semiquantitative information available immediately after the scan. This also facilitates better monitoring of response to therapy. FDG-PET/CT has high sensitivity and high negative predictive value (NPV). Its poor specificity makes differentiation of infection, inflammation, and malignancy difficult at times.

### $^{18}$F NaF PET/Computed Tomography Scan

The mechanism of skeletal uptake of $^{18}$F-NaF is based on ion exchange.[5] Bone tissue is continuously renewing itself through remodeling at the bone surface. F-18 ions exchange with hydroxyl ions (-OH) on the surface of the hydroxyapatite to form fluoroapatite.[6] This exchange occurs at a rapid rate; however, the actual incorporation of F-18 ions into the crystalline matrix of bone may take days or weeks. Uptake of $^{18}$F-NaF is a function of osseous blood flow and bone remodeling. F-18-NaF uptake on PET images are interpreted as processes that increase exposure of the surface of bone and provide a higher availability of binding sites, such as osteolytic and osteoblastic processes.[7] These characteristics make $^{18}$F-NaF scan extremely sensitive for studying bone remodeling secondary to infection/inflammation.

### $^{18}$F Fluorodeoxyglucose-Labeled Leukocyte Scan

For more specific imaging of infection, leukocytes have been labeled with F-18-FDG. However, short half-life of 110 minutes for F-18, off-site labeling, and absence of delayed imaging are its shortcomings. Furthermore, labeling efficiency of FDG is variable and lower than that of In-111-oxine. Also observed is rapid elution of FDG from leukocytes.[8] The labeling takes time. It is ex vivo technique with its potential hazards. Leukocyte accumulation is seen at the site of sterile inflammation, making it less specific for infection. However, availability of necessary components, lack of toxicity or adverse effects, and possibility of repeating examination make it a desired infection imaging agent. Overall, FDG-labeled leukocyte

PET/CT is a promising technique with high sensitivity and specificity.[9,10]

## Ga-68-Citrate PET/Computed Tomography Scan

Imaging characteristics of Ga-68-citrate are definitely superior to those of Ga-67. The uptake mechanisms remain same. Disadvantages of Ga-67, such as uptake in inflammation, trauma, and tumor, also apply to Ga-68-citrate. High background activity of Ga-68-citrate in the thorax and upper abdomen at 60 minutes postinjection may interfere with detecting lesions in these regions; therefore, Ga-68-PET is more suitable for imaging lesions in the lower abdomen and the extremities. The short half-life of Ga-68 ($T_{1/2}$ = 68 minutes) may be advantageous because of low dosimetry to patients, but disadvantageous for longer periods of study. Because Ga-68-Citrate is capable of detecting infection within 60 minutes, the need for imaging for longer periods may not be warranted.[11]

## I-124-Fialuridine PET/Computed Tomography Scan

I-124-Fialuridine is a specific substrate of bacterial thymidine kinase. Because fialuridine is incorporated into bacteria rather than inflammatory cells, it should be specific for the infectious process. In a pilot study by Luis and coworkers,[12] all eight patients with musculoskeletal infection demonstrated I-124-fialuridine accumulation in the infection. There was no abnormal uptake in the control subjects. However, results of subsequent investigations were disappointing.[13,14]

## INDICATIONS
### Osteomyelitis

The literature evidence on diagnosis of OM using FDG-PET/CT establishes this modality as one of the most promising imaging modalities with sensitivity and specificity more than 90% in most of the studies.[15–17] FDG-PET/CT is sensitive for detection of infection with high NPV. However, its specificity may be low in the immediate postoperative setting because postoperative inflammation persists up to 4 to 6 weeks after the procedure. In a meta-analysis done by Termaat and colleagues,[18] FDG-PET showed the highest accuracy in diagnosing and excluding chronic OM, with a sensitivity of 96% and a specificity of 91%, compared with 78% and 84% with combined bone and leukocyte scintigraphy and 84% and 60% with MR imaging. Guhlmann and colleagues[19] reported sensitivity and specificity of 100% and 92%,

respectively, for FDG-PET for diagnosing chronic OM in the axial and peripheral skeleton. de Winter and colleagues[16] reported sensitivity, specificity, and accuracy of 100%, 88%, and 93%, respectively, for FDG-PET in patients suspected of having chronic musculoskeletal infection.

In head-to-head comparison of FDG-PET/CT and MR imaging by Demirev and colleagues,[20] the investigators observed that both were accurate for diagnosis of active OM. They concluded that MR imaging can be considered the primary imaging modality for uncomplicated unifocal cases of OM, whereas in cases of suspected multifocal disease or contraindications for MR imaging, FDG-PET/CT should be preferred. This combined sequential strategy worked well particularly for the equivocal cases.

FDG-PET/CT may play an important role in patients with chronic OM, especially in those patients with previously documented OM and suspected recurrence, or presenting with symptoms of OM for more than 6 weeks (chronic OM).[21] In children with suspected OM, dissemination in multiple bones has to be kept in mind, for which FDG-PET/CT is suitable. However, to avoid radiation exposure, pediatricians tend to perform MR imaging rather than FDG-PET/CT in cases of suspected OM.[22] As in oncology, PET/CT is useful for initiating and monitoring therapy in patients with OM. In a retrospective study, FDG-PET/CT had a strong impact on the clinical management (initiation or prolongation of antibiotic therapy or recourse to surgical intervention) in 52% of patients with an infection.[23] In an interesting study done in children by Warmann and colleagues,[24] FDG-PET/CT was found superior in distinguishing between infection and reparative activity within the musculoskeletal system after treatment of acute OM, and termination of antibiotic treatment of children after acute OM seemed justified when laboratory parameters and clinical parameters are normal, and FDG-PET/CT is unsuspicious (**Fig. 1**).

## Infectious Spondylodiskitis

Infectious spondylodiskitis comprises of about 2% to 4% of OM cases and is mostly seen in patients with fever of unknown origin or as metastatic complication in bacteremia.[25] CT scan or MR imaging may be difficult to interpret because of inability to differentiate severe degenerative changes and infection. Also, artifacts secondary to metallic implants limit visibility in CT scan and same are contraindicated in MR imaging. Preliminary studies reported the diagnostic sensitivities of FDG-PET/CT to approach 100% and specificities of 75% to 100%, both at 100% for

## MIP PET scan

## MIP Fused PET/CT scan

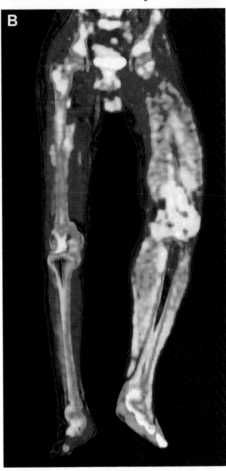

**Fig. 1.** Maximum Intensity Projection (MIP) image. A 29-year-old man with gunshot wound in the lower extremity since about 6 months and complicated left femur fracture. FDG-PET/CT undertaken in the context of recent pain: there is diffusely increased FDG uptake intramedullary distal femur and surrounding soft tissues, indicating infection that meets criteria for osteomyelitis in PET (A) and fused PET/CT (B) scans.

discriminating degenerative changes from disk space infection and thereby far surpassing MR imaging sensitivity of only 50% (**Figs. 2** and **3**).[26,27] Gratz and colleagues[28] reported that FDG-PET was superior to MR imaging for low-grade spondylitis/diskitis. Skanjeti and colleagues[29] reported that FDG-PET/CT was more accurate than MR imaging (90% vs 61.5%) for assessing treatment response.

However, there are false-positive findings seen on FDG-PET secondary to tumor or focal inflammation. Significant focal FDG uptake is seen occasionally in degenerative spine diseases.[8] Foreign body reaction around uninfected spinal implants may also cause increased uptake.[30]These problems could be solved by use of PET/CT to some extent. Meta-analysis done by Prodromou[31] and colleagues from 12 pooled studies found the

sensitivity and specificity of FDG-PET/CT to be 97% and 88%, respectively, with excellent ability to rule out the diagnosis with a low negative likelihood ratio of less than 0.1. Importantly, implants and other confounding factors did not affect the diagnostic efficacy when combined FDG-PET/CT was used. Data on Ga-68-citrate in spondylodiskitis are limited. Nanni and colleagues[32] reported that the test was 100% sensitive and 76% specific.

### Diabetic Foot

Diabetic foot is a foot infection caused by diabetic neuropathy or peripheral vascular disease and frequently a combination of both. Another important entity in the context of diabetes is neuro-osteoarthropathy or Charcot arthropathy, where

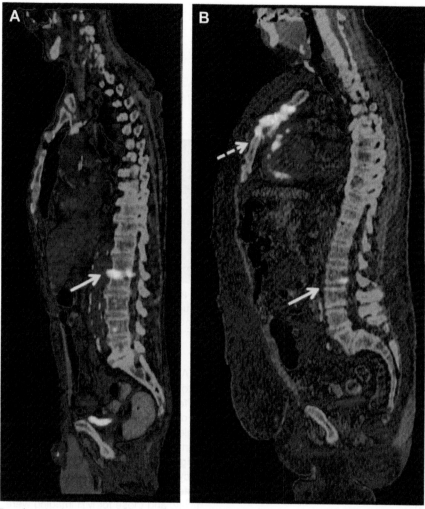

**Fig. 2.** (*A*) Fused sagittal FDG-PET/CT in a patient presenting with fever of unknown origin showing markedly increased FDG uptake consistent with L1/L2 spondylodiskitis (*arrow*). (*B*) Fused sagittal FDG-PET/CT in a patient with bacteremia of unknown origin showed increased FDG uptake consistent with L2/L3 spondylodiskitis (*solid arrow*) and sternal osteomyelitis (*dotted arrow*). (*From* Basu S, Kwee TC, Hess S. FDG-PET/CT imaging of infected bones and prosthetic joints. Curr Mol Imag 3(3):226; with permission.)

noninfectious soft tissue inflammation is associated with rapidly progressive destruction of joints and bone. Patients with diabetes carry significant risk of developing these diseases. When it comes to soft tissue infection, MR imaging with its excellent soft tissue delineation is the modality of choice. In a meta-analysis undertaken by Dinh and colleagues,[33] they compared role of exposed bone or probe-to-bone test, plain film radiography (PFR), MR imaging, bone scan, and leukocyte scan in detection of infection in diabetic foot. They concluded the presence of exposed bone or a positive probe-to-bone test result is moderately predictive of OM and MR imaging is the most accurate imaging test for diagnosis of OM.

FDG-PET has already established as a sensitive modality in imaging bone infection. Hence combination of PET/CT and MR imaging or PET/MR imaging has potential to become the best imaging combination for suspected OM in diabetic foot. One of the largest studies done by Nawaz and colleagues[34] reported results from 110 prospectively investigated patients with diabetes. In this study, head-to-head comparison was made between FDG-PET, MR imaging, and PFR of the feet. They obtained promising results with FDG-PET, which correctly diagnosed OM in 21 of 26 patients and correctly excluded it in 74 of 80, with sensitivity, specificity, positive predictive value (PPV), NPV, and accuracy of 81%, 93%, 78%, 94%, and 90%, respectively. MR imaging

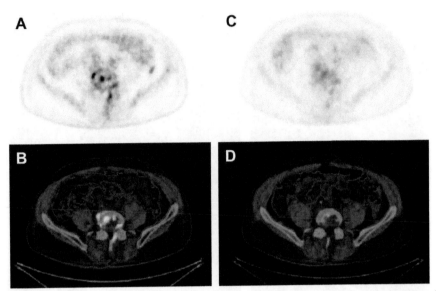

**Fig. 3.** Response evaluation in spondylodiskitis. Axial PET and PET/CT at baseline (*A, B*) and after 4 weeks of intravenous antibiotics (*C, D*). SUVmax decreased to half of its value at baseline (from 9.1 to 4.4 g/mL). (*From* Basu S, Kwee TC, Hess S. FDG-PET/CT imaging of infected bones and prosthetic joints. Curr Mol Imag 3(3):227; with permission.)

had sensitivity, specificity, PPV, NPV, and accuracy of 91%, 78%, 56%, 97%, and 81%, respectively, whereas PFR had sensitivity, specificity, PPV, NPV, and accuracy of 63%, 87%, 60%, 88%, and 81%, respectively. The investigators concluded that FDG-PET is a highly specific imaging modality for the diagnosis of OM in the diabetic foot and, therefore, should be considered to be a useful complementary imaging modality with MR imaging.

Clinically it is important to differentiate between OM and Charcot arthropathy because management of these two conditions is vastly different. Hopfner and colleagues[35] studied the role of FDG-PET for preoperative identification of neuropathic joints in patients with diabetes. The test correctly identified 95% (37/39) of the lesions, including 22 of 24 bone lesions and all 15 joint/soft tissue lesions. These investigators reported that the sensitivity of the test was not affected by blood glucose levels. Although none of the patients in this investigation had OM, these investigators suggested that, because of the low Maximum standardized uptake value (SUV max) is the ratio of the image derived radioactivity concentration and the whole body concentration of the injected radioactivity and gives semi-quantitative information about tracer dynamics (e.g. glucose metabolism in case of FDG), max in the uninfected neuropathic joints, and because of the high SUV max expected in OM, FDG-PET could differentiate OM from neuropathic disease.

A prospective study by Basu and colleagues[36] showed promising results in diagnosing OM and differentiating it from Charcot foot. A low degree of diffuse FDG uptake that was clearly distinguishable from that of normal joints was observed in joints of patients with Charcot osteoarthropathy (**Figs. 4** and **5**). The overall sensitivity and accuracy of FDG-PET in the diagnosis of Charcot osteoarthropathy were 100% and 93.8%, respectively, and those for MR imaging were 76.9% and 75.0%, respectively. The investigators concluded that these results underscored the valuable role of FDG-PET in the setting of Charcot neuroarthropathy by reliably differentiating it from OM, in general and when foot ulcer is present. Shagos and colleagues[37] reported that [18]F FDG-PET was more specific than bone scintigraphy for OM, whereas bone scintigraphy was more sensitive than [18]F FDG-PET for the neuropathic joint.

Familiari and colleagues[38] compared FDG-PET/CT with planar [99m]Tc-exametazime-labeled leukocyte imaging for diagnosing pedal OM in 13 patients with diabetes, all of whom had a high pretest likelihood of infection, including seven who presented with exposed bone. These investigators found that the highest accuracy for FDG-PET/CT (54%) was achieved when the SUVmax was greater than or equal to 2.0 at 1 and 2 hours after injection and increased over time. Accuracy improved to 62% when CT findings were included. The accuracy of planar [99m]Tc-exametazime-labeled leukocyte imaging, in contrast, was 92%.

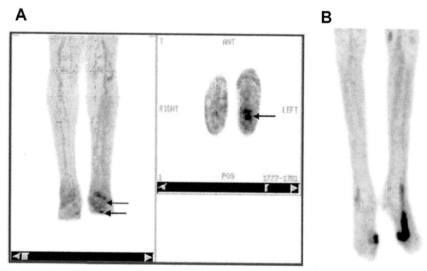

**Fig. 4.** (*A*) FDG-PET in a patient with diabetes mellitus demonstrating focal uptake in an ulcer (*arrows*) in the transaxial images and low-grade diffuse uptake in neuropathic osteoarthropathy (*arrows*) are clearly distinguishable from the uptake observed on the unaffected contralateral limb by visual inspection. (*B*) High-grade FDG uptake clearly distinctive from that of Charcot neuroarthopathy. (*From* Basu S, Chryssikos T, Houseni M, et al. Potential role of FDG-PET in the setting of diabetic neuroosteoarthropathy: can it differentiate uncomplicated Charcot's neuropathy from osteomyelitis and soft tissue infection? Nucl Med Commun 2007;28:468; with permission.)

The authors concluded that FDG-PET/CT is not accurate, and cannot replace labeled leukocyte imaging, for diagnosing pedal OM in patients with diabetes. Treglia and colleagues,[39] in a meta-analysis, reported a sensitivity and specificity of 74% and 91% for [18]F FDG. They concluded that large, multicenter studies using bone biopsy as the gold standard are warranted.

### Prosthetic Joint Infections

Differentiation between prosthetic joint loosening and infection is difficult because symptoms and conventional investigations are noncontributory in most of the cases. Radionuclide imaging with bone scan, Ga-67, and so forth has limited success. Labeled leukocyte/marrow imaging, with an accuracy of about 90%, currently is the best imaging test available. All the published studies confirm high specificity; nearly all also indicate high sensitivity.[40] Single-photon emission CT has further added exact localization and better resolution giving better results.

Zhuang and colleagues[41] reported that [18]F FDG-PET was 89.5% and 77.8% accurate for hip and knee arthroplasty infection, respectively. Correct diagnosis depended on location, not intensity, of uptake. Reinartz and colleagues[42] reported that [18]F FDG-PET was 95% accurate for hip arthroplasty infection. Basu and colleagues[43] reported sensitivity and specificity of 81.8% and 93.1%, respectively, for hip arthroplasty infection and

Axial PET scan    Coronal PET scan    Sagittal PET scan

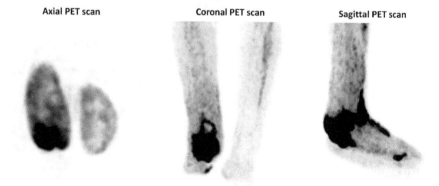

**Fig. 5.** A 72-year-old man with right diabetic foot demonstrating intense FDG uptake in the soft tissues in the tarsal region that was consistent with active soft tissue infection.

94.7% and 88.2%, respectively, for knee arthroplasty infection. Some investigators reported that [18]F FDG uptake around the femoral head and neck is not specific for infection; others reported that this pattern indicates synovitis plus infection (**Figs. 6 and 7**).[44,45]

However, other investigations showed less satisfactory results.[46–50] Van Acker and colleagues[46] reported 100% sensitivity and 73% specificity for prosthetic knee infection. Stumpe and colleagues[47] reported that [18]F FDG-PET was 69% accurate for prosthetic hip infection. García-Barrecheguren and colleagues[48] found that the test was neither sensitive (64%) nor specific (67%) for prosthetic hip infection. Love and colleagues[49] reported that F-[18]F FDG was 71% accurate for lower extremity prosthetic joint infection. Delank and colleagues[50] concluded that [18]F FDG-PET was not specific for lower extremity joint arthroplasty infection.

Comparative investigations of [18]F FDG and bone or labeled leukocyte imaging have been contradictory. Pill and colleagues[51] reported that [18]F FDG-PET was 95% sensitive and 93% specific for infection. In a subgroup, the sensitivity and specificity of labeled leukocyte/marrow imaging were 50% and 95.1%, respectively. Love and colleagues[49] found that labeled leukocyte/marrow imaging was more accurate than [18]F FDG (95% vs 71%). Kwee and colleagues,[52] in a meta-analysis, reported that the sensitivity and specificity of FDG-PET for diagnosing prosthetic joint infection were 82% and 87%, respectively. In a recent meta-analysis, the pooled sensitivity and specificity of [18]F FDG-PET and PET/CT for lower extremity prosthetic join infection both were 86%.[53]

## Septic Arthritis

Infectious organisms reach the joint through direct inoculation, hematogenous spread, or contiguous spread from an adjacent intra-articular site of infection. Ultrasound and MR imaging are the

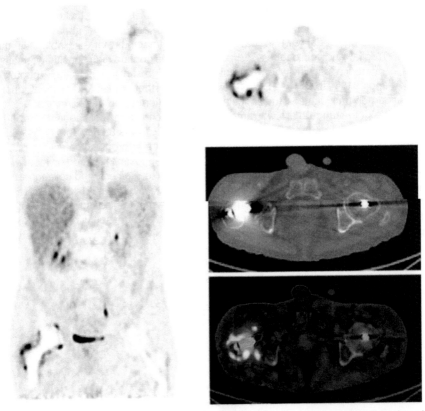

**Fig. 6.** Infected hip prosthesis. Coronal PET (*left column*) and axial PET, CT, and fused PET/CT (*right column*) show focally increased FDG uptake at the prosthesis-bone interfaces of the right hip prosthesis. Also noted are metal-induced artifacts on CT and the normal FDG distribution around the right-sided femur marrow nail. (*From* Basu S, Kwee TC, Hess S. FDG-PET/CT imaging of infected bones and prosthetic joints. Curr Mol Imag 3(3):227; with permission.)

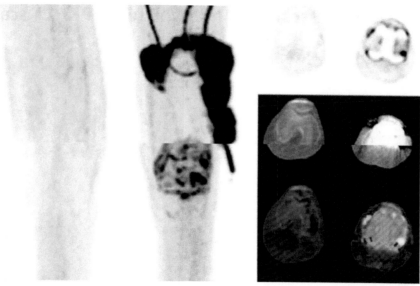

**Fig. 7.** Infected knee prosthesis. Coronal PET (*left column*) and axial PET, CT, and fused PET/CT (*right column*) show focally increased FDG uptake at the prosthesis-bone interfaces of the knee prosthesis and more diffuse distribution consistent with synovitis. Also noted are severe metal artifacts on CT. (*From* Basu S, Kwee TC, Hess S. FDG-PET/CT imaging of infected bones and prosthetic joints. Curr Mol Imag 3(3):228; with permission.)

principal imaging studies used for evaluating the suspected septic joint and show changes before radiography. Bone scan findings in septic arthritis and OM are overlapping.[54] Neither gallium nor labeled leukocyte imaging reliably separate infective from inflammatory arthritis.[55,56] Data about the role of FDG-PET in septic arthritis are limited. Like gallium and labeled leukocytes, FDG accumulates in infective and inflammatory processes. Consequently, the role of FDG-PET and PET/CT for diagnosing septic arthritis likely to be limited.

## Rheumatoid Arthritis

Rheumatoid arthritis (RA) is an autoimmune disease is associated with systemic and chronic inflammation of the joints, resulting in synovitis and pannus formation, both leading to increased FDG uptake. Several clinical studies have evaluated the role of FDG-PET in patients with RA.[57–60] The degree of FDG uptake in affected joints reflects the disease activity of RA.[57] FDG uptake correlates with clinical parameters, including the disease activity score, swelling and tenderness, ultrasonography (US) findings for synovitis and synovial thickening, power Doppler studies for neovascularization, erythrocyte sedimentation rate, and C-reactive protein.[58] FDG-PET was able to identify joints with active RA with higher sensitivity than clinical symptoms **(Fig. 8).**[57]

Few studies have evaluated FDG-PET/CT for therapy evaluation. Beckers and colleagues[61] assessed 16 patients with active RA in the knee joint using FDG-PET, dynamic MR imaging, and US at baseline and 4 weeks after the initiation of anti–tumor necrosis factor-α treatment. Significant differences in the MR imaging and US findings were observed between the FDG-PET positive and FDG-PET negative patients. Changes in the SUV after 4 weeks were correlated with changes in the MR imaging parameters, but not with the changes in synovial thickness observed by US. This suggests metabolic changes are preceding morphologic changes in patients with RA.

Goerres and colleagues[62] used a visual assessment total joint score, that is, the sum of all scores based on FDG uptake intensity between zero and four in 28 joints, in seven patients with active RA before and after infliximab treatment. The reduction of FDG joint uptake in the follow-up scans correlated significantly with clinical evaluation of disease activity. An association was found between changes in FDG joint uptake between baseline and after 2 weeks of infliximab treatment and the clinical outcome on long term. Early changes in FDG uptake in joints during infliximab treatment may predict clinical outcome.[63] In a recent study Kumar and colleagues[64] assessed the role of FDG-PET/CT in the evaluation of treatment response to disease-modifying antirheumatic drug therapy in patients with RA. They concluded that FDG-PET/CT-based assessment

## MIP PET scan

## MIP fused PET/CT scan

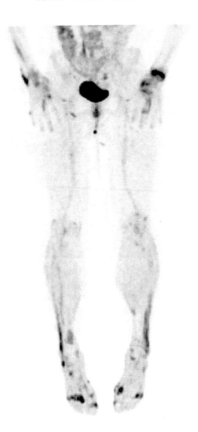 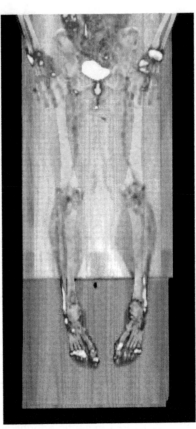

**Fig. 8.** A 65-year-old woman with history of rheumatoid arthritis. There are multiple foci of increased uptake in the wrists, hands, and feet bilaterally, representing an inflammatory/arthritic cause.

of inflammatory activity noted in the joints of RA with quantitative parameters is a promising approach for the whole-body assessment of RA disease activity and treatment response assessment, especially in inconclusive cases, and correlates well with other parameters. However, there is insufficient evidence to support the use of FDG-PET for the routine use in patients with RA. To better define the role of FDG-PET in patients with RA, larger patient studies are warranted.

### Osteoarthritis and Other Inflammatory Arthritic Diseases

Osteoarthritis (OA) is the commonest arthritis worldwide. Hip and knee are the most common large joints involved. OA is characterized by degradation and loss of articular cartilage, and remodeling of underlying bone. Currently, conventional radiography is the standard method for diagnosis and evaluation of severity of OA. A standing anteroposterior view is commonly used to assess articular degradation expressed as joint space width.[65,66]

In study of FDG-PET/CT in OA, 15 patients were studied by Nakamura and colleagues.[66] They found that FDG generally accumulated in periarticular lesions and was absent in the articular cartilage. They concluded that FDG uptake was upregulated in OA and generally accumulated in periarticular lesions. Increased uptake was found in the intercondylar notch extending along the PCL, periosteophytic lesions, and bone marrow.

In more recent study, Parsons and colleagues[67] compared the metabolic activity of the knee joints of a group of subjects with painful knees clinically (as recurrent joint pain, joint instability, and functional limitations) consistent with OA and those of another group of patients without such complaints, using FDG-PET imaging. They suggested that increased FDG uptake as measured by PET imaging was associated with pain in joints thought to be affected by OA. Thus, FDG-PET imaging may hold an application as a noninvasive diagnostic tool to detect knee joint inflammation and to assess disease severity in the clinical setting (Fig. 9).

[18]F NaF PET can assess the metabolic activity of subchondral bone remodeling. Increased bone remodeling has been implicated as a mechanism of OA progression that leads to changes in bone and adjacent cartilage.[68] Hence [18]F NaF scan can be used as an early marker to detect subchondral bone changes in OA. High [18]F NaF uptake has also been observed in degenerative and arthritic knees during evaluation of skeletal metastases. [18]F NaF PET may also be useful in the detection of bone remodeling in early stage OA of the temporomandibular and hip joints.[7,69]

There are case reports of synovitis, acne, pustulosis, hyperostosis, and osteitis syndrome[70] in which FDG-PET was of diagnostic value. Findings in other types of arthritis also suggest a valuable role of FDG-PET imaging in clinical diagnosis, including psoriatic arthritis,[71] collagen vascular diseases–associated arthritis,[72] juvenile idiopathic arthritis,[73] ankylosing spondylitis,[74] and reactive arthritis.[75]

## Myositis

Inflammatory muscle diseases are a group of muscle disorders characterized by muscle weakness, fatigue, and an association with malignancy and paraneoplastic syndrome. The diagnosis of idiopathic inflammatory myopathy is suggested by abnormal myometry and rising creatine kinase, but tissue diagnosis is also needed. MR imaging helps localize the appropriate site of biopsy, demonstrate the extent of muscle involvement, and monitor the response to therapy. However, the sensitivity of MR imaging is limited, and whole-body imaging is still far from routine. Chronic idiopathic inflammatory myopathies can occur as an isolated myositis or be associated with extramuscular features, such as skin, lung, esophageal, and cardiac involvement, or with another defined inflammatory connective tissue disease, such as mixed connective tissue disease, RA, Sjögren syndrome, systemic sclerosis, or systemic lupus erythematosus.[76]

US is widely available, low cost, and free from radiation. However, it is highly operator dependent. Early studies have shown good sensitivity of 83% in detecting polymyositis (PM), which correlates well with electromyography and creatine kinase but shows less specificity[77] and less sensitivity than MR imaging in showing muscular edema.[78] Weber and colleagues[79] compared contrast-enhanced intermittent power Doppler US with MR imaging in 35 patients with PM or dermatomyositis (DM) to quantify perfusion in clinically affected muscles. Contrast-enhanced US showed improved specificity, but the sensitivity

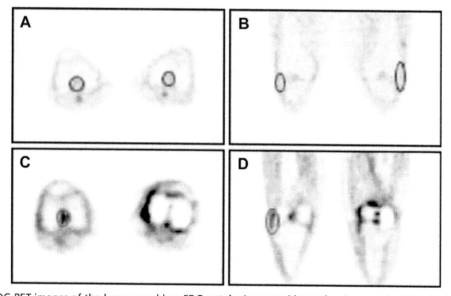

**Fig. 9.** FDG-PET images of the knee reveal low FDG uptake in control knees but increased uptake in the painful knees. (*A, B*) FDG uptake in a typical control knee (with no pain). (*C, D*) FDG uptake in a painful knee (patient had bilateral chronic knee pain and left-side prosthesis placement). Both axial (*A, C*) and coronal (*B, D*) images of knee are shown. (*From* Parsons MA, Moghbel M, Saboury B, et al. Increased 18F-FDG uptake suggests synovial inflammatory reaction with osteoarthritis: preliminary in-vivo results in humans. Nucl Med Commun 2015;36(12):1215–9; with permission.)

and NPV were reduced compared with MR imaging.

MR imaging is increasingly used as the imaging tool of choice for assessing disease activity and biopsy guidance in inflammatory myopathy. Areas with inflammatory edema show higher signal on T2-weighted images unlike normal muscles. Because fat can interfere with the interpretation of these changes, newer techniques including T2-weighted images with fat suppression and short TI inversion recovery sequence with long time to echo were introduced to eliminate fat signal.

Tomasová Studynková and colleagues[80] found that MR imaging–guided muscle biopsy samples contained significantly more inflammatory cells than the biopsy taken from areas that were negative on MR imaging. However, they found that inflammatory cells can still be found in a muscle or parts of muscles that look unaffected on MR images. In addition, they observed that the signal intensity on MR images decrease significantly after treatment, but the inflammation detected histologically did not change substantially. Whole-body MR imaging using the fat-suppressed short TI inversion recovery protocol was used in a group of seven patients with clinical PM and was found helpful in facilitating a global overview of the extent and symmetry of muscular involvement.[81] However, this technique remains difficult to implement in routine use because of the time consumed for the procedure. Also, lack of surface coil during acquisition may reduce resolution leading to reduced detection of small lesions.

In a well-prepared patient undergoing an FDG-PET scan, skeletal muscles do not show significant uptake of the tracer. This is possible because the metabolic rate is kept low by complete muscle relaxation during uptake phase of around 60 minutes post-FDG injection. The patient is instructed not to perform any muscular activity including talking and chewing during this period. Patients are instructed to have nothing by mouth for 4 to 6 hours before the injection of the tracer and are monitored for blood glucose levels in the physiologically acceptably low range. Physical exercise shortly before or during this period, and food intake or the use of insulin, can produce extensive muscle uptake that may render the scan nondiagnostic, a situation termed "muscle scan."[82] When FDG uptake in muscles is seen even in controlled conditions, then it is suggestive of muscular inflammation (**Fig. 10**).

Agriantonis and colleagues[83] presented a case of intense and diffuse muscle uptake in a 35-year-old man as part of chronic graft-versus-host disease manifestation. Early detection of graft-

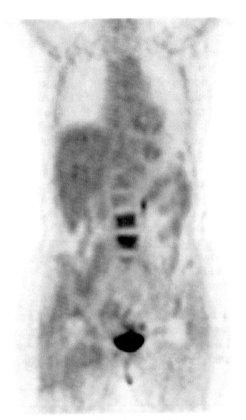

**Fig. 10.** Coronal whole-body FDG-PET image reveals significant uptake of FDG in the muscles on the right side involving the buttock, psoas muscle, and upper thigh. This finding was interpreted to represent dermatomyositis in this patient. (*From* Basu S, Zhuang H, Torigian DA, et al. Functional imaging of inflammatory diseases using nuclear medicine techniques. Semin Nucl Med 2009;39(2):142; with permission.)

versus-host disease–associated PM is vital because it is readily treatable with immunosuppressive therapy, without which devastating consequences, notably myoglobin-induce renal failure, may ensue. Similarly, Liau and colleagues[84] presented a case of a man with DM in which PET/CT imaging revealed diffuse proximal muscle hypermetabolism, in keeping with the inflammatory nature of DM, and was instrumental in the diagnosis of an underlying adenocarcinoma involving the mediastinum.

PM and DM are potential paraneoplastic diseases that require cancers screening.[85] Finding the right tool for such screening remains a problem, and FDG-PET is increasingly used for the detection of occult tumors as shown in several case reports[84,86] and in a cohort of patients with paraneoplastic syndrome that included cases of DM.[87] A review by Selva-O'Callaghan and co-workers[88] recommends yearly PET/CT study for at least 3 to 5 years in patients with PM (the risk of associated cancer is moderate) and DM (the risk of associated cancer is high) especially those with positive anti-p155 autoantibodies.

MR imaging is the imaging modality of choice in delineating the extent of disease and biopsy guidance. MR imaging involves no radiation exposure. However, it has low sensitivity and whole-body MR imaging acquisition is difficult in routine clinical practice. Although hyperintensity on T2-weighted imaging frequently represents edema and is an early sign of myositis, it may be misleading because it is not specific to myositis and can also be found in metabolic and traumatic myopathies, infection, diabetic muscle infarction, rhabdomyolysis, and even after physical exercise.[89] Hence final diagnosis is confirmed only in correlation with clinical data and laboratory data (especially muscle biopsy).

With its ability of whole-body imaging of metabolism, FDG-PET/CT can play a significant role in the diagnosis, in determining the site of muscle biopsy, and in the evaluation of disease activity and grading severity of PM/DM. In addition, higher sensitivity of PET/CT in detection of malignancy is useful to detect occult malignancy in this patient group. Information about interstitial lung disease is obtained in the same scan. Hence FDG-PET/CT is possibly an important tool with the ability to provide a multitude of information in patients with possible PM/DM. Combined PET/MR imaging would reduce the radiation exposure of patients and provide possibly the best combination for diagnosis and treatment monitoring in PM/DM patients.

## PET/MR IMAGING SCAN

PET/MR imaging systems combine high-resolution MR imaging with simultaneous molecular information from PET to study the multifaceted processes involved in numerous musculoskeletal disorders. Because MR imaging does not produce any ionizing radiation, replacing CT with MR imaging can reduce the radiation dose to patients undergoing hybrid PET imaging by up to 80%.[90] In addition to a lack of ionizing radiation, MR imaging offers superior soft tissue contrast to CT, such as in cartilage and muscle. MR imaging can also provide additional information regarding tissue biochemistry, diffusion, and perfusion.

MR imaging has been used to noninvasively study and understand many of the complex disease processes involved in joint arthritis. However, structural degenerative changes observed on MR imaging are likely at a late stage in the disease process when tissue loss has already occurred and

treatments are unlikely to be effective. Hybrid PET/MR imaging systems allow for comprehensive imaging of the whole joint, including soft tissues and bone, which is necessary to study complex disease processes in arthritis. PET imaging with $^{18}$F fluoride and $^{18}$F FDG offers metabolic information regarding bone remodeling and inflammatory processes, respectively.

## IMAGING OF PAIN-RELATED NOCICEPTIVE ACTIVITY

Pain, acute and chronic, is the most common reason patients seek medical attention. However, diagnosis and characterization of pain is challenging. Clinical assessment of pain is usually dependent on a patient's self-analysis, which is highly subjective. Current clinical imaging of pain relies on identifying anatomic abnormalities that may be producing a patient's clinical symptoms. However, structural abnormalities are often nonspecific and are often present in asymptomatic patients with a similar prevalence.[91,92] Hence, there is a great need for imaging tools that can identify pain-related nociceptive activity.

FDG-PET imaging can image the increased glucose metabolism used by inflamed or overactive neurons as a marker of neural activity. Studies in a rat model that used unilateral injury to induce neuropathic limb pain showed increased FDG uptake in injured nerves, but no increase in FDG uptake in the contralateral limb or in control asymptomatic animals.[93] Additionally, in a human subject presenting with progressive difficulty in walking, increased FDG uptake was observed in his lower spinal cord and sciatic nerves.[94] Biopsy of the tissues confirmed the pathologic signs of neuropathy.

MR imaging has been used to identify entrapment neuropathies, plexus lesions, and nerve compression syndromes.[95,96] However, although MR imaging can provide high-resolution imaging of peripheral nerve abnormalities, it has low specificity to identify the inciting nerve inflammation or injury. Early experiences with hybrid PET/MR imaging in patients suffering from chronic lower extremity neuropathic pain showed FDG uptake could be localized to affected nerves and impacted clinical management of their pain.[97]

## SUMMARY

FDG-PET/CT seems to be a promising tool in imaging various infective and inflammatory processes in the musculoskeletal system. It outperforms established diagnostic modalities with its high sensitivity, specificity, and whole-body imaging capability. The procedure is simple, less time consuming, noninvasive, and is well tolerated by the patient. Apart from FDG, $^{18}$F NaF, FDG-labelled leukocytes, and Ga-68 citrate may be used for infection/inflammation imaging. Newer tracers, such as I-124-fialuridine, are being explored for the same. FDG-PET/CT seems to be useful not only in imaging of various skeletal and joint infections, but also for various inflammatory diseases affecting muscles and nerves. PET/MR imaging fusion has added strength of metabolic imaging to MR imaging, which is already an established modality for imaging finer details of cartilage, muscles, and nerves. As more data become available, PET seems to be the front runner in imaging of musculoskeletal infection and inflammation.

# REFERENCES

1. Biswal S, Resnick DL, Hoffman JM, et al. Molecular imaging: integration of molecular imaging into the musculoskeletal imaging practice. Radiology 2007; 244:651–71.

2. Wilmot A, Gieschler S, Behera D, et al. Molecular imaging: an innovative force in musculoskeletal radiology. AJR Am J Roentgenol 2013;201: 264–77.

3. van der Horst G, van der Pluijm G. Preclinical imaging of the cellular and molecular events in the multistep process of bone metastasis. Future Oncol 2012;8:415–30.

4. Love C, Tomas MB, Tronco GG, et al. Imaging infection and inflammation with 18F-FDG-PET. Radiographics 2005;25:1357–68.

5. Czernin J, Satyamurthy N, Schiepers C. Molecular mechanisms of bone 18F-NaF deposition. J Nucl Med 2010;51:1826–9.

6. Schiepers C, Nuyts J, Bormans G, et al. Fluoride kinetics of the axial skeleton measured in vivo with fluorine-18-fluoride PET. J Nucl Med 1997;38: 1970–6.

7. Kobayashi N, Inaba Y, Tateishi U, et al. New application of 18F-fluoride PET for the detection of bone remodeling in early-stage osteoarthritis of the hip. Clin Nucl Med 2013;38:379–83.

8. Palestro CJ. Radionuclide imaging of osteomyelitis. Semin Nucl Med 2015;45:32–46.

9. Dumarey N, Egrise D, Blocklet D, et al. Imaging infection with F-18-FDG labelled leukocyte PET/CT: initial experience in 21 patients. J Nucl Med 2006; 47:625–32.

10. Rini JN, Bhargava KK, Tronco GG, et al. PET with FDG labelled leukocytes versus scintigraphy with In-111-oxine-labeled leukocytes for detection of infection. Radiology 2006;238:978–87.

11. Kumar V, Boddeti DK. (68)Ga-radiopharmaceuticals for PET imaging of infection and inflammation. Recent Results Cancer Res 2013;194:189–219.

12. Diaz LA, Foss CA, Thornton K, et al. Imaging of musculoskeletal bacterial infections by [I-124] FIAU-PET/CT. PLoS One 2007;2:1007.

13. [I-124] FIAU-PET/CT scanning in patients with pain in a prosthetic knee or hip joint (PJI). ClinicalTrials.gov website. 2012. Available at: https://clinicaltrials.gov/ct2/show/NCT01705496. Updated February 8, 2016. Accessed July 12, 2016.

14. FIAU-PET/CT scanning in diagnosing osteomyelitis in patients with diabetic foot infection. 2013. Available at: https://clinicaltrials.gov/ct2/show/NCT01764919. Updated April 6, 2016. Accessed July 12, 2016.

15. Bleeker-Rovers CP, Vos FJ, Corstens FH, et al. Imaging of infectious diseases using [$^{18}$F] fluorodeoxyglucose PET. Q J Nucl Med Mol Imaging 2008; 52(1):17–29.

16. de Winter F, van de Wiele C, Vogelaers D, et al. Fluorine-18 fluorodeoxyglucose-position emission tomography: a highly accurate imaging modality for the diagnosis of chronic musculoskeletal infections. J Bone Joint Surg Am 2001;83-a(5): 651–60.

17. Hartmann A, Eid K, Dora C, et al. Diagnostic value of 18F-FDG PET/CT in trauma patients with suspected chronic osteomyelitis. Eur J Nucl Med Mol Imaging 2007;34(5):704–14.

18. Termaat MF, Raijmakers PG, Scholten HJ, et al. The accuracy of diagnostic imaging for the assessment of chronic osteomyelitis: a systematic review and metaanalysis. J Bone Joint Surg Am 2005;87(11): 2464–71.

19. Guhlmann A, Brecht-Krauss D, Suger G, et al. Chronic osteomyelitis: detection with FDG PET and correlation with histopathologic findings. Radiology 1998;206:749–54.

20. Demirev A, Weijers R, Geurts J, et al. Comparison of [$^{18}$F] FDG PET/CT and MRI in the diagnosis of active osteomyelitis. Skeletal Radiol 2014;43(5):665–72.

21. Glaudemans AW, Signore A. FDG-PET/CT in infections: the imaging method of choice? Eur J Nucl Med Mol Imaging 2010;37(10):1986–91.

22. Darge K, Jaramillo D, Siegel MJ. Whole-body MRI in children: current status and future applications. Eur J Radiol 2008;68(2):289–98.

23. Ito K, Kubota K, Morooka M, et al. Clinical impact of $^{18}$F-FDG PET/CT on the management and diagnosis of infectious spondylitis. Nucl Med Commun 2010; 31(8):691–8.

24. Warmann SW, Dittmann H, Seitz G, et al. Follow-up of acute osteomyelitis in children: the possible role of PET/CT in selected cases. J Pediatr Surg 2011; 46(8):1550–6.

25. Vos FJ, Kullberg BJ, Sturm PD, et al. Metastatic infectious disease and clinical outcome in

Staphylococcus aureus and Streptococcus species bacteremia. Medicine 2012;91(2):86–94.

26. Schmitz A, Risse JH, Grunwald F, et al. Fluorine-18 fluorodeoxyglucose positron emission tomography findings in spondylodiscitis: preliminary results. Eur Spine J 2001;10(6):534–9.

27. Stumpe KD, Zanetti M, Weishaupt D, et al. FDG positron emission tomography for differentiation of degenerative and infectious endplate abnormalities in the lumbar spine detected on MR imaging. AJR Am J Roentgenol 2002;179(5):1151–7.

28. Gratz S, Dorner J, Fischer U, et al. F-18-FDG hybrid PET in patients with suspected spondylitis. Eur J Nucl Med Mol Imaging 2002;29:516–24.

29. Skanjeti A, Penna D, Douroukas A, et al. PET in the clinical work-up of patients with spondylodiscitis: a new tool for the clinician? Q J Nucl Med Mol Imaging 2012;56:569–76.

30. De Winter F, Gemmel F, Van de Wiele C, et al. 18-fluorine fluorodeoxyglucose positron emission tomography for the diagnosis of infection in the postoperative spine. Spine 2003;28:1314–9.

31. Prodromou ML, Ziakas PD, Poulou LS, et al. FDG PET is a robust tool for the diagnosis of spondylodiscitis: a meta-analysis of diagnostic data. Clin Nucl Med 2014;39(4):330–5.

32. Nanni C, Errani C, Boriani L, et al. 68Ga-citrate PET/CT for evaluating patients with infections of the bone: preliminary results. J Nucl Med 2010;51: 1932–6.

33. Dinh MT, Abad CL, Safdar N. Diagnostic accuracy of physical examination and imaging tests for osteomyelitis underlying diabetic foot ulcers: meta analysis. Clin Infect Dis 2008;47(4):519–27.

34. Nawaz A, Torigian DA, Siegelman ES, et al. Diagnostic performance of FDG-PET, MRI, and plain film radiography (PFR) for the diagnosis of osteomyelitis in the diabetic foot. Mol Imaging Biol 2010;12: 335–42.

35. Hopfner S, Krolak C, Kessler S, et al. Preoperative imaging of Charcot neuroarthropathy in diabetic patients: comparison of ring PET, hybrid PET, and magnetic resonance imaging. Foot Ankle Int 2004;25: 890–5.

36. Basu S, Chryssikos T, Houseni M, et al. Potential role of FDG-PET in the setting of diabetic neuroosteoarthropathy: can it differentiate uncomplicated Charcot's neuropathy from osteomyelitis and soft tissue infection? Nucl Med Commun 2007;28:465–72.

37. Shagos GS, Shanmugasundaram P, Varma AK, et al. 18-F fluorodeoxy glucose positron emission tomography-computed tomography imaging: a viable alternative to three phase bone scan in evaluating diabetic foot complications? Indian J Nucl Med 2015;30:97–103.

38. Familiari D, Glaudemans AWJM, Vitale V, et al. Can sequential ¹⁸F-FDG-PET/CT imaging replace WBC imaging in the diabetic foot? J Nucl Med 2011;52: 1012–9.

39. Treglia G, Sadeghib R, Annunziata S, et al. Diagnostic performance of fluorine-18-fluorodeoxyglucose positron emission tomography for the diagnosis of osteomyelitis related to diabetic foot: a systematic review and a meta-analysis. Foot (Edinb) 2013;23:140–8.

40. Palestro CJ. Nuclear medicine and the failed joint replacement: past, present, and future. World J Radiol 2014;6:446–58.

41. Zhuang H, Duarte PS, Pourdehnad M, et al. The promising role of ¹⁸F-FDG PET in detecting infected lower limb prosthesis implants. J Nucl Med 2001;42: 44–8.

42. Reinartz P, Mumme T, Hermanns B, et al. Radionuclide imaging of the painful hip arthroplasty: positron-emission tomography versus triple-phase bone scanning. J Bone Joint Surg Br 2005;87: 465–70.

43. Basu S, Kwee TC, Saboury B, et al. FDG PET for diagnosing infection in hip and knee prostheses: prospective study in 221 prostheses and subgroup comparison with combined ¹¹¹In-labeled leukocyte/99mTc-sulfur colloid bone marrow imaging in 88 prostheses. Clin Nucl Med 2014;39: 609–15.

44. Chacko TK, Zhuang H, Stevenson K, et al. The importance of the location of fluorodeoxyglucose uptake in periprosthetic infection in painful hip prostheses. Nucl Med Commun 2002;23:851–5.

45. Manthey N, Reinhard P, Moog F, et al. The use of [¹⁸F] fluorodeoxyglucose positron emission tomography to differentiate between synovitis, loosening and infection of hip and knee prostheses. Nucl Med Commun 2002;23:645–53.

46. Van Acker F, Nuyts J, Maes A, et al. FDG-PET, 99mTc-HMPAO white blood cell SPET and bone scintigraphy in the evaluation of painful total knee arthroplasties. Eur J Nucl Med 2001;28:1496–504.

47. Stumpe KD, Nötzli HP, Zanetti M, et al. FDG PET for differentiation of infection and aseptic loosening in total hip replacements: comparison with conventional radiography and three-phase bone scintigraphy. Radiology 2004;231:333–41.

48. García-Barrecheguren E, Rodríguez Fraile M, Toledo Santana G, et al. FDG-PET: a new diagnostic approach in hip prosthetic replacement. Rev Esp Med Nucl 2007;26:208–20.

49. Love C, Marwin SE, Tomas MB, et al. Diagnosing infection in the failed joint replacement: a comparison of coincidence detection fluorine-18 FDG and indium-111-labeled leukocyte/technetium-99m-sulfur colloid marrow imaging. J Nucl Med 2004;45: 1864–71.

50. Delank KS, Schmidt M, Michael JW, et al. The implications of ¹⁸F-FDG PET for the diagnosis of endoprosthetic loosening and infection in hip and knee

arthroplasty: results from a prospective, blinded study. BMC Musculoskelet Disord 2006;7:20.

51. Pill SG, Parvizi J, Tang PH, et al. Comparison of fluorodeoxyglucose positron emission tomography and 111indium-white blood cell imaging in the diagnosis of periprosthetic infection of the hip. J Arthroplasty 2006;21:91–7.

52. Kwee TC, Kwee RM, Alavi A. FDG-PET for diagnosing prosthetic joint infection: systematic review and metaanalysis. Eur J Nucl Med Mol Imaging 2008;35:2122–32.

53. Jin H, Yuan L, Li C, et al. Diagnostic performance of FDG PET or PET/CT in prosthetic infection after arthroplasty: a meta-analysis. Q J Nucl Med Mol Imaging 2014;58:85–93.

54. Palestro CJ, Love C, Miller TT. Imaging of musculoskeletal infections. Best Pract Res Clin Rheumatol 2006;20:1197–218.

55. Uno K, Matsui N, Nohira K, et al. Indium-111 leukocyte imaging in patients with rheumatoid arthritis. J Nucl Med 1986;27:339–44.

56. Palestro CJ, Vega A, Kim CK, et al. Appearance of acute gouty arthritis on indium-111 labeled leukocyte scintigraphy. J Nucl Med 1990;31:682–7.

57. Kubota K, Ito K, Morooka M, et al. FDG PET for rheumatoid arthritis: basic considerations and whole-body PET/CT. Ann N Y Acad Sci 2011;1228(1):29–38.

58. Palmer WE, Rosenthal DI, Schoenberg OI, et al. Quantification of inflammation in the wrist with gadolinium-enhanced MR imaging and PET with 2-[F-18]-fluoro-2-deoxy-D-glucose. Radiology 1995;196(3):647–55.

59. Kubota K, Ito K, Morooka M, et al. Whole-body FDG PET/CT on rheumatoid arthritis of large joints. Ann Nucl Med 2009;23(9):783–91.

60. McBride HJ. Nuclear imaging of autoimmunity: focus on IBD and RA. Autoimmunity 2010;43(7):539–49.

61. Beckers C, Ribbens C, André B, et al. Assessment of disease activity in rheumatoid arthritis with 18F-FDG PET. J Nucl Med 2004;45(6):956–64.

62. Goerres GW, Forster A, Uebelhart D, et al. F-18 FDG whole body PET for the assessment of disease activity in patients with rheumatoid arthritis. Clin Nucl Med 2006;31(7):386–90.

63. Elzinga EH, van der Laken CJ, Comans EFI, et al. [18]F FDG PET as a tool to predict the clinical outcome of infliximab treatment of rheumatoid arthritis: an explorative study. J Nucl Med 2011;52(1):77–80.

64. Kumar NS, Shejul Y, Asopa R, et al. Quantitative metabolic volumetric product on fluorine-2fluoro-2-deoxy-D-glucose-positron emission tomography/computed tomography in assessing treatment response to disease-modifying antirheumatic drugs in rheumatoid arthritis: multiparametric analysis integrating American College of Rheumatology/

European League Against Rheumatism criteria. World J Nucl Med 2017;16(4):293–302.

65. Zhang Y, Jordan JM. Epidemiology of osteoarthritis. Clin Geriatr Med 2010;26:355–69 [PubMed: 20699159].

66. Nakamura H, Masuko K, Yudoh K. Positron emission tomography with [18]F-FDG in osteoarthritic knee. Osteoarthritis Cartilage 2007;15:673–81.

67. Parsons MA, Moghbel M, Saboury B. Increased FDG uptake suggests synovial inflammatory reaction with osteoarthritis: preliminary in vivo results in humans. Nucl Med Commun 2015;36(12):1215–9.

68. Kurata S, Shizukuishi K, Tateishi U, et al. Age-related changes in pre- and postmenopausal women investigated with [18]F-fluoride PET–a preliminary study. Skeletal Radiol 2012;41:947–53.

69. Lee JW, Lee SM, Kim SJ, et al. Clinical utility of fluoride-18 positron emission tomography/CT in temporomandibular disorder with osteoarthritis: comparisons with [99m]Tc-MDP bone scan. Dentomaxillofac Radiol 2013;42(2):29292350.

70. Pichler R, Weiglein K, Schmekal B, et al. Bone scintigraphy using Tc-99m-DPD and F18-FDG in a patient with SAPHO syndrome. Scand J Rheumatol 2003;32:58–60.

71. Takata T, Taniguchi Y, Ohnishi T, et al. 18)FDG PET/CT is a powerful tool for detecting subclinical arthritis in patients with psoriatic arthritis and/or psoriasis vulgaris. J Dermatol Sci 2011;64:144–7.

72. Okabe T, Shibata H, Shizukuishi K, et al. F-18 FDG uptake patterns and disease activity of collagen vascular diseases-associated arthritis. Clin Nucl Med 2011;36:350–4.

73. Lord M, Allaoua M, Ratib O. Positron emission tomography findings in systemic juvenile idiopathic arthritis. Rheumatology 2011;50:1177.

74. Strobel K, Fischer DR, Tamborrini G, et al. [18]F-fluoride PET/CT for detection of sacroiliitis in ankylosing spondylitis. Eur J Nucl Med Mol Imaging 2010;37:1760–5.

75. Taniguchi Y, Kumon Y, Nakayama S, et al. F-18 FDG PET/CT provides the earliest findings of enthesitis in reactive arthritis. Clin Nucl Med 2011;36:121–3.

76. Al-Nahhas A, Jawad ASM. PET/CT imaging in inflammatory myopathies. Ann N Y Acad Sci 2011;1228:39–45.

77. Reimers CD, Fleckenstein JL, Witt TN, et al. Muscular ultrasound in idiopathic inflammatory myopathies of adults. J Neurol Sci 1993;116:82–92.

78. Reimers CD, Finkenstaedt M. Muscle imaging in inflammatory myopathies. Curr Opin Rheumatol 1997;9:75–85.

79. Weber MA, Jappe U, Essig M, et al. Contrast enhanced ultrasound in dermatomyositis and polymyositis. J Neurol 2006;253:1625–32.

80. Tomasová Studynková J, Charvát F, Jarosová K, et al. The role of MRI in the assessment of

polymyositis and dermatomyositis. Rheumatology 2007;46:1174–9.

81. O'Connell MJ, Powell T, Brennan D, et al. Whole body MR imaging in the diagnosis of polymyositis. AJR Am J Roentgenol 2002;179:967–71.

82. Yeung HW, Grewal RK, Gonen M, et al. Patterns of (18)F-FDG uptake in adipose tissue and muscle: a potential source of false-positives for PET. J Nucl Med 2003;44:1789–96.

83. Agriantonis DJ, Perlman SB, Longo WL. F-18 FDG PET imaging of GVHD-associated polymyositis. Clin Nucl Med 2008;33:688–9.

84. Liau N, Ooi C, Reid C, et al. F-18 FDG PET/CT detection of mediastinal malignancy in a patient with dermatomyositis. Clin Nucl Med 2007;32:304–5.

85. Selva-O'Callaghan A, Grau JM, Gámez-Cenzano C, et al. Conventional cancer screening versus PET/CT in dermatomyositis/polymyositis. Am J Med 2010; 123:558–62.

86. Muñoz MA, Conejo-Mir JS, Congregado-Loscertales M, et al. The utility of positron emission tomography to find an occult neoplasm in a patient with dermatomyositis. J Eur Acad Dermatol Venereol 2007;21:1418–9.

87. Berner U, Menzel C, Rinne D, et al. Paraneoplastic syndromes: detection of malignant tumors using [(18)F]FDG-PET. Q J Nucl Med 2003;47:85–9.

88. Selva-O'Callaghan A, Trallero-Araguas E, Grau-Junyent JM, et al. Malignancy and myositis: novel autoantibodies and new insights. Curr Opin Rheumatol 2010;22:627–32.

89. Maillard SM, Jones R, Owens C, et al. Quantitative assessment of MRI T2 relaxation time of thigh muscles in juvenile dermatomyositis. Rheumatology (Oxford) 2004;43(5):603–8.

90. Hirsch FW, Sattler B, Sorge I, et al. PET/MR in children. Initial clinical experience in paediatric oncology using an integrated PET/MR scanner. Pediatr Radiol 2013;43:860–75.

91. Jensen MC, Brant-Zawadzki MN, Obuchowski N, et al. Magnetic resonance imaging of the lumbar spine in people without back pain. N Engl J Med 1994;331:69–73.

92. Sher JS, Uribe JW, Posada A, et al. Abnormal findings on magnetic resonance images of asymptomatic shoulders. J Bone Joint Surg Am 1995;77:10–5.

93. Behera D, Jacobs KE, Behera S, et al. (18)F-FDG PET/MRI can be used to identify injured peripheral nerves in a model of neuropathic pain. J Nucl Med 2011;52:1308–12.

94. Cheng G, Chamroonrat W, Bing Z, et al. Elevated FDG activity in the spinal cord and the sciatic nerves due to neuropathy. Clin Nucl Med 2009;34:950–1.

95. Ohana M, Moser T, Moussaouï A, et al. Current and future imaging of the peripheral nervous system. Diagn Interv Imaging 2014;95:17–26.

96. Stoll G, Bendszus M, Perez J, et al. Magnetic resonance imaging of the peripheral nervous system. J Neurol 2009;256:1043–51.

97. Biswal S, Behera D, Yoon DH, et al. [18F] FDG PET/MRI of patients with chronic pain alters management: early experience. EJNMMI Phys 2015;2:A84.

# Clinical Applications of Positron Emission Tomography in the Evaluation of Spine and Joint Disorders

Abdullah Al-Zaghal, MD[1], Cyrus Ayubcha, MD[1],
Esha Kothekar, MD,
Abass Alavi, MD, MD (Hon), PhD (Hon), DSc (Hon)*

## KEYWORDS

- Low back pain • Osteoarthritis • Osteoporosis • Prosthetic joints • FDG • NaF • Molecular imaging
- PET

## KEY POINTS

- Fluorodeoxyglucose (FDG) remains a powerful radiotracer for assessing synovial inflammation and complicated prosthetic joints.
- Sodium fluoride (NaF) PET is highly sensitive for the detection of the earliest osteoblastic changes and has a promising role in the evaluation of osteoporosis and monitoring treatment response in skeletal disorders.
- NaF PET and FDG-PET have a potential to play an important role in the evaluation of low back pain.

## INTRODUCTION

Over the last decade, major advances have been made in PET imaging, including the introduction of hybrid PET/computed tomography (CT) and PET/MR imaging systems, facilitating a better understanding of the pathophysiology underlying a vast array of human diseases. PET has not only remained the clinical standard for most oncological disorders but also emerged as a potentially viable modality in nononcological disorders, including many musculoskeletal pathologies. As such, this review examines the relevant applications of fluorodeoxyglucose (FDG)- and fluorine-18 sodium fluoride (NaF)-PET in the assessment of common spine disorders: low back pain, degenerative disorders, postsurgical outcomes, and osteoporosis. The authors also reviewed the recent advancements of PET in the evaluation of knee osteoarthritis (OA) and prosthetic knee joints and its complications.[1,2]

## SPINE DISORDERS

Perhaps the most complex structure in the entire musculoskeletal system, the spine consists of multisegmented osseous vertebrae separated by soft tissue in the form of discs. Traditional structural imaging modalities, such as CT and MR imaging, have long been used for the diagnosis, monitoring, and study of various disorders. Molecular imaging has yet to encompass the clinical evaluation of many nononcological disorders of the spine. However, recent research has increasingly supported the application of PET in such areas.

MR imaging and CT have been useful in determining structural changes related to degeneration,

Conflicts of Interest: Authors have no conflicts to declare.
Department of Radiology, Hospital of University of Pennsylvania, 3400 Spruce Street, Philadelphia, PA 19104, USA
[1] Co-first authors.
* Corresponding author.
E-mail address: abass.alavi@uphs.upenn.edu

PET Clin 14 (2019) 61–69
https://doi.org/10.1016/j.cpet.2018.08.011
1556-8598/19/© 2018 Elsevier Inc. All rights reserved.

whether it be decreased disc height, osteophyte formation, or Modic disc alteration.[3] However, the metabolic data derived from PET has proved to be distinctly useful in this domain. Although structural imaging modalities are limited to the resultant physical structures, PET provides an opportunity to examine the preceding metabolic processes that result in the degenerative morphologic structures.

Four areas of significant potential involve back pain, degenerative disorder, osteoporosis, and postoperative assessment. Although the current standard of care for these conditions may not involve PET imaging, it would be useful for nuclear medicine physicians to be aware of the growing body of evidence demonstrating the value of PET in these applications.

## Pain Syndromes

Issues regarding pain syndrome are exceedingly common in the spine region. Lower back pain and neck pain are 2 of the most prevalent issues in the world. Diagnosis, treatment, and management costs of back pain are alarmingly high worldwide.[4,5] The difficulty of treatment and management in pain disorders lies in etiologic determinations. Common clinical procedure involves structural MR imaging or CT imaging to uncover acute abnormalities causing pain (eg, herniated discs or ankylosing spondylitis). However, other disorders may be more difficult to diagnose. To address these inadequacies, studies have made preliminary headway in determining the relevance of metabolic PET data in the context of structural CT data in the diagnosis of acute disorders that result in pain (**Fig. 1**).

Byrnes and colleagues[6] conducted a study with 58 patients reportedly suffering from neck pain. In 49 cases, a subsequent NaF PET scan showed increased uptake in the regions of pain, only some of which could be visualized by conventional imaging modalities. The imaging was clinically useful in most cases, especially in neck pain with radiculopathy, although less so in postoperative cases. In the cases where PET was irrelevant, background uptake due to intense degeneration complicated analyses.

Similarly, Gamie and El-Maghraby[7] assessed 67 patients with lower back pain where structural imaging had been unhelpful in determining the source of pain and demonstrated that 56 of these patients showed increased NaF uptake in the spine. The scans were noted to be specifically useful in determining the source of pain within the postoperative cohort (eg, lumbar fusion or laminectomy); elevated uptake often occurred in facet joints or discs. Seifen and colleagues[8] identified 38

cases of suspected spondylodiscitis that lacked a clear diagnosis on initial structural imaging. FDG accumulation as measured through $SUV_{max}$ was found to be abnormal in spondylodiscitis cases, allowing for 34 of 38 cases to be accurately diagnosed with FDG-PET/CT. Similarly, a study of spondylitis performed by Grantz and colleagues demonstrated that elevated FDG activity accurately localized inflammation related to spondylitis.

## Degenerative Process

Disc degeneration is another spinal pathology that can underlie idiopathic back pain. The degenerative process begins, like most other OA processes, with nonosseous disorders or specifically disc disorders (eg, compression, herniation), which result in high levels of disc inflammation.[9–11] The proceeding effects are observed in the vertebrae, where increased pressure on individual vertebra or contact between vertebrae result in abnormal bone formation (eg, osteophytes, spondylolysis). This process of degeneration is known as spondylosis.

Current studies have noted that elevated NaF and FDG uptake in the spine is seen with increased age and weight.[12,13] Furthermore, the magnitude of localized FDG uptake has been shown to align with the qualitative degree of morphologic degeneration.[14] NaF activity can indicate the formation of abnormal osseous morphologies, whereas FDG activity can visualize inflammation in the discs and bone (**Fig. 2**). In older populations, metabolically active osseous diseases such as osteoporosis can complicate the use of NaF in evaluating degenerative disease.[13]

## Postoperative Assessment

Spinal orthopedics is another useful aspect of PET imaging. Postsurgical infections are a significant concern given the potential for proliferation and sepsis. Accordingly, studies have used FDG-PET to image infections via its inflammatory consequences.[15] Inanami and colleagues'[16] case-control study of postoperative posterior lumbar interbody fusion surgery found that elevated FDG activity at the surgical site aligned with clinical data to effectively indicate a surgical site infection. Nakahara and colleagues[17] similarly found that FDG-PET accurately localized active infection in the spine post-surgery. In fact, Nakahara and colleagues reported a sensitivity and specificity of 100% and 79%, respectively, for FDG-PET/CT, which was superior to those of MR imaging, 76% and 42%.

Alternatively, PET has been studied in the context of monitoring patients' progress from a

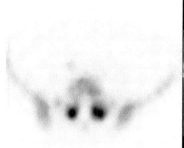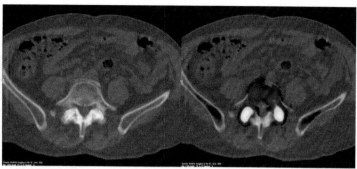

**Fig. 1.** Transaxial PET, CT, and fused PET/CT images of a 71-year-old woman showing focal hypermetabolic activity of 18F-NaF at the facet joint in the lower back. Facet joint arthrosis is a common cause of low back pain in the general population.

surgical perspective. Multiple studies have determined that NaF PET is highly accurate, sensitive, and specific in determining the various sources underlying postoperative back pain. Seifen examined the NaF PET scans of patients who had undergone intervertebral fusion stabilization but complained of persistent pain.[18] NaF PET was found to be accurate in determining both screw loosening and screw breakage, likely causes of the reported discomfort, as well as in confirming a normal surgical site. In a similar vein, Quon and colleagues[19] examined the NaF scans of patients complaining of recurrent back pain after a spinal fusion surgery and found that NaF PET accurately determined lesions (screws, rods, cages) worthy of further surgical intervention in 15 of the 16 patients (1 false-positive abnormality). Peters and colleagues[20] measured uptake in the vertebral end plates and discs of patients who had undergone spinal fusion surgery and reported painful pseudarthrosis. The degree of uptake correlated with the clinical measure of pain reported by the patient. Such a finding may indicate the usefulness of PET in assessing postoperative pain and thus better determining appropriate treatment.

## Osteoporosis

In the context of osteoporosis, NaF has proved to be an ideal tracer. The present diagnostic criteria for osteoporosis involve a DEXA scan to determine bone mineral density (BMD). On the other hand, NaF PET can reflect the metabolic activity required to maintain a normal BMD. As such, decreased NaF uptake demonstrates the metabolic derangements that occur in osteoporosis before the resultant decrease in BMD is observed.[21] Accordingly, many studies seeking to examine the metabolic aspect of osteoporosis have segmented spinal NaF uptake.[22,23] Frost and colleagues[24,25] conducted studies assessing the effects of various

treatments on the basis of NaF uptake in the spine. Treatments such as alendronate and risedronate were confirmed to effectively alter the local metabolism in the spine. Many relevant skeletal structures, such as the femoral neck, are similarly useful in assessing osteoporosis via NaF uptake.

## SACROILIAC JOINT

Sacroiliitis, inflammation of the sacroiliac joint (SIJ), is the hallmark of ankylosing spondylitis (AS) and can be observed in the course of a variety of other rheumatological and non-rheumatological disorders as well. MR imaging is currently the imaging modality of choice for evaluating pathologies of the sacroiliac joint. However, the sensitivity of MR imaging in showing active inflammation is limited to approximately 70%.[26,27] As such, FDG-PET/CT can serve as a useful additional tool for the diagnosis of enthesitis in AS patients.[28]

In a study by Rose and colleagues[29] in which they evaluated 65 patients with psoriasis and psoriatic arthritis, they reported a positive association between vascular inflammation and sacroiliitis as measured by FDG-PET.

Buchbender and colleagues[30] investigated the utility of 18F-labeled fluoride PET and MR imaging in the evaluation of AS and found that bone marrow edema rather than chronic changes were associated with an increase in osteoblastic activity, whereas the combination of bone marrow edema and fat deposition showed the highest 18F-F uptake. By contrast, Fischer and colleagues[31] found that increased 18F-fluoride uptake in PET/CT is only modestly associated with bone marrow edema on MR imaging in the spine and SIJ of patients with AS, suggesting different aspects of bone involvement in AS.

A study by Strobel and colleagues[32] found an overall NaF PET sensitivity of 80% for the

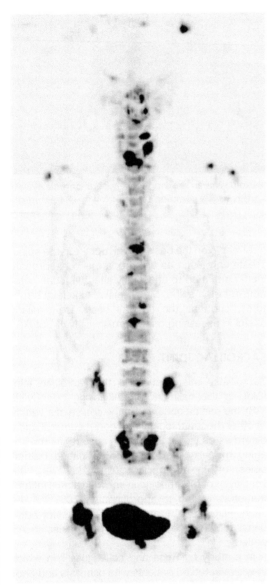

**Fig. 2.** Maximum intensity projection PET image showing the focal accumulation of 18F-NaF in the spine, hip, shoulder, and wrist joints. Sites of increased metabolic activity represent an increase in osteoblastic activity and reactive bone formation due to degenerative joint disease.

diagnosis of sacroiliitis and explained the superiority of 18F-fluoride PET/CT over scintigraphy due to its rapid blood clearance with high and quick bone uptake, resulting in a better lesion-to-background ratio than 99mTc-labeled phosphonates (**Fig. 3**).

In a study that included 31 patients with possible spondyloarthritis not meeting ASAS criteria, Darrieutort-Laffite and colleagues[33] found that the positive predictive value of NaF PET for diagnosing spondyloarthritis or predicting a response to TNF-α antagonist therapy seems very low.

An additional study examined performance of 18F-fluoride PET/CT in 10 patients with nonradiographic axial spondyloarthritis and 5 patients with AS; PET/CT was reported as positive in all AS patients and negative in all nrAxSpA patients, further suggesting specificity of this imaging for bone formation, rather than for inflammation.[34]

## Knee

### Degenerative process

OA is a degenerative joint disease with a multifactorial cause, including aging, obesity, genetic predisposition, and prior joint injury or surgery. Symptomatic OA affects about 12.1% of the US population and is a leading musculoskeletal cause of impaired mobility in the elderly. Its prevalence and incidence are expected to increase with the worldwide increase in life expectancy.[35–37] Joint inflammation plays an important role in the pathophysiology of OA, and it has been suggested that age-related proinflammatory changes are among the early triggers of the disease.[38] Obesity has been also found to promote synovial and soft tissue inflammation by both local and systemic factors.[39] Imaging plays an important role in OA research, including hybrid PET/CT and PET/MR imaging.[40]

FDG is highly sensitive for the early detection of inflammatory processes in many organ disorders. In a retrospective study, Parsons and colleagues[41] reported higher FDG uptake in the knee joints of symptomatic subjects than of those in controls. Saboury and colleagues[42] retrospectively studied FDG-PET scans of 64 subjects and reported an association between aging and global knee joint inflammation as measured by FDG-PET. Hong and Kong[43] also reported a significant correlation between aging and FDG uptake in the knees of OA patients, where FDG uptake also correlated with the severity of the disease. Savic and colleagues[44] found a significant correlation between cartilage degeneration and subchondral bone remolding as detected by NaF PET/MR imaging images in the knee joints of symptomatic subjects. Al-Zaghal and colleagues used a novel CT-segmentation methodology to assess the metabolic activity of the knee joint compartments and reported a positive correlation between body mass index and knee joint inflammation as well as bone turnover as measured using FDG and NaF PET. They also reported a positive association between FDG activities in the soft tissue compartment of the knee with aging.[45] **Fig. 4** shows the synovial FDG uptake in an obese subject in comparison with normal-weight subject.

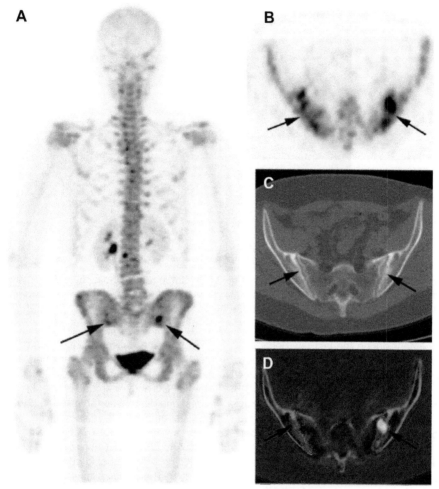

**Fig. 3.** A 49-year-old woman patient with ankylosing spondylitis. 18F-Fluoride PET/CT with increased uptake (*arrows*) in both SIJs with more uptake in the left joint. MIP image (*A*), axial PET (*B*), CT (*C*), and fused PET/CT images (*D*) demonstrate the morphologically severely altered joints with sclerosis and multiple erosions on both sides (*arrows*). (*From* Strobel K, Fischer DR, Tamborrini G, et al. 18F-Fluoride PET/CT for detection of sacroiliitis in ankylosing spondylitis. Eur J Nucl Med Mol Imaging 2010;37(9):1763; with permission.)

It has been reported that NaF PET can identify early osteoblastic activity before morphologic changes become evident on MR imaging. Kogan and colleagues[46] investigated the knees of 22 subjects with a history of knee pain by using hybrid 3T PET/MR imaging and NaF PET imaging. They found significantly higher standardized uptake values in osseous lesions, osteophytes, and sclerotic lesions than in normal bone. They also observed some active lesions on PET that had normal morphologic features on MR imaging.[47–49] Draper and colleagues[50] compared the MR imaging and NaF PET/CT scans of 22 patients with knee pain and found that not all active bone lesions on NaF PET correspond with structural damage on MR imaging. They did a lesion-based analysis and found that 49% of the abnormal regions consisted of increased tracer uptake detected by PET alone, whereas 12% of all abnormal regions were detected by MR imaging alone. The remaining 39% of the abnormal regions were localized by both PET and MR imaging.

Jonnakuti and colleagues[51] investigated the feasibility of quantifying global disease activity in the knee joints of 18 patients with rheumatoid arthritis using NaF PET and found that patients with higher NaF uptake demonstrated greater knee deterioration on plain radiographs.

### Prosthetic infections

The number of primary total knee and hip arthroplasties is increasing due to an aging population across the world. Kremers and colleagues[52] studied the epidemiology of individuals who had total

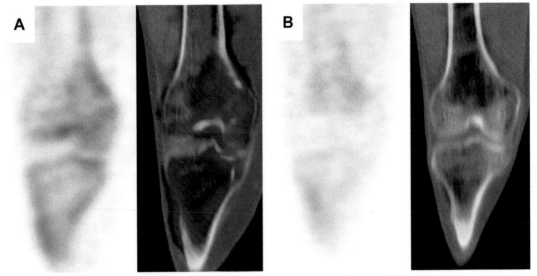

**Fig. 4.** Coronal FDG-PET and fused PET/CT images of the knee joint in a 36-year-old obese man (*A*) and a 36-year-old man with normal weight (*B*). Extensive FDG uptake is noted in the joint of the obese subject in comparison with the normal physiologic tracer distribution in the nonobese subject.

knee replacement during the last few decades in the United States and reported a prevalence of 1.52% of the population in 2010 compared with 0.13% in 1980. Postsurgical complications are not uncommon and include aseptic loosening, infection, dislocation, and fractures. Although infection occurs in less than 2% of all arthroplasties, it is the most serious and life-threatening complication. Clinicians face major challenges in differentiating aseptic loosening, the most common complication of arthroplasty, from infection, because both pathologies have similar clinical manifestations.

The application of FDG-PET/CT in the assessment prosthesis joint infection holds a great deal of promise but requires further evaluation. FDG-PET has an excellent sensitivity for detection of infections. Although both prosthesis joint infection and aseptic loosening may demonstrate periprosthetic FDG activity around the neck, periprosthetic uptake is diagnostic for infection (**Fig. 5**).[53,54] The results of a recent meta-analysis of 11 studies with a total of 635 lower extremity prostheses show that FDG-PET achieves a pooled sensitivity of 82.1% and a pooled specificity of 86.6%.[55] A study by Basu and colleagues[56] evaluated the utility of FDG-PET and radiolabeled leukocytes and bone marrow scintigraphy (LS/BMS) in the diagnosis of infection in 88 painful prosthetic joints and reported a sensitivity and specificity of 81.8% and 93.1% for FDG-PET and 38.5% and 95.7% for LS/BMS.

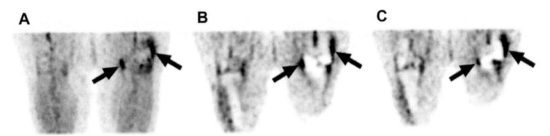

**Fig. 5.** In this patient with proven infected left knee prosthesis, the maximum intensity projection image (*A*) reveals intense uptake of FDG in the medial and upper lateral aspect (*arrows*) of the prosthesis, which are typical of prosthetic joint infection. Tomographic images (*B, C*) show the exact locations of these sites at the bone-prosthesis interface (*arrows*). (*From* Basu S, Kwee TC, Saboury B, et al. FDG-PET for diagnosing infection in hip and knee prostheses: prospective study in 221 prostheses and subgroup comparison with combined (111)In-labeled leukocyte/(99m)Tc-sulfur colloid bone marrow imaging in 88 prostheses. Clin Nucl Med 2014;39(7):612; with permission.)

Many studies have described the use of LS/ BMS in diagnosing prosthetic joint infections and shown it to have greater accuracy in this domain than FDG-PET. However, FDG-PET imaging has many practical advantages over combined LS/ BMS, including its routine availability, the requirement for only a single radiotracer injection, completion of the test within a brief period of time, outstanding safety record (lack of pathogens in the final product based on existing Food and Drug Administration records), and substantially lower radiation exposure and costs. Moreover, PET provides significantly superior spatial resolution and high-quality/quantitative imaging data unachievable by LS/BMS.

## SUMMARY

In summary, NaF PET is highly sensitive for the detection of the earliest osteoblastic changes and has a promising role in the evaluation of low back pain, OA, postsurgical assessment, bone minerality, and osteoporosis. FDG-PET remains the best radiotracer to evaluate synovial inflammation, osteomyelitis, and complications of orthopedic devices. Prospective trials with well-defined endpoints are encouraged to evaluate the multiple facets of these emerging imaging tools in the management of joint disorders.

## REFERENCES

1. Wong KK, Piert M. Dynamic bone imaging with 99mTc-labeled diphosphonates and 18F-NaF: mechanisms and applications. J Nucl Med 2013; 54(4):590–9.
2. Bastawrous S, Bhargava P, Behnia F, et al. Newer PET application with an old tracer: role of 18F-NaF skeletal PET/CT in oncologic practice. Radiographics 2014;34(5):1295–316.
3. Chen L, Hu X, Zhang J, et al. Modic changes in the lumbar spine are common aging-related degenerative findings that parallel with disk degeneration. Clin Spine Surg 2018. https://doi.org/10.1097/BSD. 0000000000000662.
4. Patrick N, Emanski E, Knaub MA. Acute and chronic low back pain. Med Clin North Am 2014;98(4): 777–89.
5. Buchbinder R, Blyth FM, March LM, et al. Placing the global burden of low back pain in context. Best Pract Res Clin Rheumatol 2013;27(5):575–89.
6. Byrnes TJ, Xie W, Al-Mukhailed O, et al. Evaluation of neck pain with 18F-NaF PET/CT. Nucl Med Commun 2014;35(3):298–302.
7. Gamie S, El-Maghraby T. The role of PET/CT in evaluation of Facet and Disc abnormalities in patients

with low back pain using (18)F-Fluoride. Nucl Med Rev Cent East Eur 2008;11(1):17–21.
8. Seifen T, Rettenbacher L, Thaler C, et al. Prolonged back pain attributed to suspected spondylodiscitis. The value of 18F-FDG PET/CT imaging in the diagnostic work-up of patients. Nuklearmedizin 2012; 51(5):194–200.
9. Jarman JP, Arpinar VE, Baruah D, et al. Intervertebral disc height loss demonstrates the threshold of major pathological changes during degeneration. Eur Spine J 2015;24(9):1944–50.
10. Sun Z, Zhang M, Zhao XH, et al. Immune cascades in human intervertebral disc: the pros and cons. Int J Clin Exp Pathol 2013;6(6):1009–14.
11. Wade KR, Robertson PA, Thambyah A, et al. How healthy discs herniate: a biomechanical and microstructural study investigating the combined effects of compression rate and flexion. Spine (Phila Pa 1976) 2014;39(13):1018–28.
12. Win AZ, Aparici CM. Normal SUV values measured from NaF18- PET/CT bone scan studies. PLoS One 2014;9(9):e108429.
13. Ayubcha C, Zadeh MZ, Rajapakse CS, et al. Effects of age and weight on the metabolic activities of the cervical, thoracic and lumbar spines as measured by fluorine-18 fluorodeoxyglucose-positron emission tomography in healthy males. Hell J Nucl Med 2018; 21(1):2–6.
14. Rosen RS, Fayad L, Wahl RL. Increased 18F-FDG uptake in degenerative disease of the spine: characterization with 18F-FDG PET/CT. J Nucl Med 2006;47(8):1274–80.
15. Basu S, Chryssikos T, Moghadam-Kia S, et al. Positron emission tomography as a diagnostic tool in infection: present role and future possibilities. Semin Nucl Med 2009;39(1):36–51.
16. Inanami H, Oshima Y, Iwahori T, et al. Role of 18F-fluoro-D-deoxyglucose PET/CT in diagnosing surgical site infection after spine surgery with instrumentation. Spine (Phila Pa 1976) 2015;40(2):109–13.
17. Nakahara M, Ito M, Hattori N, et al. 18F-FDG PET/CT better localizes active spinal infection than MRI for successful minimally invasive surgery. Acta Radiol 2015;56(7):829–36.
18. Seifen T1, Rodrigues M, Rettenbacher L, et al. The value of (18)F-fluoride PET/CT in the assessment of screw loosening in patients after intervertebral fusion stabilization. Eur J Nucl Med Mol Imaging 2015;42(2):272–7.
19. Quon A, Dodd R, Iagaru A, et al. Initial investigation of 18F-NaF PET/CT for identification of vertebral sites amenable to surgical revision after spinal fusion surgery. Eur J Nucl Med Mol Imaging 2012;39(11):1737–44.
20. Peters M, Willems P, Weijers R, et al. Pseudarthrosis after lumbar spinal fusion: the role of 18F-fluoride PET/CT. Eur J Nucl Med Mol Imaging 2015;42(12): 1891–8.

21. Frost ML, Blake GM, Fogelman I. (18)F-Fluoride PET in osteoporosis. PET Clin 2010;5(3):259–74.

22. Blake GM, Siddique M, Frost ML, et al. Imaging of site specific bone turnover in osteoporosis using positron emission tomography. Curr Osteoporos Rep 2014;12(4):475–85.

23. Blake GM, Siddique M, Frost ML, et al. Quantitative PET Imaging using (18)F sodium fluoride in the assessment of metabolic bone diseases and the monitoring of their response to therapy. PET Clin 2012;7(3):275–91.

24. Frost ML, Cook GJ, Blake GM, et al. A prospective study of risedronate on regional bone metabolism and blood flow at the lumbar spine measured by 18F-fluoride positron emission tomography. J Bone Miner Res 2003;18(12):2215–22.

25. Frost ML, Siddique M, Blake GM, et al. Regional bone metabolism at the lumbar spine and hip following discontinuation of alendronate and risedronate treatment in postmenopausal women. Osteoporos Int 2012;23(8):2107–16.

26. Jans L, Coeman L, Van Praet L, et al. How sensitive and specific are MRI features of sacroiliitis for diagnosis of spondyloarthritis in patients with inflammatory back pain ? JBR-BTR 2014;97(4):202–5.

27. Rudwaleit M, van der Heijde D, Landewé R, et al. The development of Assessment of SpondyloArthritis international Society classification criteria for axial spondyloarthritis (part II): validation and final selection. Ann Rheum Dis 2009;68(6):777–83.

28. Taniguchi Y, Arii K, Kumon Y, et al. Positron emission tomography/computed tomography: a clinical tool for evaluation of enthesitis in patients with spondyloarthritides. Rheumatology (Oxford) 2010;49(2): 348–54.

29. Rose S, Dave J, Millo C, et al. Psoriatic arthritis and sacroiliitis are associated with increased vascular inflammation by 18-fluorodeoxyglucose positron emission tomography computed tomography: baseline report from the Psoriasis Atherosclerosis and Cardiometabolic Disease Initiative. Arthritis Res Ther 2014;16(4):R161.

30. Buchbender C, Ostendorf B, Ruhlmann V, et al. Hybrid 18F-labeled fluoride positron emission tomography/Magnetic Resonance (MR) imaging of the sacroiliac joints and the spine in patients with axial spondyloarthritis: a pilot study exploring the link of MR bone pathologies and increased osteoblastic activity. J Rheumatol 2015;42(9):1631–7.

31. Fischer DR, Pfirrmann CW, Zubler V, et al. High bone turnover assessed by 18F-fluoride PET/CT in the spine and sacroiliac joints of patients with ankylosing spondylitis: comparison with inflammatory lesions detected by whole body MRI. EJNMMI Res 2012;2(1):38.

32. Strobel K, Fischer DR, Tamborrini G, et al. 18F-Fluoride PET/CT for detection of sacroiliitis in ankylosing spondylitis. Eur J Nucl Med Mol Imaging 2010;37(9): 1760–5.

33. Darrieutort-Laffite C, Ansquer C, Maugars Y, et al. Sodium (18)F-sodium fluoride PET failed to predict responses to TNFα antagonist therapy in 31 patients with possible spondyloarthritis not meeting ASAS criteria. Joint Bone Spine 2015; 82(6):411–6.

34. Toussirot E, Caoduro C, Ungureanu C, et al. 18F-fluoride PET/CT assessment in patients fulfilling the clinical arm of the ASAS criteria for axial spondyloarthritis. A comparative study with ankylosing spondylitis. Clin Exp Rheumatol 2015;33(4):588.

35. Fransen M, Simic M, Harmer AR. Determinants of MSK health and disability: lifestyle determinants of symptomatic osteoarthritis. Best Pract Res Clin Rheumatol 2014;28(3):435–60.

36. Nguyen US, Zhang Y, Zhu Y, et al. Increasing prevalence of knee pain and symptomatic knee osteoarthritis: survey and cohort data. Ann Intern Med 2011; 155(11):725–32.

37. Luyten FP, Denti M, Filardo G, et al. Definition and classification of early osteoarthritis of the knee. Knee Surg Sports Traumatol Arthrosc 2012;20(3): 401–6.

38. Greene MA, Loeser RF. Aging-related inflammation in osteoarthritis. Osteoarthritis Cartilage 2015; 23(11):1966–71.

39. Berenbaum F, Eymard F, Houard X. Osteoarthritis, inflammation and obesity. Curr Opin Rheumatol 2013;25(1):114–8.

40. Hayashi D, Roemer FW, Guermazi A. Imaging of osteoarthritis-recent research developments and future perspective. Br J Radiol 2018;91(1085): 20170349.

41. Parsons MA, Moghbel M, Saboury B, et al. Increased 18F-FDG uptake suggests synovial inflammatory reaction with osteoarthritis: preliminary in-vivo results in humans. Nucl Med Commun 2015;36(12):1215–9.

42. Saboury B, Parsons MA, Moghbel M, et al. Quantification of aging effects upon global knee inflammation by 18F-FDG PET. Nucl Med Commun 2016; 37(3):254–8.

43. Hong YH, Kong EJ. 18F-Fluoro-deoxy-D-glucose uptake of knee joints in the aspect of age-related osteoarthritis: a case-control study. BMC Musculoskelet Disord 2013;14:141.

44. Savic D, Pedoia V, Seo Y, et al. Imaging bone–cartilage interactions in osteoarthritis using [18F]-NaF PET-MRI. Mol Imaging 2016;15:1–12.

45. Al-Zaghal A, Yellanki DP, Ayubcha C, et al. CT-based tissue segmentation to assess knee joint inflammation and reactive bone formation assessed by 18F-FDG and 18F-NaF PET/CT: effects of age and BMI. Hell J Nucl Med 2018. https://doi.org/10.1967/s002449910801.

46. Kogan F, Fan AP, McWalter EJ, et al. PET/MRI of metabolic activity in osteoarthritis: a feasibility study. J Magn Reson Imaging 2017;45(6):1736–45.

47. Jadvar H, Desai B, Conti PS. Sodium 18F-fluoride PET/CT of bone, joint, and other disorders. Semin Nucl Med 2015;45(1):58–65.

48. Raynor W, Houshmand S, Gholami S, et al. Evolving role of molecular imaging with 18F-sodium fluoride PET as a biomarker for calcium metabolism. Curr Osteoporos Rep 2016;14(4):115–25.

49. Hafezi-Nejad N, Demehri S, Guermazi A, et al. Osteoarthritis year in review 2017: updates on imaging advancements. Osteoarthritis Cartilage 2018;26(3): 341–9.

50. Draper CE, Quon A, Fredericson M, et al. Comparison of MRI and $^{18}$F-NaF PET/CT in patients with patellofemoral pain. J Magn Reson Imaging 2012; 36(4):928–32.

51. Jonnakuti VS, Raynor WY, Taratuta E. A novel method to assess subchondral bone formation using [18F]NaF PET in the evaluation of knee degeneration. Nucl Med Commun 2018;39(5):451–6.

52. Kremers MH, Larson DR, Crowson CS, et al. Prevalence of total hip and knee replacement in the United States. J Bone Joint Surg Am 2015;97(17): 1386–97.

53. Love C, Marwin SE, Tomas MB, et al. Diagnosing infection in the failed joint replacement: a comparison of coincidence detection 18F-FDG and 111In-labeled leukocyte/99mTc-sulfur colloid marrow imaging. J Nucl Med 2004;45(11):1864–71.

54. Stumpe KD, Notzli HP, Zanetti M, et al. FDG PET for differentiation of infection and aseptic loosening in total hip replacements: comparison with conventional radiography and three-phase bone scintigraphy. Radiology 2004;231(2):333–4.

55. Kwee TC, Kwee RM, Alavi A. FDG PET for diagnosing prosthetic joint infection: systematic review and meta-analysis. Eur J Nucl Med Mol Imaging 2008;35(11):2122–32.

56. Basu S, Kwee TC, Saboury B, et al. FDG PET for diagnosing infection in hip and knee prostheses: prospective study in 221 prostheses and subgroup comparison with combined (111)In-labeled leukocyte/(99m)Tc-sulfur colloid bone marrow imaging in 88 prostheses. Clin Nucl Med 2014;39(7): 609–15.

# Evolving Role of PET/CT-MRI in Assessing Muscle Disorders

Esha Kothekar, MD[a], William Y. Raynor, BS[a,b],
Abdullah Al-Zaghal, MD[a], Venkata S. Jonnakuti, BS[a,c],
Thomas J. Werner, MSe[a],
Abass Alavi, MD, MD (Hon), PhD (Hon), DSc (Hon)[a,*]

## KEYWORDS

- PET/CT-MRI • FDG • Muscle disorders • Inflammatory muscle disorders
- Musculoskeletal malignancies

## KEY POINTS

- Following a standardized patient preparation protocol for FDG-PET imaging is essential for optimal quantification.
- FDG PET/CT is the most sensitive imaging modality to identify and characterize inflammatory myopathies.
- The use of FDG PET/CT is vital in management of musculoskeletal malignancies.

## INTRODUCTION

The glucose transporter (GLUT) family of facilitative glucose transporter proteins allows passive diffusion of glucose and glucose analogs down their concentration gradients owing to a high degree of stereoselectivity. The GLUT4 isoform, which is present in the heart, skeletal muscle, and adipose tissue, plays a major role in insulin-responsive transport of glucose in adulthood. It translocates from intracellular vesicles to the plasma membrane in response to insulin and is almost completely responsible for insulin-stimulated glucose transport.[1,2] In a healthy adult, skeletal muscle accounts for approximately 70% to 80% of insulin-stimulated glucose utilization in vivo.[3]

2-deoxy-2-[18F]fluoroglucose (FDG) is a radioactive glucose analog created by the substitution of the 2'-hydroxyl moiety in a glucose molecule with fluorine 18, which decays by positron emission.[4] Much like conventional glucose, FDG enters cells via the same facilitative GLUT proteins and shares similar whole-body biodistribution.[5] Intracellular

FDG is subsequently phosphorylated into FDG-6-phosphate, which exhibits poor membrane permeability and is unable to enter downstream glycolytic metabolic pathways. Consequently, FDG is effectively trapped within cells.[6] It is only able to exit a cell when the effect of hexokinase is reversed by glucose-6-phosphatase, which dephosphorylates FDG-6-phosphate and converts it back to FDG.[7,8] Hence, the accumulation of FDG depends on the level of glucose-6-phosphatase, which varies depending on the metabolic activity of the cell. It has been observed that there are higher enzyme concentration and activity in normal and benign cells compared with malignant cells.[9] In inflammatory conditions, increased FDG uptake can be attributed to an increase in the number of GLUTs, with an increased expression of these transporters by the inflammatory cells.[10]

FDG-PET has been traditionally used to detect malignant tumors because cancerous cells exhibit increased glucose metabolism due to a combination of increased activity/expression of

[a] Department of Radiology, University of Pennsylvania, 3400 Spruce Street, Philadelphia, PA 19104, USA;
[b] Department of Radiology, Drexel University College of Medicine, 230 N Broad Street, Philadelphia, PA 19102, USA; [c] 1 Baylor Plaza, Houston, TX 77030, USA
* Corresponding author. 3400 Spruce Street, Philadelphia, PA 19104.
*E-mail address:* abass.alavi@uphs.upenn.edu

PET Clin 14 (2019) 71–79
https://doi.org/10.1016/j.cpet.2018.08.010

GLUT transporters, increased intracellular glucose phosphorylation, decreased phosphatase activity on glucose-6-phosphate, and a shift in cellular metabolism from the efficient aerobic metabolism to the inefficient anaerobic glycolytic pathway.[11,12] More recent studies have suggested the use of this imaging modality to assess glucose transport in skeletal and cardiac muscle.[13] For example, studies have used FDG-PET to examine the effects of free fatty acids, age, duration of physical training, and modality of exercise on insulin sensitivity in muscular tissue.[14–19]

FDG-PET can be combined with CT and MR imaging to evaluate molecular activity with anatomic data.[20] Superior soft tissue contrast and lack of ionizing radiation burden in MR imaging represent major advantages compared with CT. FDG-PET/CT and FDG–PET/MR imaging have been used to assess rhabdomyosarcoma (RMS),[21–24] leiomyosarcoma,[25–30] and myositis.[31–35] The focus of this review is limited to the evaluation of diseases that affect muscle uptake of glucose, inflammatory and infectious myopathies, and primary and secondary tumors of muscle by PET/CT and PET/MR imaging in humans.

## PHYSIOLOGIC UPTAKE OF 2-DEOXY-2-[$^{18}$F] FLUOROGLUCOSE

It is extremely important to differentiate between pathologic and physiologic skeletal uptake. Glucose transport in skeletal muscle is primarily mediated by insulin-dependent GLUT4. In the resting state, GLUT4 is mostly sequestered in vesicles, and fatty acid oxidation serves as the primary source of energy.[36] With increased plasma insulin, such as after eating, GLUT4-containing vesicles translocate to the plasma membrane, increasing the rate of glucose uptake. Accordingly, FDG uptake in skeletal muscle is increased in a postprandial state compared with a resting state. In general, physiologic skeletal uptake is symmetric, regular, and mild to moderate in intensity. Asymmetric skeletal muscle uptake is seen, however, in unilateral surgery, radiation therapy, paresis, spasms, and improper positioning of the patient.[37] For these reasons, proper patient preparation is essential. Avoidance of chewing, talking, and other movements in the postinjection waiting period, insulin and oral hypoglycemic drugs in diabetic patients, and strenuous exercise before FDG administration along with fasting for at least 4 hours to 6 hours are warranted (**Fig. 1**).[38] Hence, it is ideal that patients are in a comfortable and relaxed position to avoid tensing of muscle groups.[39]

Elevated glucose levels can compete with FDG for GLUT proteins and subsequent tissue uptake,

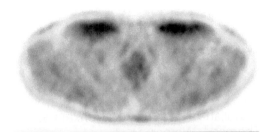

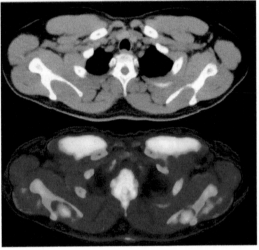

**Fig. 1.** Axial PET *(upper)*, CT *(middle)*, fused PET/CT *(lower)* showing uptake in the anterior chest wall muscles; the patient had exercised the day before his examination.

ultimately affecting biodistribution of FDG and potentially lowering both the resolution and diagnostic sensitivity of the FDG-PET imaging modality.[40] Diabetes mellitus is clinically characterized as dysfunction in glucose metabolism that leads to a range of chronic and acute complications. In cancer patients with mild to moderate diabetes mellitus, the overall sensitivity, specificity, positive/negative predictive values, and diagnostic accuracy of FDG-PET are not significantly impacted. Many groups hypothesize that sufficiently high FDG uptake occurs in tumors to allow reliable visual clinical diagnosis in most cases.[41] Some studies have reported, however, decreased FDG uptake in the cardiac muscle of patients with type 2 diabetes mellitus, with glucose levels greater than 150 mg/dL at the time of tracer injection.[42] Although fatty acids are the primary metabolic substrate for myocardiocytes, approximately 30% of myocardial ATP is generated from glucose transported via GLUT4 proteins.[43] Mutations within and reduced expression of these GLUT proteins have been associated with insulin resistance and diabetes.[44] Taken together, these findings suggest that insulin deficiency or peripheral insulin resistance explains the decreased

FDG uptake in the hearts of most patients with type 2 diabetes mellitus.

Exogenous insulin therapies have been shown to acutely increase muscular, adipose, and hepatic glucose (and FDG) uptake (**Fig. 2**).[45] The timing of insulin and FDG administration is, therefore, crucial when attempting to optimize the quality of the PET image. Intravenous administration of insulin at least an hour prior to FDG administration can effectively decrease serum glucose levels in diabetic patients without significantly affecting muscular FDG uptake.[46] Additionally, studies have suggested that ultra–short-acting insulin can improve blood glucose distribution and PET imaging resolution in patients with poorly controlled diabetes (blood glucose levels >180 mg/dL).[47] Similar to insulin, oral hypoglycemic agents result in increased glucose uptake within tissues. Drugs like metformin achieve this result by operating through a variety of interactions to suppress hepatic gluconeogenesis, increase insulin sensitivity, and ultimately reduce serum glucose levels.[48–50] Yet, the impact of these oral hypoglycemic agents on FDG uptake is poorly understood. A recent study has indicated that a metformin dose less than 24 hours prior to

FDG-PET imaging results in abnormally increased muscular, adipose, and intestinal FDG uptake, limiting diagnostic quality of the imaging modality.[51] Standardized protocols and strategies to optimize conditions for the paired use of oral hypoglycemic agents and FDG imaging, therefore, are critical for this particularly vulnerable patient demographic.

Active use of expiratory muscles is seen in patients with chronic obstructive pulmonary disease (COPD), resulting in increased physiologic FDG uptake (**Fig. 3**). Kothekar E and collegues of this communication have generated preliminary data in 28 male patients (age 66.4 years ± 8.0 years; range 51–81 years) diagnosed with emphysema and 35 male nonsmoker control subjects (age 43.9 years ± 13.4 years; range 22–69 years). After FDG-PET/CT images were acquired, a region of interest was manually delineated around the rectus abdominis muscle. The metabolic activity of the rectus abdominis muscle was quantified by averaging the standardized uptake values (SUVs) in all voxels within the region of interest, and an unpaired $t$ test was used to assess differences between the groups. It was found that the FDG uptake in the rectus abdominis muscle of

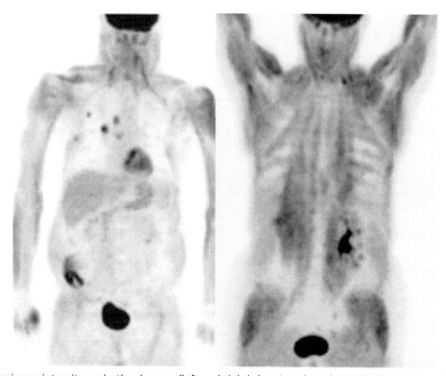

**Fig. 2.** Maximum intensity projection images *(left and right)* showing altered FDG biodistribution with diffuse homogenous increase in FDG uptake in body muscles. This patient had a fasting glucose level of greater than 10 mmol/L and intravenous short-acting insulin was administered. (*From* Roy FN, Beaulieu S, Boucher L, et al. Impact of intravenous insulin on 18F-FDG PET in diabetic cancer patients. J Nucl Med 2009;50(2):180; with permission.)

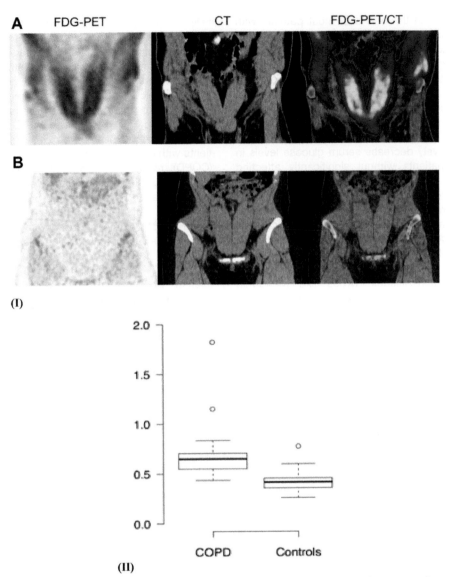

**Fig. 3.** (I) FDG- Rectus abdominis muscle visible in this coronal slice of the abdomen of a patient diagnosed with emphysema (A) *(upper)* reveals a clear increase in FDG uptake compared with a control subject (B) *(middle)*, which does not show significant uptake in the rectus abdominis muscle. (II) *(lower)* Preliminary data generated by the authors' group found that the rectus abdominus muscle in patients diagnosed with emphysema had significantly higher meta- bolic activity as measured by FDG PET compared with healthy controls (P<.0001C).

the emphysema group was significantly higher (P<.0001) than that of the control group. This observation is consistent with the known physiologic changes in the muscle of respiration in patients with COPD.

## INFLAMMATORY MYOPATHY

Inflammatory myopathies are a group of disorders characterized by chronic progressive, symmetric muscle weakness with a presence of mononuclear inflammatory cell infiltrate and include polymyositis (PM), dermatomyositis (DM), and inclusion body myositis.[52] The activation of nicotinamide adenine dinucleotide phosphate oxidase required for oxidative burst results in up-regulation of GLUT1 and GLUT3. This allows increased glucose transport to meet metabolic demand, reflected by increased FDG uptake (**Fig. 4**). DM and PM are both autoimmune in origin, which can be evidenced by their association with other autoimmune diseases, certain HLA alleles, presence of autoantibodies, and maternal microchimerism in the juvenile types.[53] Cytotoxicity due to infiltration by T lymphocytes

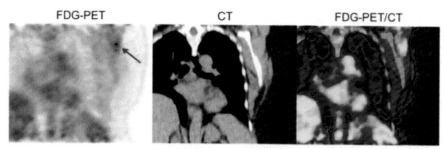

**Fig. 4.** A 62 year old with a history of DM. The arrow shows proximal muscle uptake in the left arm (left). Whereas it is difficult to identify the disorder on the CT (middle), fused FDG-PET/CT image (right) shows anatomic and metabolic characteristics of the inflammatory disorder.

and macrophages, damage of the muscles fibers due to indirect effect of cytokines or disturbance, and involvement of the microcirculation could be possible pathophysiologies that lead to PM and DM.[54] Both PM and DM are clinically characterized by proximal muscle weakness, elevation of creatine kinase, abnormalities on myopathic electromyogram, degeneration followed by regeneration, and sometimes even atrophy of the involved muscles. Although a biopsy is required for an accurate diagnosis, it could be difficult in some cases to approach a muscle due to heterogeneity or inaccessibility. The site of biopsy can be assessed with FDG-PET/CT based on the metabolic activity in the muscle or muscle group and lead toward establishing an accurate diagnosis.[54]

A study by Sun and colleagues[31] showed that FDG-PET/CT is diagnostic for PM/DM and has the ability to identify severity of inflammation in the different muscle groups. Although MR imaging detects inflammatory edema, FDG-PET/CT picks up abnormal signals from active inflammatory cells, which is more accurate for diagnosis. This study also proved that PET/CT can detect areas not routinely screened by conventional methods, like the paraspinal muscle inflammation in the aforementioned study. PET/CT is also superior to other conventional imaging (CI) modalities because it can detect malignancy associated with DM in a single scan, for example, by detecting lung cancer in 1 of the patients.

## GRANULOMATOUS MYOPATHY

Tuberculosis (TB) is a common infective disease in the developing world. It is caused by *Mycobacterium tuberculosis* and is characterized by the formation of granulomas. It usually involves the lymph nodes, bones, and bowel. Muscle involvement is rare and could be attributed to lack of lymphoid tissue, high lactate content, and rich blood supply. The prevalence of muscle involvement is found in only 3% of TB cases.[55]

In a study by Stelzmueller and colleagues,[56] the investigators showed that FDG-PET/CT is more accurate than CT for initial patient-based as well as lesion-based assessment and also for therapy response in the follow-up period in TB. Although more investigation is required, this study indicated that FDG-PET/CT could be useful in determining treatment duration in TB.

Sarcoidosis is a chronic multisystem granulomatous disease without an identifiable cause. It is characterized by noncaseating granuloma and commonly involves lungs, intrathoracic lymph nodes, eyes, and skin. The involvement of skeletal muscles in sarcoidosis is common and has a predilection for proximal thigh muscles. Clinically, muscular sarcoid lesion presents with myalgia, myositis, and palpable nodular lesions.[57–59] FDG-PET/CT shows a characteristic tiger man appearance in areas of increased uptake.[60]

Results of a study by Umeda and colleagues,[61] which calculated SUVs at the 2 time points, indicated that retention index–SUV has higher accuracy for diagnosis of persistent lung inflammation in sarcoidosis compared with single-time FDG-PET and 67Ga scanning at 1 year. In both TB and sarcoidosis, FDG-PET/CT can be used to evaluate treatment and management strategies in patients by providing structural as well as metabolic detail.[62]

## MALIGNANCY

Since its introduction of FDG-PET, this molecular imaging modality has been essential in diagnosing cancers and improving diagnostic accuracy significantly. Because it is complementary to the conventional anatomic imaging techniques, such as CT and MR, PET is increasingly used for staging and restaging cancers. Due to its accuracy in detecting residual and recurrent disease, it also has the potential for assessing therapy response.[63]

RMS is a malignant tumor that is believed to arise from the skeletal muscle cell lineage, meaning it is mesenchymal in origin. It is the most common soft tissue sarcoma of childhood. It is commonly sporadic but can be associated with neurofibromatosis and Li-Fraumeni syndrome. Common sites of tumor location are the head and neck, extremities, and genitourinary tract.[64] FDG-PET/CT can identify the most aggressive site of tumor activity based on metabolic activity and help guide biopsy for tumor grading.[65,66] A study by Tateishi and colleagues[24] compared FDG-PET/CT with CI in their role of staging RMS. They showed that FDG-PET/CT has higher accuracy of overall staging and M staging than CI modalities. Eleven of their study patients had distant metastases, which was picked up on FDG-PET/CT but not with CI. Whole-body FDG-PET/CT can be used to stage and restage RMS with higher accuracy than CI.

Multiple myeloma (MM) is a malignant disorder characterized by clonal plasma cell proliferation. Clinically it presents with hypercalcemia, renal abnormalities, anemia, and diffuse bone pain. Plasma cells are derived from B cells and produce immunoglobulins. MM is caused due to cytogenetic abnormalities that lead to translocations of oncogenes to the immunoglobulin heavy chain region on chromosome 14. These factors lead to uncontrolled proliferation and cause cells to escape apoptosis and evade the immune system.[67] Uncommonly, MM can involve muscle, presenting as a painless intramuscular mass in the paraspinal, thigh, iliopsoas, or calf muscles. Rarely, it can present as generalized myopathy with elevated creatinine kinase levels.[68–71] FDG-PET/CT can differentiate skeletal lesions from extramedullary disease and distinguish active myeloma from monoclonal myopathy of undetermined significance (MGUS) or smoldering disease; MGUS is generally FDG-negative whereas myeloma is FDG-positive.[69]

Hodgkin lymphoma and non-Hodgkin lymphoma (NHL) are malignant lymphomas arising from clonal expansion of lymphocytes.[72] Extranodal forms of lymphoma are rare and have a predilection for gluteal and pelvic muscle involvement. The spread of disease is either contiguous from an involved lymph node or lymphatic or hematogenous in nature.[38] Due to an increase in the prevalence of lymphoma, extranodal forms are becoming increasingly common. FDG-PET/CT has become an imaging technique of choice for staging and follow-up of lymphoma.[73] This could be attributed to the finding of skeletal muscle lesions in NHL being isointense with normal muscles on CT and T1-weighted MR images.[74,75] Because presence of extranodal lymphoma changes treatment and management strategies,

it is critical not to overlook these lesions. According to 1 study, NHL was upstaged with FDG-PET/CT in 31% of cases and downstaged in 1% relative to CT findings. Hodgkin disease was upstaged with FDG-PET/CT in 32% of cases and downstaged in 15%.[76] The diagnostic accuracy for extranodal lymphoma can be increased with suspicion for these lesions and after standard PET/CT protocol. Only biopsy is confirmatory.[73]

Although rare, skeletal muscle metastases occurs hematogenously, commonly originating from the lung, kidney, and colon.[77] The low incidence of skeletal muscle metastases could be related to high levels of lactic acid during exertion.[78] A study by Magee and Rosenthal[79] suggested that skeletal muscle injury may cause alterations in muscle physiology and increase risk of development of metastatic disease. Skeletal muscle metastasis clinically presents with local pain, erythema, and swelling.[80] FDG-PET/CT showed 100% sensitivity in contrast to CT, which showed 61% sensitivity in detecting skeletal muscle metastases.[81] The low sensitivity could be attributable to the lesions being isodense on CT.[65] High suspicion should be maintained with increased uptake without any anatomic or morphologic abnormalities.[38]

## SUMMARY

In summary, FDG uptake in muscle is influenced by many normal physiologic processes and can also indicate pathology. Variability in physiologic uptake can be reduced with proper patient preparation, allowing for a better determination of abnormal activity. Although malignant diseases, such as RMS and skeletal muscle metastasis, are clear applications of FDG-PET/CT, there may be additional applications in infection and benign inflammatory disorders that warrant further research.

## REFERENCES

1. Zorzano A, Palacin M, Guma A. Mechanisms regulating GLUT4 glucose transporter expression and glucose transport in skeletal muscle. Acta Physiol Scand 2005;183(1):43–58.
2. Medina RA, Owen GI. Glucose transporters: expression, regulation and cancer. Biol Res 2002;35(1): 9–26.
3. Olefsky JM. Insulin-stimulated glucose transport minireview series. J Biol Chem 1999;274(4):1863.
4. Yu S. Review of F-FDG synthesis and quality control. Biomed Imaging Interv J 2006;2(4):e57.
5. Ahmad Sarji S. Physiological uptake in FDG PET simulating disease. Biomed Imaging Interv J 2006; 2(4):e59.

6. Moadel RM, Nguyen AV, Lin EY, et al. Positron emission tomography agent 2-deoxy-2-[18F]fluoro-D-glucose has a therapeutic potential in breast cancer. Breast Cancer Res 2003;5(6):R199–205.

7. Vallabhajosula S. (18)F-labeled positron emission tomographic radiopharmaceuticals in oncology: an overview of radiochemistry and mechanisms of tumor localization. Semin Nucl Med 2007;37(6): 400–19.

8. Macheda ML, Rogers S, Best JD. Molecular and cellular regulation of glucose transporter (GLUT) proteins in cancer. J Cell Physiol 2005;202(3): 654–62.

9. Basu S, Kung J, Houseni M, et al. Temporal profile of fluorodeoxyglucose uptake in malignant lesions and normal organs over extended time periods in patients with lung carcinoma: implications for its utilization in assessing malignant lesions. Q J Nucl Med Mol Imaging 2009;53(1):9–19.

10. Palestro CJ. FDG-PET in musculoskeletal infections. Semin Nucl Med 2013;43(5):367–76.

11. Hawkins RA, Hoh C, Dahlbom M, et al. PET cancer evaluations with FDG. J Nucl Med 1991;32(8): 1555–8.

12. Yonekura Y, Benua RS, Brill AB, et al. Increased accumulation of 2-deoxy-2-[18F]Fluoro-D-glucose in liver metastases from colon carcinoma. J Nucl Med 1982;23(12):1133–7.

13. Kelley DE, Price JC, Cobelli C. Assessing skeletal muscle glucose metabolism with positron emission tomography. IUBMB Life 2001;52(6):279–84.

14. Bai X, Wang X, Zhuang H. Long-lasting FDG uptake in the muscles after strenuous exercise. Clin Nucl Med 2015;40(12):975–6.

15. Reichkendler MH, Auerbach P, Rosenkilde M, et al. Exercise training favors increased insulin-stimulated glucose uptake in skeletal muscle in contrast to adipose tissue: a randomized study using FDG PET imaging. Am J Physiol Endocrinol Metab 2013;305(4):E496–506.

16. Lyall A, Capobianco J, Strauss HW, et al. Treadmill exercise inducing mild to moderate ischemia has no significant effect on skeletal muscle or cardiac 18F-FDG uptake and image quality on subsequent whole-body PET scan. J Nucl Med 2012;53(6):917–21.

17. Shimada H, Sturnieks D, Endo Y, et al. Relationship between whole body oxygen consumption and skeletal muscle glucose metabolism during walking in older adults: FDG PET study. Aging Clin Exp Res 2011;23(3):175–82.

18. Gondoh Y, Tashiro M, Itoh M, et al. Evaluation of individual skeletal muscle activity by glucose uptake during pedaling exercise at different workloads using positron emission tomography. J Appl Physiol (1985) 2009;107(2):599–604.

19. Fujimoto T, Kemppainen J, Kalliokoski KK, et al. Skeletal muscle glucose uptake response to exercise in trained and untrained men. Med Sci Sports Exerc 2003;35(5):777–83.

20. Al-Zaghal A, Yellanki DP, Ayubcha C, et al. T-based tissue segmentation to assess knee joint inflammation and reactive bone formation assessed by (18)F-FDG and (18)F-NaF PET/CT: effects of age and BMI. Hell J Nucl Med 2018. https://doi.org/10.1967/s002449910801.

21. Natarajan A, Puranik A, Purandare N, et al. An infrequent case of adult alveolar rhabdomyosarcoma with pancreatic metastases detected in F-18 FDG PET/CT. Indian J Nucl Med 2017;32(3):227–9.

22. Yi J, Zhou DA, Huo JR, et al. Primary intratesticular rhabdomyosarcoma: a case report and literature review. Oncol Lett 2016;11(2):1016–20.

23. Armeanu-Ebinger S, Griessinger CM, Herrmann D, et al. PET/MR imaging and optical imaging of metastatic rhabdomyosarcoma in mice. J Nucl Med 2014;55(9):1545–51.

24. Tateishi U, Hosono A, Makimoto A, et al. Comparative study of FDG PET/CT and conventional imaging in the staging of rhabdomyosarcoma. Ann Nucl Med 2009;23(2):155–61.

25. Makis W, Brimo F, Probst S. Primary renal leiomyosarcoma presenting with subcutaneous and osseous metastases: staging and follow-up with 18F-FDG PET/CT. Nucl Med Mol Imaging 2018; 52(1):69–73.

26. Xie P, Zhuang H. FDG PET/CT findings of primary hepatic leiomyosarcoma in an immunocompetent pediatric patient. Clin Nucl Med 2017;42(4): 323–4.

27. Gauthe M, Testart Dardel N, Nascimento C, et al. Uterine leiomyosarcoma metastatic to thyroid shown by (18)F-FDG PET/CT imaging. Rev Esp Med Nucl Imagen Mol 2017;36(2):113–5.

28. Milanetto AC, Liço V, Blandamura S, et al. Primary leiomyosarcoma of the pancreas: report of a case treated by local excision and review of the literature. Surg Case Rep 2015;1(1):98.

29. Singh N, Shivdasani D, Karangutkar S. Rare case of primary inferior vena cava leiomyosarcoma on F-18 fluorodeoxyglucose positron emission tomography-computed tomography scan: differentiation from nontumor thrombus in a background of procoagulant state. Indian J Nucl Med 2014;29(4):246–8.

30. Payne MJ, Macpherson RE, Bradley KM, et al. Trabectedin in advanced high-grade uterine leiomyosarcoma: a case report illustrating the value of (18) FDG-PET-CT in assessing treatment response. Case Rep Oncol 2014;7(1):132–8.

31. Sun L, Dong Y, Zhang N, et al. [(18)F]Fluorodeoxyglucose positron emission tomography/computed tomography for diagnosing polymyositis/dermatomyositis. Exp Ther Med 2018;15(6):5023–8.

32. Bai X, Tie N, Wang X, et al. Intense muscle activity due to polymyositis incidentally detected in a patient

evaluated for possible malignancy by FDG PET/CT imaging. Clin Nucl Med 2017;42(8):647–8.

33. Chen SJ, Wang XY, Hua FC, et al. Detection of multiple muscle involvement in eosinophilic myositis with (1)(8)F-FDG PET/CT. Eur J Nucl Med Mol Imaging 2013;40(8):1297.

34. Tomita H, Kita T, Hayashi K, et al. Radiation-induced myositis mimicking chest wall tumor invasion in two patients with lung cancer: a PET/CT study. Clin Nucl Med 2012;37(2):168–9.

35. Clarencon F, Larousserie F, Babinet A, et al. FDG PET/CT findings in a case of myositis ossificans circumscripta of the forearm. Clin Nucl Med 2011; 36(1):40–2.

36. Felig P, Wahren J. Fuel homeostasis in exercise. N Engl J Med 1975;293(21):1078–84.

37. Abouzied MM, Crawford ES, Nabi HA. 18F-FDG imaging: pitfalls and artifacts. J Nucl Med Technol 2005;33(3):145–55 [quiz: 162–3].

38. Karunanithi S, Soundararajan R, Sharma P, et al. Spectrum of physiologic and pathologic skeletal muscle (18)F-FDG uptake on PET/CT. AJR Am J Roentgenol 2015;205(2):W141–9.

39. Engel H, Steinert H, Buck A, et al. Whole-body PET: physiological and artifactual fluorodeoxyglucose accumulations. J Nucl Med 1996;37(3):441–6.

40. Lindholm P, Minn H, Leskinen-Kallio S, et al. Influence of the blood glucose concentration on FDG uptake in cancer–a PET study. J Nucl Med 1993;34(1):1–6.

41. Martin J, Saleem N. 18F-FDG PET-CT scanning and diabetic patients: what to do? Nucl Med Commun 2014;35(12):1197–203.

42. Israel O, Weiler-Sagie M, Rispler S, et al. PET/CT quantitation of the effect of patient-related factors on cardiac 18F-FDG uptake. J Nucl Med 2007; 48(2):234–9.

43. Bryant NJ, Govers R, James DE. Regulated transport of the glucose transporter GLUT4. Nat Rev Mol Cell Biol 2002;3(4):267–77.

44. Karim S, Adams DH, Lalor PF. Hepatic expression and cellular distribution of the glucose transporter family. World J Gastroenterol 2012;18(46):6771–81.

45. Roy FN, Beaulieu S, Boucher L, et al. Impact of intravenous insulin on 18F-FDG PET in diabetic cancer patients. J Nucl Med 2009;50(2):178–83.

46. Turcotte E, Leblanc M, Carpentier A, et al. Optimization of whole-body positron emission tomography imaging by using delayed 2-deoxy-2-[F-18]fluoro-D: -glucose Injection following I.V. Insulin in diabetic patients. Mol Imaging Biol 2006;8(6):348–54.

47. Song HS, Yoon JK, Lee SJ, et al. Ultrashort-acting insulin may improve on 18F-FDG PET/CT image quality in patients with uncontrolled diabetic mellitus. Nucl Med Commun 2013;34(6):527–32.

48. An H, He L. Current understanding of metformin effect on the control of hyperglycemia in diabetes. J Endocrinol 2016;228(3):R97–106.

49. Capitanio S, Marini C, Sambuceti G, et al. Metformin and cancer: technical and clinical implications for FDG-PET imaging. World J Radiol 2015;7(3): 57–60.

50. Inzucchi SE, Bergenstal RM, Buse JB, et al. Management of hyperglycemia in type 2 diabetes: a patient-centered approach: position statement of the American Diabetes Association (ADA) and the European Association for the Study of Diabetes (EASD). Diabetes Care 2012;35(6):1364–79.

51. Morris M, Saboury B, Chen W, et al. Finding the sweet spot for metformin in 18F-FDG-PET. Nucl Med Commun 2017;38(10):875–80.

52. Amato AA, Greenberg SA. Inflammatory myopathies. Continuum (Minneap Minn) 2013;19(6 Muscle Disease):1615–33.

53. Dalakas MC, Hohlfeld R. Polymyositis and dermatomyositis. Lancet 2003;362(9388):971–82.

54. Al-Nahhas A, Jawad AS. PET/CT imaging in inflammatory myopathies. Ann N Y Acad Sci 2011;1228: 39–45.

55. Trikha V, Gupta V. Isolated tuberculous abscess in biceps brachii muscle of a young male. J Infect 2002;44(4):265–6.

56. Stelzmueller I, Huber H, Wunn R, et al. 18F-FDG PET/CT in the initial assessment and for follow-up in patients with tuberculosis. Clin Nucl Med 2016; 41(4):e187–94.

57. Moore SL, Teirstein AE. Musculoskeletal sarcoidosis: spectrum of appearances at MR imaging. Radiographics 2003;23(6):1389–99.

58. Otake S, Ishigaki T. Muscular sarcoidosis. Semin Musculoskelet Radiol 2001;5(2):167–70.

59. Matsuo M, Ehara S, Tamakawa Y, et al. Muscular sarcoidosis. Skeletal Radiol 1995;24(7):535–7.

60. Soussan M, Augier A, Brillet PY, et al. Functional imaging in extrapulmonary sarcoidosis: FDG-PET/CT and MR features. Clin Nucl Med 2014;39(2): e146–59.

61. Umeda Y, Demura Y, Morikawa M, et al. Prognostic value of dual-time-point 18F-fluorodeoxyglucose positron emission tomography in patients with pulmonary sarcoidosis. Respirology 2011;16(4): 713–20.

62. Nishiyama Y, Yamamoto Y, Fukunaga K, et al. Comparative evaluation of 18F-FDG PET and 67Ga scintigraphy in patients with sarcoidosis. J Nucl Med 2006;47(10):1571–6.

63. Kelloff GJ, Hoffman JM, Johnson B, et al. Progress and promise of FDG-PET imaging for cancer patient management and oncologic drug development. Clin Cancer Res 2005;11(8):2785–808.

64. Dagher R, Helman L. Rhabdomyosarcoma: an overview. Oncologist 1999;4(1):34–44.

65. Emmering J, Vogel WV, Stokkel MP. Intramuscular metastases on FDG PET-CT: a review of the literature. Nucl Med Commun 2012;33(2):117–20.

66. Eary JF, Conrad EU. Imaging in sarcoma. J Nucl Med 2011;52(12):1903–13.

67. Al-Farsi K. Multiple myeloma: an update. Oman Med J 2013;28(1):3–11.

68. Walker RC, Brown TL, Jones-Jackson LB, et al. Imaging of multiple myeloma and related plasma cell dyscrasias. J Nucl Med 2012;53(7):1091–101.

69. Healy CF, Murray JG, Eustace SJ, et al. Multiple myeloma: a review of imaging features and radiological techniques. Bone Marrow Res 2011;2011: 583439.

70. Surov A, Holzhausen HJ, Arnold D, et al. Intramuscular manifestation of non-Hodgkin lymphoma and myeloma: prevalence, clinical signs, and computed tomography features. Acta Radiol 2010;51(1):47–51.

71. Islam A, Myers K, Cassidy DM, et al. Malignancy: case report: muscle involvement in multiple myeloma: report of a patient presenting clinically as polymyositis. Hematology 1999;4(2):123–5.

72. Matasar MJ, Zelenetz AD. Overview of lymphoma diagnosis and management. Radiol Clin North Am 2008;46(2):175–98, vii.

73. Paes FM, Kalkanis DG, Sideras PA, et al. FDG PET/CT of extranodal involvement in non-Hodgkin lymphoma and Hodgkin disease. Radiographics 2010; 30(1):269–91.

74. Chong J, Som PM, Silvers AR, et al. Extranodal non-Hodgkin lymphoma involving the muscles of mastication. AJNR Am J Neuroradiol 1998;19(10):1849–51.

75. Harnsberger HR, Bragg DG, Osborn AG, et al. Non-Hodgkin's lymphoma of the head and neck: CT evaluation of nodal and extranodal sites. AJR Am J Roentgenol 1987;149(4):785–91.

76. Raanani P, Shasha Y, Perry C, et al. Is CT scan still necessary for staging in Hodgkin and non-Hodgkin lymphoma patients in the PET/CT era? Ann Oncol 2006;17(1):117–22.

77. Damron TA, Heiner J. Distant soft tissue metastases: a series of 30 new patients and 91 cases from the literature. Ann Surg Oncol 2000;7(7):526–34.

78. Seely S. Possible reasons for the high resistance of muscle to cancer. Med Hypotheses 1980;6(2): 133–7.

79. Magee T, Rosenthal H. Skeletal muscle metastases at sites of documented trauma. AJR Am J Roentgenol 2002;178(4):985–8.

80. Surov A, Hainz M, Holzhausen HJ, et al. Skeletal muscle metastases: primary tumours, prevalence, and radiological features. Eur Radiol 2010;20(3): 649–58.

81. So Y, Yi JG, Song I, et al. Detection of skeletal muscle metastasis: torso FDG PET-CT versus contrast-enhanced chest or abdomen CT. Acta Radiol 2015;56(7):860–6.

# PET Imaging of Peripheral Nerve Tumors

Majid Assadi, MD[a], Erik Velez, MD[b], Mohammad Hosein Najafi, MD[c], George Matcuk, MD[a], Ali Gholamrezanezhad, MD, FEBNM, DABR[b],*

## KEYWORDS

• PET • Malignant peripheral nerve sheath tumor (MPSNT) • PET/CT imaging • PET/MR imaging

## KEY POINTS

- Malignant peripheral nerve sheath tumors (MPNST) are the sixth most frequent soft tissue sarcoma (STS), consisting of 5% to 10% of cases.
- Traditionally, MR imaging has been the main imaging modality to evaluate the extent and involvement of MPNT.
- The potential value of PET and PET/CT in regards to diagnosis, biopsy guidance, staging, and therapy response of MPNT are presented in the literature.
- Multimodality imaging with multiparametric hybrid PET/MR has also shown some utility in the management of peripheral nerve tumors (PNTs).
- Quantitative FDG-PET imaging used in combination with CT or MR imaging has shown great potential to discriminate benign from malignant PNTs.

## INTRODUCTION

Peripheral nerve tumors (PNT) are a heterogeneous category of neoplasms that are very rare in the population. The classification of theses tumors is variable, as most of these tumors have more than one name. Furthermore, peripheral nerve sheath tumors encompass a variety of cell types, some of which are not yet completely characterized. Common classification systems are based on the presence or absence of neoplasia, whether the neoplasm is benign or malignant, and the cellular origin of the primary neoplasia.[1,2]

Malignant peripheral nerve sheath tumors (MPNST) are the sixth most frequent soft tissue sarcoma (STS), consisting of 5% to 10% of cases.[3–5] Approximately 50% of all MPNST develop sporadically, whereas the other 50% are associated with neurofibromatosis type 1

(NF1).[6–8] Patients with NF1 have an 8% to 13% lifetime risk of developing MPNST, with an incidence of 1:3500, compared with the incidence of 1:100,000 among the general population.[6] Approximately 30% of NF1-associated MPNST arise from a deeply located neurofibroma, with most of the tumors developing in the proximal upper and lower limbs.[9] Patients can present with a variety of symptoms, which may include pain, paresthesia, and neurologic deficits.[10] MPNST have a poor prognosis, with overall 5-year survival rates ranging from 20% to 50% for high-grade MPNST and a mortality of up to 75%.[11]

Diagnostic imaging of PNT is crucial for proper characterization and management. Traditionally, MR imaging has been the main imaging modality to evaluate the extent and involvement of PNT. Ultrasound and computed tomography (CT) can also be of value in select patients and may be

[a] Department of Molecular Imaging and Radionuclide Therapy (MIRT), The Persian Gulf Nuclear Medicine Research Center, Bushehr Medical University Hospital, Bushehr University of Medical Sciences, Moallem Street, Bushehr 3631, Iran; [b] Department of Diagnostic Radiology, Keck School of Medicine, University of Southern California (USC), 1520 San Pablo Street, Suite L1600, Los Angeles, CA 90033, USA; [c] Department of Cardiology, Tehran Medical Unit, Azad University, Shariati Street, Tehran 1916893813, Iran
* Corresponding author. 1520 San Pablo Street, Suite L1600, Los Angeles, CA 90033.
E-mail addresses: gholamre@med.usc.edu; a.gholamrezanezhad@yahoo.com

PET Clin 14 (2019) 81–89
https://doi.org/10.1016/j.cpet.2018.08.013

used for image-guided biopsies.[12] Furthermore, bone scintigraphy may be useful to evaluate for osseous involvement.[13]

Over recent years, PET has been gaining increasing traction in the assessment of musculoskeletal tumors. The use of PET to assess disease biology at an individual level is now playing a pivotal role in personalized clinical decision making and further clinical management.[14–16] However, although the use of PET/CT is being increasingly used in patients with MPNST, its definite role within the clinical routine is still not delineated, partially because of the rarity of these tumors hindering prospective investigations with large patient groups. Here, the authors discuss the role and potential value of PET and PET/CT in regards to diagnosis, biopsy guidance, staging, and therapy response of PNT.

## DIAGNOSIS AND DIFFERENTIATION BETWEEN BENIGN AND MALIGNANT PERIPHERAL NERVE TUMORS WITH FLUDEOXYGLUCOSE-PET

The diagnosis of MPNST and their distinction from benign tumors remain a clinical challenge, because the symptoms of the 2 conditions demonstrate substantial overlap. At present, CT, MR imaging, and PET are the main imaging tools used to assess and diagnose MPNST. Both CT and MR imaging are useful to define the anatomic tumor size and local invasiveness of MPNST.[17] In addition, several investigations have developed diagnostic criteria to help aid in the discrimination between benign and malignant PNT using CT and MR imaging. However, these criteria have not been reliable in distinguishing between benign and malignant PNTs, especially when tumors are inhomogeneous.[18] Thus, the main shortcoming of both CT and MR imaging is the inability to efficiently confirm malignant transformation of lesions.[17]

To address this issue, several studies have assessed the ability of fludeoxyglucose (FDG)-PET with or without CT to distinguish benign from malignant primary PNT based on a tumor's metabolic activity.[17,19–22] In general, benign PNTs depict no or low FDG uptake, whereas malignant PNTs demonstrate moderate to high FDG accumulation. In these studies, standard uptake values (SUV), a quantitative amount of FDG uptake, range between 1.0 and 3.99 in benign PNTs and between 3.1 and 21.4 in malignant PNTs.[17,23–26] In a systematic review by Tovmassian and colleagues,[19] summarizing 796 tumors from 13 various reports, FDG-PET demonstrated noteworthy difference regarding the distinction of

benign from malignant PNTs (mean SUVmax: 1.93 vs 7.48) with a mean accuracy across the studies of 83.5%. Receiver operating characteristic analysis was carried out in several of the studies to determine optimal SUVmax cutoff. These values yielded cutoffs of 3.1, 3.2, 3.5, 4.1, and 6.1 to attain maximum statistical parameters of ascertaining malignant lesions.[19] It revealed that FDG-PET/CT could be valuable in the diagnosis of malignant lesions with the sensitivities ranging from 91% to 100% and specificity ranging from 72% to 95%. However, there was significant overlap in ranges of SUVmax in these studies and inadequate evidence to admit a universal cutoff value for SUVmax (**Fig. 1**).[19]

Recently, Azizi and colleagues[27] evaluated the value of FDG-PET imaging in the detection of malignant transformation of symptomatic and asymptomatic plexiform neurofibromas in 41 children with NF1. This study demonstrated overlap between the SUVmax of malignant and benign lesions, yet no malignant lesion demonstrated FDG uptake less than 3.15 (**Fig. 2**). Asymptomatic malignant lesions were diagnosed with a sensitivity of 100%, a negative predictive value of 100%, and a specificity of 45.1%. This value highlights the utility of FDG-PET in detecting malignant transformation of plexiform neurofibromas, especially in asymptomatic patients. This issue may reveal MPNST at early stages, potentially increasing the possibility of oncologically curative resections.

Dual-time-point FDG-PET has demonstrated some potential in distinction between malignant and nonmalignant PNTs.[23,28] However, PNTs have mostly shown similar FDG uptake on delayed projection, and the implication of this protocol remains unknown.[26] Multimodality imaging with multiparametric hybrid PET/MR has also shown some utility in the management of PNTs.[29,30] A few studies have assessed the combined use of FDG-PET and MR imaging in this regard.[24,31,32] Broski and colleagues[31] carried out the largest study to date assessing the performance of FDG-PET and MR imaging in a cohort of histologically proven benign and malignant peripheral nerve sheath tumors involving 38 patients with 23 benign PNSTs and 20 malignant PNSTs. In this study, FDG PET was 90% to 100% sensitive and 52.2% to 82.6% specific for diagnosing MPNST, whereas expertly interpreted MR images had a 62.5% to 81.3% sensitivity and 94.1% to 100% specificity, thus underscoring the complementary role of PET/MR imaging in the management of PNTs. In addition, as state-of-the-art PET/MR imaging becomes more common, concurrent combined PET and MR imaging offers the potential of a "one-stop-shop" imaging modality for patients.

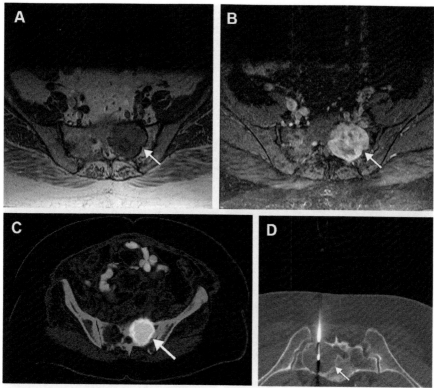

**Fig. 1.** A 70-year-old woman who initially presented with left paraspinal and lower extremity pain. Axial T1 (*A*) and T1 FS postcontrast (*B*) MR images demonstrate a 4.8-cm mass (*arrows*) centered in the left S1 neural foramen. 18F-FDG PET/CT (*C*) shows intense hypermetabolism with SUVmax of 8.9 (*arrow*). CT-guided biopsy (*D*) and subsequent resection (*arrow*) both came back as benign schwannoma despite the high SUVmax.

In conclusion, definitive imaging difference of benign and malignant PNTs remains a challenge. Quantitative FDG-PET imaging used in combination with CT or MR imaging has shown great potential to discriminate benign from malignant PNTs. Nevertheless, additional studies are needed, and the imaging and clinical characteristics of PNTs have not yet replaced histopathologic consideration as the gold standard for diagnosis.

## GRADING OF MALIGNANT PERIPHERAL NERVE SHEATH TUMORS WITH FLUDEOXYGLUCOSE-PET

Accurate histologic grading is imperative in the assessment and management of MPNST. Preoperative imaging appraisal of the histologic grade is a challenging subject, with several contradicting results between FDG uptake (SUVmax) and histopathologic grading of MPNST.

In a study by Ferner and colleagues,[28] assessing FDG-PET/CT as a diagnostic modality for MPNST in NF1 cases with symptomatic plexiform neurofibromas, a total of 116 lesions were evaluated in 105 patients, including 80 plexiform neurofibromas, 5 atypical neurofibromas, 29 MPNST, and 2 other tumors. FDG-PET and PET/CT detected NF1-associated tumors with a sensitivity of 0.89 (95% confidence interval [CI] 0.76 to 0.96) and a specificity of 0.95 (CI 0.88–0.98); however, the SUVmax level did not predict tumor grade. Kim and colleagues[33] retrospectively investigated CT (n = 14), MR imaging (n = 16), and 18F-FDG PET/CT (n = 5) imaging characteristics of 18 different MPNST of the head and neck in 17 patients. 18F-FDG PET/CT images acquired for 5 cases depicted homogeneous (n = 3) or heterogeneous (n = 2) hypermetabolic foci with a mean SUVmax of 7.16 ± 4.57 (range, 3.2–14.6). In this study, the SUVmax correlated well with the histologic grade of the tumors: 2 with SUVmax of 3.2 and 3.9 were histologically categorized as low grade; one with SUVmax of 6.1 as intermediate grade; and 2 with SUVmax of 8.0 and 14.6 as high grade (**Fig. 3**). Warbey and colleagues[23] assessed 69 patients with NF1 with 85 lesions, including 10 atypical neurofibromas and 21 MPNST. In this study, FDG-PET was very sensitive (97%) and specific (87%) in the diagnosis of

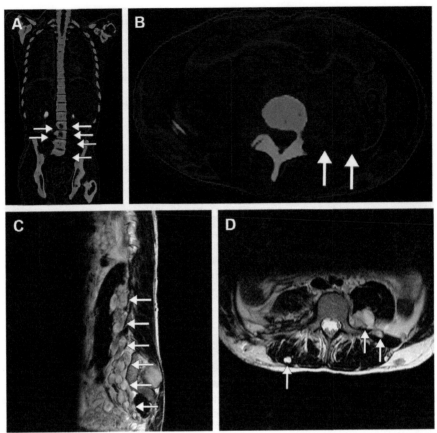

**Fig. 2.** A 24-year-old man with history of NF1. Coronal (*A*) and axial (*B*) 18F-FDG PET/CT and sagittal (*C*) and axial (*D*) T2-weighted MR images demonstrate numerous paraspinal masses (*arrows*). The SUVmax was 3 or less for all of these masses, indicating that these are all benign neurofibromas without need for further workup at this time.

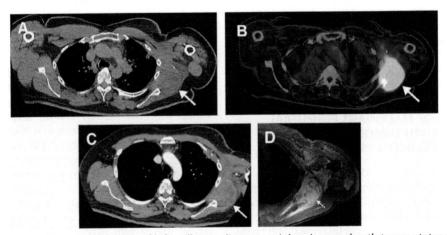

**Fig. 3.** A 44-year-old man with history of left axillary malignant peripheral nerve sheath tumor, status postresection with positive margins and adjuvant radiation therapy. A recent biopsy of a left chest wall mass demonstrated fibrosis on pathology. Axial noncontrast CT (*A*) demonstrates an ill-defined left chest wall periscapular mass (*arrow*). 18F-FDG PET/CT (*B*) shows intense hypermetabolism with SUVmax of 23.5 (*arrow*). Axial contrast-enhanced CT (*C*) and axial STIR MR imaging (*D*) show heterogeneous enhancement and signal intensity within this recurrent high-grade MPNST (*arrows*).

MPNST. Cardona and colleagues[34] demonstrated that MPNST have considerably higher FDG uptake in their assessment of 25 neurogenic STS.

Furthermore, schwannomas should be included in the differential diagnosis of peripheral nerve sheath tumors with low, intermediate, or high SUVs.[35] Given the considerable overlap in the SUVmax between low- and high-grade MPNST, further studies using new tracers and parameters may be helpful in discriminating high- and low-grade MPNST.[28,36]

In summary, although higher-grade tumors are typically more metabolically active than lower-grade tumors, there is currently a lack of evidence for the ability of FDG-PET to assess tumor grade in PNTs. Further studies evaluating SUV parameters and tumor grade of PNTs are needed, and biopsies with histologic analysis should be routinely performed to accurately ascertain tumor grade.

## BIOPSY GUIDANCE AND STAGING OF MALIGNANT PERIPHERAL NERVE SHEATH TUMORS WITH FLUDEOXYGLUCOSE-PET/COMPUTED TOMOGRAPHY

The standard management of MPNST requires biopsy before surgical resection. One way to improve biopsy results is to leverage the metabolic data afforded by PET imaging to efficiently target and sample tissues, especially when other modalities such as radiograph, CT, or ultrasound do not clearly identify the abnormality. PET/CT-guided biopsy combines the well-established worth of anatomic information from CT with the metabolic information from FDG-PET. In a study of 26 NF1 patients with a clinical suspicion of MPNST and suspect lesion on PET/CT scan, Brahmi and colleagues[37] demonstrated a diagnostic accuracy rate of 96% with PET/CT-guided percutaneous biopsies (**Fig. 4**).

The exact role of PET-guided biopsy is not yet well established, but may be of most benefit in patients with previous inconclusive biopsy findings or findings discordant with the overall clinical and imaging data. Furthermore, large malignant lesions can be heterogeneous, and PET/CT functional imaging-driven biopsy may be of great benefit for guiding biopsies.[38,39] Last, in the case of local tumor recurrence, whereby it can be difficult to distinguish between posttreatment changes and local recurrence, PET/CT-guided biopsies may be of value.

Accurate staging of MPNST is important for treatment planning and prognostic stratification. It has been demonstrated that most MPNST are high-grade sarcomas, with a high probability of local recurrence and distant metastasis. In total, 40% to 65% of MPNST cases experience local recurrence and 30% to 60% develop metastases.[40–42] Approximately 65% of MPNST metastases are to the lungs, with the liver, brain, bones, and adrenal glands also being common sites of distant spread. Regional lymph node involvement is infrequent, and for this reason, lymph node dissection should not be regularly done.[4]

Overall, PET/CT has a noteworthy effect on staging and restaging sarcomas particularly for lymph nodal metastases, distant metastases, and local relapse. Local recurrence can often be difficult to distinguish from posttreatment changes. In a study of 47 patients with MPNST, Khiewvan and colleagues[43] demonstrated 100% sensitivity for PET/CT to detect locally recurrent disease compared with 86% with conventional CT imaging. Furthermore, the PET/CT scans detected significantly more distant sites of disease, resulting in treatment changes in 31% of patients undergoing initial staging examinations. However, the sensitivity has been shown to be lower for lung metastases; thus, nodules found on diagnostic CT should be suspect in the appropriate clinical setting, even in the absence of increased metabolically activity. In conclusion, PET/CT can more accurately stage and restage

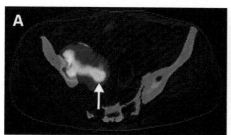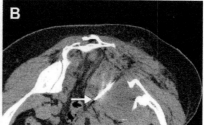

**Fig. 4.** A 34-year-old female patient with history of NF1 and pelvic mass. 18F-FDG PET/CT (*A*) shows heterogeneous hypermetabolism of the right pelvis mass (*arrow*) with an SUVmax of 12.3 and erosion of the right ilium. CT-guided biopsy (*B*) targeted the most hypermetabolic medial aspect of the mass (*arrow*), which was diagnosed to be an MPNST.

patients with PNT and may result in a paradigm shift in patient management strategy.

## THERAPY RESPONSE ASSESSMENT AND PROGNOSIS OF MALIGNANT PERIPHERAL NERVE SHEATH TUMORS WITH FLUDEOXYGLUCOSE-PET/COMPUTED TOMOGRAPHY

The literature addressing the utility of FDG-PET/CT for therapy response assessment and prognosis for MPNST is scarce. At present, most STS cases, particularly those with intermediate and high grades, are treated with neoadjuvant chemotherapy or radiotherapy before surgical resection.[44] Precise noninvasive evaluation of therapy response would be of great value for STS treatment to better guide therapeutic decisions and avoid ineffective chemotherapy or radiation treatment. The RECIST criteria for solid tumors have been shown to be ineffective for sarcoma treatment response evaluation.[45,46] This demerit is due to the fact that most of these tumors encompass structural parts, hindering tumor shrinkage after cytotoxic therapy. Therefore, several reports have revealed that metabolic imaging with FDG-PET/CT is superior to morphologic imaging such as MR imaging or CT in therapy response evaluation in STS.[47–49]

In patients with STS, it is imperative to identify prognostic parameters to delineate the best management strategy and follow-up examinations. Although factors such as large tumor size and intermediate- or high-grade histology are associated with reduced survival, numerous studies have focused on the relation between tumor FDG uptake and tumor necrosis, with higher levels of tumor necrosis a strong predictor of long-term therapy response.[44,50–52]

Moreover, as noted above, it is frequently problematic to diagnose local recurrence of STS due to changes in the normal anatomy by prior manipulations such as surgery or radiotherapy. Based on the small number of reports regarding this issue, PET imaging has demonstrated a high sensitivity for the revealing of local recurrence in high-grade STS, although diagnosis of recurrences of low-grade tumors cannot be anticipated from FDG-PET.[43,53,54] Despite the potential implication of FDG-PET/CT in the diagnosis of STS recurrence, the application of FDG-PET into the follow-up strategy of STS patients is not yet well characterized.

## NEW PARAMETERS AND RADIOTRACERS

Novel parameters such as metabolic tumor volume and total lesion glycolysis have been used

in prior studies with promising results.[19,31,55,56] In addition, Derlin and colleagues[24] have evaluated the utility of the Homogeneity Index SUV, incorporating the metabolic homogeneity of a lesion, which has resulted in increasing specificity between benign and malignant lesions. However, SUVmax remains the most supported parameter in the literature, and further investigations into these novel parameters are required to elucidate their clinical significance. In view of multitracer PET imaging, it has been demonstrated that intertumoral and intratumoral heterogeneity of blood flow and angiogenesis, hypoxia, necrosis, cellular proliferation, gene mutation, and expression of specific receptors can be evaluated with FDG and non-FDG-PET radiotracers, potentially assisting in medical decision making in the era of personalized medicine.[52,57,58]

In a study of 22 patients with schwannomas, Ahmed and colleagues[59] compared 18F FDG-PET to 18F-fluoro-α-methyl tyrosine (18FMT), an amino acid tracer that monitors protein metabolism, and concluded that 18FMT-PET is more accurate for distinction between benign schwannoma and malignancy than 18FDG-PET. In addition, prostate-specific membrane antigen (PSMA), a transmembrane glycoprotein primarily expressed by prostate cells and other tissues (eg, small intestine, renal tubules, or salivary glands),[60] was noted in the endothelium of tumor-associated neovasculature in some solid cancers such as MPNST, possibly due to the effect of tumor-associated angiogenic factors.[61–64] Somatostatin receptor agonists such as DOTA-TATE have also been proven to have valuable effects on the management of neuroendocrine cancers, indicating value for these radiotracers in the clinical management of somatostatin-avid cancers,[65] such as PNTs.[66–69] Furthermore, PSMA and DOTA-TATE also can be bound with radionuclides such as gallium-68 and lutetium-177 to develop radiopharmaceuticals for both PET imaging and radionuclide therapy.

## SUMMARY

In conclusion, FDG-PET, especially in conjunction with CT, is a useful imaging modality for patients with PNT with many advantages over conventional imaging. This modality can aid in the diagnosis, staging, and restaging of PNT as well as in image-guided biopsy. Furthermore, FDG-PET may serve a role in the grading of PNT and assist in determining prognosis and treatment response, although additional data are needed. The use of FDG-PET/CT for PNT can significantly affect clinical management and enables the implementation of precision medicine, an emerging theme for future clinical practice. In addition, a growing body of evidence supports the use of hybrid PET-MR imaging and alternative radiotracers in PNT.

This overview provides insights into the usefulness of PET in peripheral nerve oncology and how it can assist in providing optimal patient care. However, additional studies evaluating FDG-PET and the development of more specific radiotracers are still needed to improve the performance of PET in the assessment of PNT.

## REFERENCES

1. De Luca-Johnson J, Kalof AN. Peripheral nerve sheath tumors: an update and review of diagnostic challenges. Diagn Histopathol 2016;22(11):447–57.
2. Gilchrist JM, Dona hue JE. Peripheral nerve tumors. Riverwoods (IL): UpToDate; 2018. Available at: https://www.uptodate.com/contents/peripheral-nerve-tumors/print.
3. Grobmyer SR, Reith JD, Shahlaee A, et al. Malignant Peripheral Nerve Sheath Tumor: molecular pathogenesis and current management considerations. J Surg Oncol 2008;97(4):340–9.
4. James AW, Shurell E, Singh A, et al. Malignant peripheral nerve sheath tumor. Surg Oncol Clin N Am 2016;25(4):789–802.
5. Lin CT, Huang TW, Nieh S, et al. Treatment of a malignant peripheral nerve sheath tumor. Onkologie 2009;32(8–9):503–5.
6. Bradtmoller M, Hartmann C, Zietsch J, et al. Impaired Pten expression in human malignant peripheral nerve sheath tumours. PLoS One 2012; 7(11):e47595.
7. Tucker T, Wolkenstein P, Revuz J, et al. Association between benign and malignant peripheral nerve sheath tumors in NF1. Neurology 2005;65(2): 205–11.
8. Ibrahim A, Asuku ME. Images in clinical medicine. Neurofibromatosis. N Engl J Med 2011;365(21): 2020.
9. Evans DG, Baser ME, McGaughran J, et al. Malignant peripheral nerve sheath tumours in neurofibromatosis 1. J Med Genet 2002;39(5):311–4.
10. Katz D, Lazar A, Lev D. Malignant peripheral nerve sheath tumour (MPNST): the clinical implications of cellular signalling pathways. Expert Rev Mol Med 2009;11:e30.
11. Hruban RH, Shiu MH, Senie RT, et al. Malignant peripheral nerve sheath tumors of the buttock and lower extremity. A study of 43 cases. Cancer 1990; 66(6):1253–65.
12. Rafailidis V, Kaziani T, Theocharides C, et al. Imaging of the malignant peripheral nerve sheath tumour

with emphasis on ultrasonography: correlation with MRI. J Ultrasound 2014;17(3):219–23.
13. Murphey MD, Smith WS, Smith SE, et al. From the archives of the AFIP. Imaging of musculoskeletal neurogenic tumors: radiologic-pathologic correlation. Radiographics 1999;19(5):1253–80.
14. Mahajan A, Azad GK, Cook GJ. PET imaging of skeletal metastases and its role in personalizing further management. PET Clin 2016;11(3):305–18.
15. Kandathil A, Subramaniam RM. PET/computed tomography and precision medicine: musculoskeletal sarcoma. PET Clin 2017;12(4):475–88.
16. Tabacchi E, Fanti S, Nanni C. The possible role of PET imaging toward individualized management of bone and soft tissue malignancies. PET Clin 2016; 11(3):285–96.
17. Benz MR, Czernin J, Dry SM, et al. Quantitative F18-fluorodeoxyglucose positron emission tomography accurately characterizes peripheral nerve sheath tumors as malignant or benign. Cancer 2010;116(2): 451–8.
18. Mautner VF, Friedrich RE, von Deimling A, et al. Malignant peripheral nerve sheath tumours in neurofibromatosis type 1: MRI supports the diagnosis of malignant plexiform neurofibroma. Neuroradiology 2003;45(9):618–25.
19. Tovmassian D, Abdul Razak M, London K. The role of [(18)F]FDG-PET/CT in predicting malignant transformation of plexiform neurofibromas in neurofibromatosis-1. Int J Surg Oncol 2016;2016:6162182.
20. Etchebehere EC, Hobbs BP, Milton DR, et al. Assessing the role of (1)(8)F-FDG PET and (1)(8)F-FDG PET/CT in the diagnosis of soft tissue musculoskeletal malignancies: a systematic review and meta-analysis. Eur J Nucl Med Mol Imaging 2016; 43(5):860–70.
21. Ren J, Yang G, Zhou J, et al. The value of 18F-FDG PET/CT in patient with neurofibromatosis type 1: a case report and literature review. Medicine 2018; 97(20):e10648.
22. Combemale P, Valeyrie-Allanore L, Giammarile F, et al. Utility of 18F-FDG PET with a semiquantitative index in the detection of sarcomatous transformation in patients with neurofibromatosis type 1. PLoS One 2014;9(2):e85954.
23. Warbey VS, Ferner RE, Dunn JT, et al. [18F]FDG PET/CT in the diagnosis of malignant peripheral nerve sheath tumours in neurofibromatosis type-1. Eur J Nucl Med Mol Imaging 2009;36(5):751–7.
24. Derlin T, Tornquist K, Munster S, et al. Comparative effectiveness of 18F-FDG PET/CT versus whole-body MRI for detection of malignant peripheral nerve sheath tumors in neurofibromatosis type 1. Clin Nucl Med 2013;38(1):e19–25.
25. Salamon J, Veldhoen S, Apostolova I, et al. 18F-FDG PET/CT for detection of malignant peripheral nerve sheath tumours in neurofibromatosis

type 1: tumour-to-liver ratio is superior to an SUV-max cut-off. Eur Radiol 2014;24(2):405–12.

26. Chirindel A, Chaudhry M, Blakeley JO, et al. 18F-FDG PET/CT qualitative and quantitative evaluation in neurofibromatosis type 1 patients for detection of malignant transformation: comparison of early to delayed imaging with and without liver activity normalization. J Nucl Med 2015;56(3):379–85.

27. Azizi AA, Slavc I, Theisen BE, et al. Monitoring of plexiform neurofibroma in children and adolescents with neurofibromatosis type 1 by [(18) F]FDG-PET imaging. Is it of value in asymptomatic patients? Pediatr Blood Cancer 2018;65(1):1–9.

28. Ferner RE, Golding JF, Smith M, et al. [18F]2-fluoro-2-deoxy-D-glucose positron emission tomography (FDG PET) as a diagnostic tool for neurofibromatosis 1 (NF1) associated malignant peripheral nerve sheath tumours (MPNSTs): a long-term clinical study. Ann Oncol 2008;19(2):390–4.

29. Rosenkrantz AB, Friedman K, Chandarana H, et al. Current status of hybrid PET/MRI in oncologic imaging. AJR Am J Roentgenol 2016;206(1):162–72.

30. Fayad LM, Wang X, Blakeley JO, et al. Characterization of peripheral nerve sheath tumors with 3T proton MR spectroscopy. AJNR Am J Neuroradiol 2014;35(5):1035–41.

31. Broski SM, Johnson GB, Howe BM, et al. Evaluation of (18)F-FDG PET and MRI in differentiating benign and malignant peripheral nerve sheath tumors. Skeletal Radiol 2016;45(8):1097–105.

32. Urban T, Lim R, Merker VL, et al. Anatomic and metabolic evaluation of peripheral nerve sheath tumors in patients with neurofibromatosis 1 using whole-body MRI and (18)F-FDG PET fusion. Clin Nucl Med 2014;39(5):e301–7.

33. Kim HY, Hwang JY, Kim HJ, et al. CT, MRI, and (18) F-FDG PET/CT findings of malignant peripheral nerve sheath tumor of the head and neck. Acta Radiol 2017;58(10):1222–30.

34. Cardona S, Schwarzbach M, Hinz U, et al. Evaluation of F18-deoxyglucose positron emission tomography (FDG-PET) to assess the nature of neurogenic tumours. Eur J Surg Oncol 2003;29(6):536–41.

35. Beaulieu S, Rubin B, Djang D, et al. Positron emission tomography of schwannomas: emphasizing its potential in preoperative planning. AJR Am J Roentgenol 2004;182(4):971–4.

36. Brenner W, Friedrich RE, Gawad KA, et al. Prognostic relevance of FDG PET in patients with neurofibromatosis type-1 and malignant peripheral nerve sheath tumours. Eur J Nucl Med Mol Imaging 2006;33(4):428–32.

37. Brahmi M, Thiesse P, Ranchere D, et al. Diagnostic accuracy of PET/CT-guided percutaneous biopsies for malignant peripheral nerve sheath tumors in neurofibromatosis type 1 patients. PLoS One 2015;10(10):e0138386.

38. Klaeser B, Mueller MD, Schmid RA, et al. PET-CT-guided interventions in the management of FDG-positive lesions in patients suffering from solid malignancies: initial experiences. Eur Radiol 2009;19(7):1780–5.

39. Kobayashi K, Bhargava P, Raja S, et al. Image-guided biopsy: what the interventional radiologist needs to know about PET/CT. Radiographics 2012;32(5):1483–501.

40. Goertz O, Langer S, Uthoff D, et al. Diagnosis, treatment and survival of 65 patients with malignant peripheral nerve sheath tumors. Anticancer Res 2014;34(2):777–83.

41. Zou C, Smith KD, Liu J, et al. Clinical, pathological, and molecular variables predictive of malignant peripheral nerve sheath tumor outcome. Ann Surg 2009;249(6):1014–22.

42. Okada K, Hasegawa T, Tajino T, et al. Clinical relevance of pathological grades of malignant peripheral nerve sheath tumor: a multi-institution TMTS study of 56 cases in Northern Japan. Ann Surg Oncol 2007;14(2):597–604.

43. Khiewvan B, Macapinlac HA, Lev D, et al. The value of (1)(8)F-FDG PET/CT in the management of malignant peripheral nerve sheath tumors. Eur J Nucl Med Mol Imaging 2014;41(9):1756–66.

44. Crush AB, Howe BM, Spinner RJ, et al. Malignant involvement of the peripheral nervous system in patients with cancer: multimodality imaging and pathologic correlation. Radiographics 2014;34(7):1987–2007.

45. Ratain MJ, Eckhardt SG. Phase II studies of modern drugs directed against new targets: if you are fazed, too, then resist RECIST. J Clin Oncol 2004;22(22):4442–5.

46. Therasse P, Arbuck SG, Eisenhauer EA, et al. New guidelines to evaluate the response to treatment in solid tumors. European Organization for Research and treatment of cancer, National cancer Institute of the United States, National cancer Institute of Canada. J Natl Cancer Inst 2000;92(3):205–16.

47. Evilevitch V, Weber WA, Tap WD, et al. Reduction of glucose metabolic activity is more accurate than change in size at predicting histopathologic response to neoadjuvant therapy in high-grade soft-tissue sarcomas. Clin Cancer Res 2008;14(3):715–20.

48. Benz MR, Allen-Auerbach MS, Eilber FC, et al. Combined assessment of metabolic and volumetric changes for assessment of tumor response in patients with soft-tissue sarcomas. J Nucl Med 2008;49(10):1579–84.

49. Sheikhbahaei S, Mena E, Pattanayak P, et al. Molecular imaging and precision medicine: PET/computed tomography and therapy response

assessment in oncology. PET Clin 2017;12(1): 105–18.

50. Iagaru A, Masamed R, Chawla SP, et al. F-18 FDG PET and PET/CT evaluation of response to chemotherapy in bone and soft tissue sarcomas. Clin Nucl Med 2008;33(1):8–13.

51. Ye Z, Zhu J, Tian M, et al. Response of osteogenic sarcoma to neoadjuvant therapy: evaluated by 18F-FDG-PET. Ann Nucl Med 2008;22(6):475–80.

52. Basu S, Alavi A. PET-based personalized management in clinical oncology: an unavoidable path for the foreseeable future. PET Clin 2016;11(3):203–7.

53. Arush MW, Israel O, Postovsky S, et al. Positron emission tomography/computed tomography with 18fluoro-deoxyglucose in the detection of local recurrence and distant metastases of pediatric sarcoma. Pediatr Blood Cancer 2007;49(7):901–5.

54. Schwarzbach MH, Dimitrakopoulou-Strauss A, Willeke F, et al. Clinical value of [18-F]] fluorodeoxyglucose positron emission tomography imaging in soft tissue sarcomas. Ann Surg 2000; 231(3):380–6.

55. Salamon J, Papp L, Toth Z, et al. Nerve sheath tumors in neurofibromatosis type 1: assessment of whole-body metabolic tumor burden using F-18-FDG PET/CT. PLoS One 2015;10(12):e0143305.

56. Van Der Gucht A, Zehou O, Djelbani-Ahmed S, et al. Metabolic tumour burden measured by 18F-FDG PET/CT predicts malignant transformation in patients with neurofibromatosis type-1. PLoS One 2016;11(3):e0151809.

57. Basu S, Kwee TC, Gatenby R, et al. Evolving role of molecular imaging with PET in detecting and characterizing heterogeneity of cancer tissue at the primary and metastatic sites, a plausible explanation for failed attempts to cure malignant disorders. Eur J Nucl Med Mol Imaging 2011;38(6):987–91.

58. Ghasemi M, Nabipour I, Omrani A, et al. Precision medicine and molecular imaging: new targeted approaches toward cancer therapeutic and diagnosis. Am J Nucl Med Mol Imaging 2016;6(6): 310–27.

59. Ahmed AR, Watanabe H, Aoki J, et al. Schwannoma of the extremities: the role of PET in preoperative planning. Eur J Nucl Med 2001;28(10):1541–51.

60. Rahbar K, Afshar-Oromieh A, Jadvar H, et al. PSMA theranostics: current status and future directions. Mol Imaging 2018;17. 1536012118776068.

61. Heitkotter B, Trautmann M, Grunewald I, et al. Expression of PSMA in tumor neovasculature of high grade sarcomas including synovial sarcoma, rhabdomyosarcoma, undifferentiated sarcoma and MPNST. Oncotarget 2017;8(3):4268–76.

62. Vamadevan S, Le K, Shen L, et al. Incidental prostate-specific membrane antigen uptake in a peripheral nerve sheath tumor. Clin Nucl Med 2017; 42(7):560–2.

63. Gulhane B, Ramsay S, Fong W. 68Ga-PSMA uptake in neurofibromas demonstrated on PET/CT in a patient with neurofibromatosis type 1. Clin Nucl Med 2017;42(10):776–8.

64. Kanthan GL, Izard MA, Emmett L, et al. Schwannoma showing avid uptake on 68Ga-PSMA-HBED-CC PET/CT. Clin Nucl Med 2016;41(9):703–4.

65. Poeppel TD, Binse I, Petersenn S, et al. 68Ga-DO-TATOC versus 68Ga-DOTATATE PET/CT in functional imaging of neuroendocrine tumors. J Nucl Med 2011;52(12):1864–70.

66. Mojtahedi A, Thamake S, Tworowska I, et al. The value of (68)Ga-DOTATATE PET/CT in diagnosis and management of neuroendocrine tumors compared to current FDA approved imaging modalities: a review of literature. Am J Nucl Med Mol Imaging 2014;4(5):426–34.

67. Makis W, McCann K, McEwan AJ. Esthesioneuroblastoma (olfactory neuroblastoma) treated with 111In-octreotide and 177Lu-DOTATATE PRRT. Clin Nucl Med 2015;40(4):317–21.

68. Sabongi JG, Goncalves MC, Alves CD, et al. Lutetium 177-DOTA-TATE therapy for esthesioneuroblastoma: a case report. Exp Ther Med 2016;12(5): 3078–82.

69. Mawrin C, Schulz S, Hellwig-Patyk A, et al. Expression and function of somatostatin receptors in peripheral nerve sheath tumors. J Neuropathol Exp Neurol 2005;64(12):1080–8.

# Management of Primary Osseous Spinal Tumors with PET

Ali Batouli, MD[a],*, Ali Gholamrezanezhad, MD[b],
David Petrov, MD[c], Scott Rudkin, MD[c],
George Matcuk, MD[b], Hossein Jadvar, MD, PhD, MPH, MBA[d,e]

## KEYWORDS

- Molecular imaging • Positron emission tomography (PET) • Spine • Spine tumor • Osseous tumors
- Standardized uptake value (SUV)

## KEY POINTS

- One of the principal ways of distinguishing spine tumors is their location within the vertebrae, with lesions originating in the posterior elements primarily benign. With the exception of hemangiomas and enostoses, lesions originating in the vertebral bodies are primarily malignant.
- Although PET/CT and PET/MR imaging can be used to distinguish benign from malignant chondral lesions, their utility in distinguishing aggressive benign lesions from malignancies of other histologic categories is not as consistent.
- 18F-sodium fluoride PET and fluorodeoxyglucose (FDG) PET can play complementary roles in the detection and diagnosis of primary spine tumors, with the latter having greater overall data and especially useful for lytic lesions and the former useful for sclerotic lesions.
- FDG PET/CT and PET/MR imaging are superior to anatomic imaging alone in predicting histologic response of osteosarcoma and Ewing sarcoma to treatment, helping to differentiate viable tumor from necrosis and sclerosis.

## INTRODUCTION

Primary spine tumors account for 5% of all osseous tumors.[1] Given the imaging overlap of many benign and malignant lesions, tumors of the vertebrae can present a diagnostic challenge. Using imaging to accurately diagnose tumors can prevent unnecessary biopsy and determine the optimal medical or surgical therapy. Prompt and accurate diagnosis is necessary because both malignant and certain benign tumors can cause mass effect on the thecal sac and lead to irreversible neurologic compromise. Primary osseous tumors of the spine are for the most part similar to osseous tumors found within the rest of the body. Although they can often be diagnosed based on anatomic imaging alone, fluorodeoxyglucose (FDG) PET can help in more challenging cases. Additionally, knowledge of the PET findings of such tumors is important because

Disclosure Statement: The authors declare that they have no disclosures.
a Department of Radiology, Division of Neuroradiology, Oregon Health and Science University, 8833 Southwest 30th Avenue, Portland, OR 97219, USA; b Department of Radiology, Division of Musculoskeletal Radiology, Keck School of Medicine, University of Southern California, 2250 Alcazar Street, CSC 102, Los Angeles, CA 90033, USA; c Department of Radiology, Allegheny Health Network, 320 East North Avenue, Pittsburgh, PA 15214, USA; d Department of Radiology, Division of Nuclear Medicine, Keck School of Medicine, University of Southern California, 2250 Alcazar Street, CSC 102, Los Angeles, CA 90033, USA; e Department of Radiology, Keck School of Medicine, University of Southern California, 2250 Alcazar Street, CSC 102, Los Angeles, CA 90033, USA
* Corresponding author.
E-mail address: dibatouli@gmail.com

PET Clin 14 (2019) 91–101
https://doi.org/10.1016/j.cpet.2018.08.002
1556-8598/19/© 2018 Elsevier Inc. All rights reserved.

they are often incidentally encountered when imaging patients for an unrelated primary neoplastic process.

The first means of differentiating tumor types is through consideration of patient demographics in combination with the location of the tumor. The greatest differentiator is simply age, with the vast majority of spine lesions presenting before 30 years of age benign, with the exception of Ewing sarcoma and osteosarcoma.[2]

Location of the lesion, vertebral body versus posterior elements, is another important differentiating factor. Lesions originating from the posterior elements are primarily benign and include osteoid osteoma, osteoblastoma, osteochondroma, and aneurysmal bone cyst (ABC). Malignant lesions of vertebral body, such as chondrosarcoma, osteosarcoma, and Ewing sarcoma, however, may extend into the posterior elements. Both benign and malignant lesions can be expansile and encroach on the thecal sac or nerve roots, causing neurologic symptoms. Many benign lesions, such as osteoblastomas or even vertebral hemangiomas, can be expansile, leading to spinal cord or nerve compression.[3] Within the vertebral body, the majority of primary lesions are benign hemangiomas or enostoses. Other lesions centered primarily within the vertebral bodies include myeloma/plasmacytoma, lymphoma, chordoma, eosinophilic granuloma, and giant cell tumor (GCT).[4]

In addition to location, certain morphologic characteristics seen on radiography and CT can help differentiate benign from aggressive lesions. In general, benign lesions demonstrate well-defined borders, which are often sclerotic, whereas aggressive tumors have a wider zone of transition to normal bone. Aggressive lesions also often have more aggressive periosteal reaction, often showing a lamellated or sunburst appearance. On MR imaging, aggressive lesions are often found to demonstrate adjacent marrow edema as well as soft tissue component and edema. In addition to these general morphologic features, specific types of lesions can often be diagnosed with very specific findings. Fluid-fluid level seen on MR imaging or CT, for example, is most often associated with ABCs in the posterior elements, although it can also be seen with telangiectatic osteosarcoma and GCTs. Chondroblastomas, although rare in the spine, also may demonstrate fluid-fluid levels. A sclerotic lesion with a central nidus is often seen with osteoid osteoma, again usually centered in the posterior elements. Lesions that clearly contain fat are most often benign, with the majority representing hemangiomas.[4] Vertebral hemangiomas demonstrate thickening of the primary vertical weight-bearing trabeculae on CT, resulting in corduroy sign on sagittal or vertical projections and polka-dot sign on axial images.

## PET/COMPUTED TOMOGRAPHY IN THE DIAGNOSIS OF BENIGN OSSEOUS SPINAL LESIONS

FDG PET can be used in conjunction with CT or MR imaging to characterize lesions that appear similar or to grade lesions as more aggressive or less aggressive. As a whole, malignancies of the vertebrae, as elsewhere in the body, have greater FDG uptake than benign lesions.[5–8] FDG PET/CT is an excellent tool for differentiating metastatic disease from benign spinal lesions, proving more sensitive and specific than CT or MR imaging alone.[9] Differentiation between lesions is most useful when comparing tumors of the similar histopathology, such as chondrosarcoma versus enchondroma.[5,6,10–12] Although cartilage lesions usually demonstrate characteristic ring and arc matrix on plain film and CT as well as high T2 signal on MR imaging, this does not necessarily indicate benignity, and differentiation between malignant and benign lesions can be difficult on the basis of anatomic imaging alone. Evaluation of glucose metabolism with FDG PET has a sensitivity of 91%, specificity of 100%, and accuracy of 97% in differentiating benign and malignant chondral lesions.[10,11] Specifically, the vast majority of malignant lesions studied demonstrate maximum standardized uptake value (SUVmax) of greater than 2, whereas all benign lesions show SUVmax of lower than 2. On the contrary, enchondromas demonstrate substantial uptake on 18F-sodium fluoride (NaF) PET due to their osteoblastic activity, potentially confusing them with chondrosarcoma.[13,14]

Despite its utility in differentiating malignant and benign chondral lesions, distinguishing between aggressive benign lesions of differing histologies and high-grade malignancies of spine by FDG PET is not always possible, as shown by a study of 202 patients by Schulte and colleagues.[5] Additionally, many benign tumors with the exact same histology can have widely varying levels of FDG uptake. Of the benign spinal column tumors, several, including fibrous dysplasia, ABC, GCT, eosinophilic granuloma, osteoid osteoma, and osteoblastoma, often exhibit substantial FDG avidity.[7,8,10,15] Many of these lesions can have the same levels of uptake as highly aggressive neoplasms, such as osteosarcoma. The only benign vertebral lesions with consistently low FDG uptake are benign cartilaginous lesions, hemangiomas, and intraosseous lipomas. Some investigators, however, argue that benign cartilaginous tumors of the spine are rare. Similar to FDG, NaF can also not be definitively used to differentiate benign from malignant spine lesions as a whole.[16–18] When combined with morphologic details provided by MR imaging or CT, however, both FDG and NaF PET can prove diagnostically useful in certain instances. Langsteger[19] studied 150 lesions in 20 patients who underwent both NaF PET/CT and FDG PET/CT to decipher whether one radiotracer was more sensitive than the other in detecting osseous metastases and found that approximately 50% of the metastatic lesions were found on both modalities, whereas approximately 20% were found on FDG PET/CT only and 20% were found on NaF PET/CT only. Specifically, FDG PET/CT was better at detecting osteolytic lesions overall and NaF PET/CT was better at detecting non–FDG-avid lesions, such as renal cell carcinoma and thyroid cancer.[19] Additional studies have also shown the superiority of NaF in the diagnosis of sclerotic lesions.[20] This sensitivity, however, also leads to a high false-positive rate in NaF.[21]

GCT is a traditionally benign lesion that can prove difficult to differentiate from aggressive malignancies on both anatomic and physiologic imaging. This benign tumor is composed of ovoid mononuclear cells and osteoclastic giant cells, occurring in skeletally mature patients. Of the 7% of GCTs affecting the spine, 90% are found in the sacrum, especially within the sacral ala.[4,22,23] Due to the prevalence of endosteal scalloping, cortical destruction and even associated soft tissue mass, it is difficult to distinguish these lesions from malignancies on anatomic imaging alone. Unfortunately, the lesions are also highly FDG avid, with a mean SUVmax of approximately 4 to 5, limiting the role of FDG PET/CT in distinguishing them from malignancy.[5–7,11] Although not well studied using NaF PET, there are reports of increased uptake on this modality, even though

the lesion is generally lytic.[13,24] Another lytic lesion that is often expansile and primarily exists within the posterior elements of the spine is an ABC. The spine can be involved in up to 20% of cases.[4,25] ABC is composed of blood-filled cavities within the bone, sometimes occurring within other primary lesions, most commonly GCT, followed by osteoblastoma and chondroblastoma.[4,25,26] They are expansile lytic lesions, often with associated cortical thinning. The characteristic finding on MR imaging or CT is multiple fluid-fluid levels within the hemorrhagic cavities. Unfortunately, telangiectatic osteosarcoma, an aggressive malignancy, can have a similar appearance on anatomic imaging. The 2 also cannot be reliably differentiated on FDG PET, because they are both often slightly hypermetabolic. ABCs typically demonstrate SUVmax ranging from 1 to 6, with a mean of approximately 3.[5,10]

Another lytic lesion, eosinophilic granuloma, is found most often in children, usually occurring before age 30.[27] Lesions are often multiple and, when within the spine, can lead to partial or complete vertebral body collapse (vertebra plana). Due to high histiocyte content, lesions are usually FDG avid, with FDG PET having been found at least as sensitive as MR imaging in lesion detection, often used as the test of choice for screening and follow-up in multifocal disease.[28] Given their FDG avidity, FDG PET is of little utility in differentiating eosinophilic granuloma from malignancy. Similarly, despite being lytic, eosinophilic granuloma can also demonstrate substantial uptake of NaF.[14]

Osteoid osteoma is a benign mainly sclerotic lesion, which often presents as painful scoliosis in the spine. On CT, the lesion has a lucent nidus, often with a central sclerotic dot representing mineralized osteoid, with surrounding reactive sclerosis, usually within the posterior elements (**Fig. 1A**). Osteoblastoma, which is usually larger in size, by definition greater than 2 cm, also

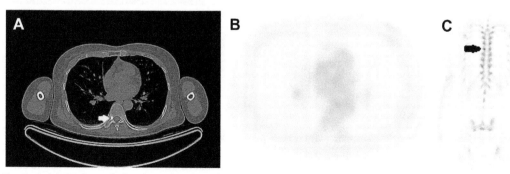

**Fig. 1.** Axial CT through the thoracic spine of a young male patient with symptomatic osteoid osteoma shows a sclerotic focus within the right pedicle of T5 (*A, white arrow*). The osteoid osteoma demonstrated no significant uptake on FDG PET (*B*). A coronal NaF PET, however, shows increased radiotracer uptake corresponding to the lesion (*C, black arrow*).

involves the posterior elements. Although osteoid osteomas usually regress, however, osteoblastomas grow and can be locally aggressive, often being confused with malignant lesions on imaging (**Fig. 2**). At times, osteoblastomas can also demonstrate malignant degeneration. Osteoblastomas are lytic and expansile with mixed sclerosis.[4,29] Both lesions demonstrate FDG uptake above background. Osteoid osteoma has a mean SUVmax between 2 and 3 whereas osteoblastoma has a minimally higher mean SUVmax slightly above 3.[5,30–32] Neither can be differentiated from a malignant lesion purely based on FDG uptake. Occasionally, osteoid osteomas are not active on FDG PET (**Fig. 1B**). In such situations, NaF PET may prove useful because these lesions have also been shown to be NaF avid (**Fig. 1C**).[18,33]

Fibrous dysplasia is another lesion that has higher than background FDG avidity. Although fibrous dysplasia has a mean SUVmax of approximately 2, many lesions have a much higher standardized uptake value (SUV) and, therefore, cannot be differentiated from malignancies, such as metastatic disease, osteosarcoma, or chondrosarcoma based on FDG uptake.[5,7,32] Fortunately, its anatomic appearance is usually more characteristic of a benign entity than more aggressive appearing lesions, such as osteoblastoma and GCT. A more aggressive appearance, however, including secondary ABC formation and cortical breakthrough, can be seen on CT.[34] Although vertebral involvement of the disease is rare, it can be seen with polyostotic forms. On CT and radiography, there is often a classic ground-glass appearance to the osseous matrix, with many lesions being expansile and demonstrating lytic components and a sclerotic rim (**Fig. 3**).[4] Given increased osteoblastic activity, fibrous dysplasia is also NaF avid, further potentially confusing it with more aggressive tumors on the basis of physiologic imaging alone.[18]

Osseous hemangiomas are common hamartomatous lesions of bone, which are composed of vessels interposed by normal marrow. They are the most common benign lesions of the spine, found frequently in middle-aged individuals.[1] Although most often clinically irrelevant, some can become expansile and compress on the spinal cord.[35] They are often simple to diagnose on both CT and MR imaging, demonstrating a classic corduroy appearance of vertical striations, with portions of fat equivalent signal on MR imaging. Expansile hemangiomas can appear more aggressive, sometimes being confused with Ewing sarcoma or other vascular lesions, such as hemangioblastoma. Fortunately, FDG PET can help distinguish these lesions because hemangiomas are classically not particularly FDG avid, with SUVmax less than 2 (**Fig. 4**).[5,7,10] Case reports of particularly FDG-avid lesions, however, have been described.[36] On NaF PET,

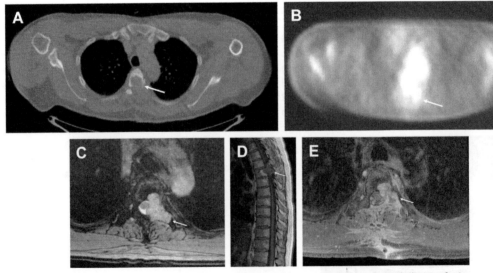

**Fig. 2.** Axial CT (*A*) through the T4 vertebrae in a 58-year-old man shows an expansile lytic soft tissue mass within the body and posterior elements (*white arrow*). The mass was somewhat FDG avid on PET (*B*), similar to the aortic arch blood pool. Axial T2-weighted (*C*), sagittal precontrast T1-weighted (*D*), and axial postcontrast T1-weighted (*E*) images better define the mildly T2 hyperintense and T1 hypointense mass with diffuse enhancement, effacing the thecal sac and causing mass effect on the thoracic spinal cord. On surgical pathology, the lesion was found to represent an osteoblastoma.

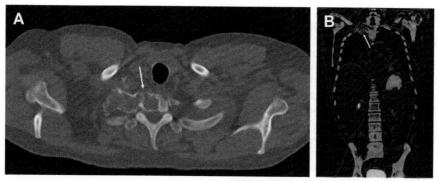

**Fig. 3.** Axial CT (A) and coronal fused FDG PET/CT (B) images in a 38-year-old man with complaints of neck and shoulder pain as well as numbness of the right fourth and fifth digits demonstrate an expansile lytic lesion of the T1 vertebral body and adjacent right first rib. There is general preserved cortex with small foci of cortical breakthrough. There are some areas of ground-glass matrix within the rib lesion. The SUVmax, found within the rib, was 8. An additional lesion was seen in the left iliac bone (not shown). The rib lesion was biopsied, allowing for diagnosis of polyostotic fibrous dysplasia.

hemangiomas can often demonstrate significant radiotracer uptake.[18]

Osteochondroma, a cartilage-covered bony excrescence, rarely involves the posterior elements of the spine. Although these lesions are not FDG avid, PET has been used in the evaluation of suspected malignant/sarcomatous transformation of these lesions.

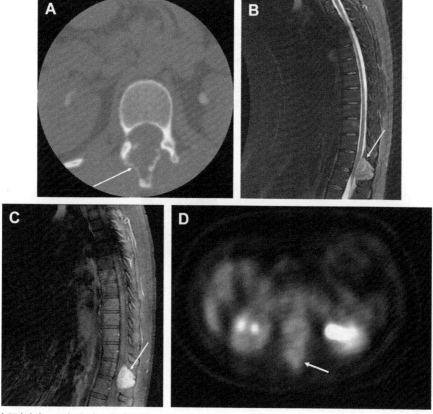

**Fig. 4.** Axial CT (A) through the level of T12 in a 37-year-old man demonstrates an expansile, osteolytic lesion involving the spinous process with mildly aggressive features and breakthrough into the posterior spinal canal. The lesion causes mass effect on the conus medullaris and demonstrates heterogeneous T2 hyperintensity (B) and avid T1 postcontrast enhancement (C). The mass demonstrates similar FDG avidity to the unaffected vertebral body seen on the same FDG PET axial image (D). On biopsy, the mass was found to represent an expansile hemangioma.

## PET/CT AND PET/MR IMAGING IN THE DIAGNOSTIC MANAGEMENT OF MALIGNANT OSSEOUS SPINAL LESIONS

The most common malignant spinal lesions aside from metastatic disease are hematologic malignancies, such as multiple myeloma (MM) and lymphoma. MM is the most common primary bone malignancy in adults and solitary plasmacytoma is one of the most common primary osseous lesions of the vertebrae and pelvis.[37] As expected, FDG PET/CT has been shown superior to FDG PET alone in detecting diffuse spiny involvement of MM and in detecting lesions less than 10 mm (**Fig. 5**).[38] Furthermore, Fonti and colleagues[39] compared FDG PET/CT with technetium sestamibi ([99]Tc-MIBI) and found that PET/CT was better at detecting focal lesions whereas [99]Tc-MIBI was superior in detecting multifocal disease. Sachpekidis and colleagues[40] similarly found that although NaF PET/CT can detect many myeloma lesions, FDG PET/CT is much more sensitive, detecting more than twice as many lesions. Although FDG PET/CT has good sensitivity for MM lesions, Breyer and colleagues[41] have described that this sensitivity is greatly increased by MR imaging when small focal lesions are present. PET/MR imaging, therefore, is a promising modality that can help to assess the extent of lesions as well as better define neural compromise.

Primary bone lymphoma, also known as reticulum cell sarcoma or osteolymphoma, is less common than secondary involvement of bone from systemic lymphoma. More commonly, they are from non-Hodgkin histologic subtypes, with only 6% of cases diagnosed as Hodgkin lymphoma. Primary bone lymphoma is distinguished from other PET-avid bone lesions as extremely FDG avid, with SUV values up to and beyond 10 compared with approximately 5 in the majority of other primary bone lesions.[41] Primary lymphoma of the spine is a rare entity and makes for difficult radiographic diagnosis because it may mimic other primary or metastatic bony spine lesions.[7] Epidural extension can occur in approximately 14% of primary lymphomatous lesions involving the vertebrae.[42,43] Because timely radiotherapy and chemotherapy can improve prognosis substantially, especially compared with other osseous malignancies, prompt and accurate diagnosis is imperative.[42–44] Lei and colleagues[45] described the utility of FDG PET/CT in the diagnosis of primary spinal lymphoplasmacytic lymphoma that had destroyed much of the thoracic and lumbar vertebrae and extended into the epidural space, causing cord compression.

The possibility of chordoma should also be raised when an FDG-avid sacrococcygeal lesion is noted on PET/CT.[46,47] Chordoma typically presents in the fifth and sixth decades, most often involving the clivus or sacrum, with other vertebral involvement less common. On MR imaging, they are classically extremely T2 hyperintense and T1 hypointense. Chordomas have heterogeneous

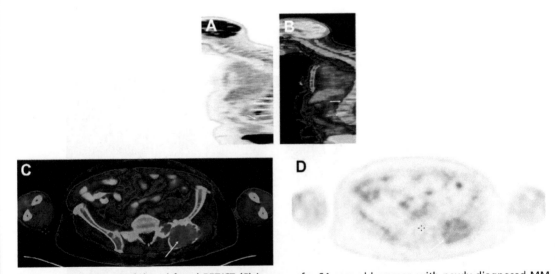

**Fig. 5.** Sagittal FDG PET (*A*) and fused PET/CT (*B*) images of a 64-year-old woman with newly diagnosed MM demonstrates numerous FDG-avid spinal lesions (*white arrows*), most prominent in the lower thoracic and lumbar spine. The most FDG-avid lesion in L4 has an SUV of 6.2. Axial fused FDG PET/CT (*C*) and PET (*D*) images through the sacrum of a 61-year-old man with MM on maintenance therapy presenting for restaging show a large FDG-avid expansile plasmacytoma involving the left sacral ala as well as the left iliac bone (white arrows) with SUVmax of 3.6.

FDG uptake and cause local bony destruction in the sacrum when present, often extending into the sacral epidural space and causing nerve root compromise.[47]

The most common nonhematologic primary vertebral malignancies are Ewing sarcoma and osteosarcoma. FDG PET/CT has been successfully used to stage and restage osteosarcoma and Ewing sarcoma.[48,49] Both tumors are generally FDG avid, allowing detection of distant metastatic disease (**Fig. 6**). In addition to providing information regarding distant metastatic disease, FDG PET/CT is an excellent prognosticating tool for these malignancies. FDG PET–based imaging can provide information on tumor response to therapy before any change is seen on anatomic imaging alone.[50] In the case of osteosarcoma, pretherapeutic and post-therapeutic FDG uptake, as well as change in uptake between the 2 scans, have all been shown to correlate with histologic tumor response, progression-free survival, and overall survival.[51–54] FDG PET is particularly adept at determining histologic response, because tumor necrosis can be differentiated

from residual metabolically active tumor in osteosarcomas. A post-therapeutic SUV of less than 2.5 and reduction in metabolic tumor volume by 50% have been found to independently correlate with tumor necrosis.[53] Evaluating response to treatment through FDG PET/CT can help alter the chemotherapeutic regimen in tumors that seem resistant to therapy. Although FDG PET/CT also allows prognostication in Ewing sarcoma, the evidence is somewhat less strong than for osteosarcoma. Favorable histologic response in Ewing sarcoma, for example, correlates with greater than 90% reduction in metabolic tumor volume, compared with 50% in osteosarcoma (**Fig. 7**). Additionally, only post-therapy FDG uptake has been found to correlate significantly with progression-free survival, with a post-therapy SUV of 2.5 or lower correlating with a 4-year progression-free survival of 72%.[51] Pretherapeutic uptake and change in uptake between pretherapy and post-therapy scans have not shown similar significance.

More recently, FDG PET/MR imaging has been used in an attempt to improve evaluation of

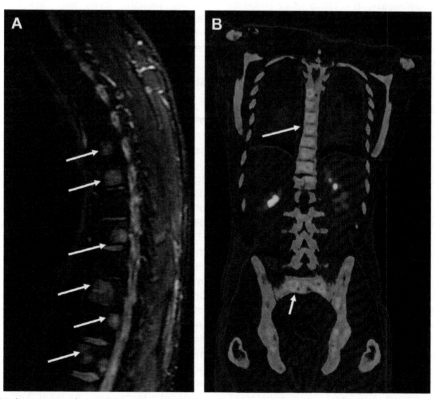

**Fig. 6.** Sagittal contrast-enhanced T1-weighted MR imaging through the thoracic spine (*A*) of a 21-year-old man with biopsy-proved Ewing sarcoma of the right anterior iliac bone shows multiple enhancing metastases throughout the visualized vertebrae (white arrows). Fused coronal PET/CT images in the same patient (*B*) demonstrate these vertebral lesions, as well as multiple sacral and bilateral iliac lesions, as having higher FDG avidity than normal marrow (white arrows).

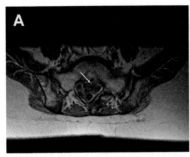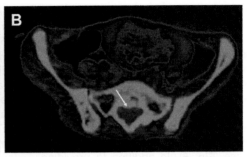

**Fig. 7.** FDG PET/CT and separate MR imaging were obtained in a 13-year-old girl with history of Ewing sarcoma, status post treatment with chemotherapy and local radiation. Residual epidural soft tissue at the L5-S1 level is seen on axial unenhanced T1-weighted MR imaging (*A, white arrow*). Because of its stability on 1-year follow-up (previous images not shown) and lack of uptake on FDG PET/CT (*B, white arrow*), the findings likely represent post-treatment changes rather than recurrent/residual disease.

therapy response in osteosarcoma. Byun and colleagues[55] obtained fused, separate acquisition PET/MR imaging images in 30 patients who had undergone 2 cycles of neoadjuvant chemotherapy for osteosarcoma. Although not focused on spine lesions, they found that this modality was also able to predict histologic response using both metabolic tumor volume and total lesion glycolysis. Specifically, in a study of 27 patients undergoing pretreatment and post-treatment sequential PET/MR imaging, both change in mean apparent diffusion coefficient and change in SUVmax was found to significantly correlate with histologic response. The combination of the 2 variables improved on the sensitivity, specificity, and accuracy of either value alone.[55] Again, using fused separate acquisition PET/MR imaging, Kong and colleagues[30] found that the percentage of tumor necrosis at the location of SUVmax correlated significantly with overall histologic response of the entire resected tumor to chemotherapy. Similar analyses attempted on PET/CT have not been as successful, presumably due to the inferior contrast differentiation between necrotic and enhancing tissue. Using hybrid PET/MR images, the same group has also found an additional benefit of the physiologic information provided by MR imaging in predicting histologic response.

As opposed to FDG PET, NaF PET evaluation of osteosarcoma has not been studied as extensively. The few reports available, however, show that NaF is potentially useful in this setting. Hoh and colleagues[53] first described osteosarcoma as an intensely NaF-avid osseous lesion. Both the primary lesion and pulmonary metastases have been shown NaF avid, with substantial reduction in NaF uptake after successful chemotherapy.[20,56,57] The level of NaF avidity of osteosarcoma is such that NaF PET is more sensitive than FDG PET in the detection of pulmonary and soft tissue metastases from osteosarcoma.[58,59] Combined NaF and FDG PET has been shown in at least 1 documented case to alter clinical management. Specifically, Brunkhorst and colleagues[60] described the case of a 15-year-old girl whose treatment changed from curative intent to palliative intent after combined NaF and FDG PET revealed greater extent of disease than initially thought. Even less has been studied regarding the uptake of NaF in Ewing sarcoma, with only a few scattered cases showing substantial radiotracer avidity.[61]

## SUMMARY

Familiarity with the PET findings of common and rare primary spine tumors is paramount for anyone who regularly reads PET studies for cancer staging. Unfortunately, there is much overlap between the FDG avidity of many benign and malignant primary osseous spinal lesions, making differentiation between the 2 entities based on physiologic imaging alone difficult. When combined with morphologic characteristics seen on CT or MR imaging, however, PET can help point the radiologist toward the correct diagnosis. PET/CT and PET/MR imaging are also of utmost importance in the follow-up of primary malignant processes of the spine, proving better than MR imaging or CT alone in assessing response to treatment. Although research on the use of alternative radiotracers, such as NaF, and alternative modalities, such as PET/MR imaging, in the diagnosis of primary spine tumors is sparse, the available data point to their utility beyond standard diagnostic techniques. As such, further research is necessary to explore and define the utility and limitations of PET/MR imaging and non-FDG PET radiotracers in the realm of spinal lesions (**Boxes 1** and **2**).

---

**Box 1**
**Diagnostic criteria of primary osseous lesions on PET/CT and PET/MR imaging**

| | |
|---|---|
| Cartilaginous lesions | Characteristic ring and arc matrix on CT and T2 hyperintense on MR imaging. SUVmax greater than 2 is a highly sensitive and specific cutoff for malignancy on FDG PET. NaF PET is not as specific. |
| Giant cell tumors | Lytic lesions, often with endosteal scalloping or even at times cortical destruction on CT. Highly FDG-avid and, therefore, not able to be distinguished from malignancy based on FDG PET. |
| ABC | Expansile lucent lesion on CT, often with hematocrit levels on MR imaging. Often FDG-avid and cannot be differentiated from malignancy on the basis of FDG PET. |
| Eosinophilic granuloma | Lucent lesion on CT found in children and can lead to vertebra plana. Both FDG and NaF avid. |
| Osteoid osteoma | Characteristic sclerotic lesion with lucent nidus and a central sclerotic dot on CT. Usually involves the posterior elements. Demonstrates surrounding T2 hyperintense marrow edema on MR imaging. Highly NaF avid with usually intermediate uptake on FDG PET, having an SUVmax of 2–3. |
| Osteoblastoma | Lytic expansile lesion of the posterior elements with mean SUVmax slightly >3. Highly NaF avid. |
| Fibrous dysplasia | Classic ground-glass matrix with usually benign morphologic characteristics on CT, including intact cortex. Variable FDG uptake, with mean SUVmax of 2. |
| Osseous hemangioma | Classic corduroy appearance on CT with fat intensity signal on MR imaging. Typically not FDG avid, with SUVmax similar or below background marrow. Often highly NaF avid. |
| Myeloma | Lucent lesion within the Marrow on CT. T2 hyperintensity, T1 hypointensity, and enhancement on MR imaging. Usually no cortical involvement unless expansile plasmacytoma. FDG has greater sensitivity than NaF PET. |
| Lymphoma | Lytic, sclerotic, or mixed lesion on CT. T2 hyperintensity, T1 hypointensity, and enhancement on MR imaging. Can be distinguished from other primary bone pathologies by its intense FDG avidity, often with SUVmax of 10 or greater. |
| Chordoma | Lytic lesion with cortical breakthrough on CT predominantly within the sacrum or clivus. Light-bulb bright signal on T2-weighted MR imaging. FDG uptake is heterogeneous and inconsistent. |
| Ewing sarcoma | Generally lytic lesion on CT with intense enhancement on MR imaging. Moderate to intense FDG avidity. Treatment response can be assessed using FDG PET. |
| Osteosarcoma | Mixed sclerotic and lytic lesion on CT with aggressive periosteal reaction and bone formation. Avidly enhancing on MR imaging. Intensely NaF avid and moderately FDG avid. Treatment response can be assessed using both FDG PET and NaF PET. |

---

**Box 2**
**What the referring physician needs to know about PET-based imaging for primary spine tumors**

- As a general rule, PET cannot definitively differentiate benign from malignant primary spine tumors of unknown histology. In general, more aggressive lesions have higher FDG uptake. There are only 3 primary spine tumors that nearly always have low FDG uptake and, therefore, can be confidently diagnosed as benign: hemangioma, enostosis, and benign cartilaginous lesions.

- Given the greater sensitivity and specificity of MR imaging, PET/MR imaging is superior to PET/CT in characterizing many primary osseous lesions.

- FDG PET/CT and PET/MR imaging are of greater utility than anatomic imaging alone in assessing treatment response in osteosarcoma and Ewing sarcoma.

- NaF PET and FDG PET can play complementary roles in the detection and diagnosis of primary spine tumors, with the former having greater overall data and especially useful for lytic lesions and the latter useful for sclerotic lesions.

## REFERENCES

1. Patnaik S, Jyotsnarani Y, Uppin SG, et al. Imaging features of primary tumors of the spine: a pictorial essay. Indian J Radiol Imaging 2016; 26:279–89.

2. Wang K, Allen L, Fung E, et al. Bone scintigraphy in common tumors with osteolytic components. Clin Nucl Med 2005;30:655–71.

3. Rich JA, Donahue TC, Mick TJ. Symptomatic expansile vertebral hemangioma causing conus medullaris compression. J Manipulative Physiol Ther 2005; 28:194–8.

4. Rodallec MH, Feydy A, Larousserie F, et al. Diagnostic imaging of solitary tumors of the spine: what to do and say. Radiographics 2008;28:1019–41.

5. Schulte M, Brecht-Krauss D, Heymer B, et al. Grading of tumors and tumorlike lesions of bone: evaluation by FDG PET. J Nucl Med 2000;41:1695–701.

6. Costelloe CM, Chuang HH, Chasen BA, et al. Bone windows for distinguishing malignant from benign primary bone tumors on FDG PET/CT. J Cancer 2013;4:524–30.

7. Aoki J, Watanabe H, Shinozaki T, et al. FDG PET of primary benign and malignant bone tumors: standardized uptake value in 52 lesions. Radiology 2001;219:774–7.

8. Tian R, Su M, Tian Y, et al. Dual-time point PET/CT with F-18 FDG for the differentiation of malignant and benign bone lesions. Skeletal Radiol 2009;38: 451–8.

9. Wafaie A, El-Liethy N, Kassem H, et al. Comparison between FDG PET/CT, CT and MRI in detection of spinal metastases and its impact on clinical management. Egypt J Nucl Med 2013;8:30–44.

10. Costelloe CM, Chuang HH, Madewell JE. FDG PET/CT of primary bone tumors. Am J Roentgenol 2014; 202:W521–31.

11. Feldman F, Heertum R, Saxena C, et al. 18FDG-PET applications for cartilage neoplasms. Skeletal Radiol 2005;34:367–74.

12. Aoki J, Watanabe H, Shinozaki T, et al. FDG-PET in differential diagnosis and grading of chondrosarcomas. J Comput Assist Tomogr 1999;23:603–8.

13. Even-Sapir E, Metser U, Flusser G, et al. Assessment of malignant skeletal disease: initial experience with 18F-fluoride PET/CT and comparison between 18F-fluoride PET and 18F-fluoride PET/CT. J Nucl Med 2004;45:272–8.

14. Beheshti M. Clinical utility of [18]F NaF PET/CT in benign and malignant disorders. PET Clin 2012;7(3):249–344.

15. Shin DS, Shon OJ, Han DS, et al. The clinical efficacy of 18F-FDG-PET/CT in benign and malignant musculoskeletal tumors. Ann Nucl Med 2008;22:603–9.

16. Segall G, Delbeke D, Stabin MG, et al. SNM practice guideline for sodium 18F-fluoride PET/CT bone scans 1.0. J Nucl Med 2010;51:1813–20.

17. Schirrmeister H. Detection of bone metastases in breast cancer by positron emission tomography. Radiol Clin North Am 2007;45:669–76.

18. Bastawrous S, Bhargava P, Behnia F, et al. Newer PET application with an old tracer: role of [18] F-NaF skeletal PET/CT in oncologic practice. Radiographics 2014;34:1295–316.

19. Langsteger W. The role of fluorodeoxyglucose, 18F-dihydroxyalanine, 18F-choline, and 18F-fluoride in bone imaging with emphasis on prostate and breast. Semin Nucl Med 2006;36:72–96.

20. Tse N, Hoh C, Hawkins R, et al. Positron emission tomography diagnosis of pulmonary metastases in osteogenic sarcoma. J Am J Clin Oncol 1994;17:22–5.

21. Jadvar H, Desai B, Ji L, et al. Prospective evaluation of 18F-NaF and 18F-FDG PET/CT in detection of occult metastatic disease in biochemical recurrence of prostate cancer. Clin Nucl Med 2012;37:637–43.

22. Hart RA, Boriani S, Biagini R, et al. A system for surgical staging and management of spine tumors. A clinical outcome study of giant cell tumors of the spine. Spine 1997;22:1773–82.

23. Laredo JD, el Quessar A, Bossard P, et al. Vertebral tumors and pseudotumors. Radiol Clin North Am 2001;39:137–63.

24. Even-Sapir E, Metser U, Mishani E, et al. The detection of bone metastases in patients with high-risk prostate cancer: 99mTc-MDP Planar bone scintigraphy, single- and multi-field-of-view SPECT, 18F-fluoride PET, and 18F-fluoride PET/CT. J Nucl Med 2006;47:287–97.

25. Suzuki M, Satoh T, Nishida J, et al. Solid variant of aneurysmal bone cyst of the cervical spine. Spine 2004;29:E376–81.

26. Kransdorf MJ, Sweet DE. Aneurysmal bone cyst: concept, controversy, clinical presentation, and imaging. Am J Roentgenol 1995;164:573–80.

27. Yeom JS, Lee CK, Shin HY, et al. Langerhans' cell histiocytosis of the spine. Analysis of twenty-three cases. Spine 1999;24:1740–9.

28. Mansberg R, Ho B, Bui C, et al. False positive F-18 FDG PET/CT of skeletal metastasis due to solitary eosinophilic granuloma. Mol Imaging Radionucl Ther 2013;22:103–5.

29. Greenspan A. Benign bone-forming lesions: osteoma, osteoid osteoma, and osteoblastoma. Clinical, imaging, pathologic, and differential considerations. Skeletal Radiol 1993;22:485–500.

30. Kong CB, Byun BH, Lim I, et al. 18F-FDG PET SUVmax as an indicator of histopathologic response after neoadjuvant chemotherapy in extremity osteosarcoma. Eur J Nucl Med Mol Imaging 2013;40:728–36.

31. Kole AC, Nieweg OE, Hoekstra HJ, et al. Fluorine-18-fluorodeoxyglucose assessment of glucose metabolism in bone tumors. J Nucl Med 1998;39:810–5.

32. Dimitrakopoulou-Strauss A, Strauss LG, Heichel T, et al. The role of quantitative (18)F-FDG PET studies

for the differentiation of malignant and benign bone lesions. J Nucl Med 2002;43:510–8.

33. Ovadia D, Metser U, Loevshitz G, et al. Back pain in adolescents: assessment with integrated 18F-fluoride positron-emission tomography-computed tomography. J Pediatr Orthop 2007;27:90–3.

34. Guler I, Nayman A, Gedik GK, et al. Fibrous dysplasia mimicking vertebral bone metastasis on 18F-FDG PET/computed tomography in a patient with tongue cancer. Spine J 2015;15:1501–2.

35. Laredo JD, Reizine D, Bard M, et al. Vertebral hemangiomas: radiologic evaluation. Radiology 1986; 161:183–9.

36. Cha JG, Yoo JH, Kim HK, et al. PET/CT and MRI of intra-osseous haemangioma of the tibia. Br J Radiol 2012;85:e94–8.

37. Hanrahan CJ, Christensen CR, Crim JR. Current concepts in the evaluation of multiple myeloma with MR imaging and FDG PET/CT. Radiographics 2010;30: 127–42.

38. Agarwal A, Chirindel A, Shah BA, et al. Evolving role of FDG PET/CT in multiple myeloma imaging and management. Am J Roentgenol 2013;200:884–90.

39. Fonti R, Salvatore B, Quarantelli M, et al. 18F-FDG PET/CT, 99mTc-MIBI, and MRI in evaluation of patients with multiple myeloma. J Nucl Med 2008;49:195–200.

40. Sachpekidis C, Goldschmidt H, Hose D, et al. PET/CT studies of multiple myeloma using 18F-FDG and 18F-NaF: comparison of distribution patterns and tracers' pharmacokinetics. Eur J Nucl Med Mol Imaging 2014;41:1343–53.

41. Breyer RJ, Mulligan ME, Smith SE, et al. Comparison of imaging with FDG PET/CT with other imaging modalities in myeloma. Skeletal Radiol 2006;35:632–40.

42. Nasiri MR, Varshoee F, Mohtashami S, et al. Primary bone lymphoma: a clinicopathological retrospective study of 28 patients in a single institution. J Res Med Sci 2011;16:814–20.

43. Zinzani P, Carrillo G, Ascani S, et al. Primary bone lymphoma: experience with 52 patients. Haematologica 2003;88:280–5.

44. Rahmat K, Wastie M, Abdullah B. Primary bone lymphoma: report of a case with multifocal skeletal involvement. Biomed Imaging Interv J 2007;3:e52.

45. Lei Y, Zi L, Long S, et al. Primary bone lymphoplasmacytic lymphoma presenting with spinal cord compression: a case report. Turk J Haematol 2013;30:409–12.

46. Farsad K, Kattapuram SV, Sacknoff R, et al. Sacral chordoma. Radiographics 2009;29:1525–30.

47. Park SA, Kim HS. F-18 FDG PET/CT evaluation of sacrococcygeal chordoma. Clin Nucl Med 2008; 33:906–8.

48. Bestic JM, Peterson JJ, Bancroft LW. Use of FDG PET in staging, restaging, and assessment of therapy response in ewing sarcoma. Radiographics 2009;29:1487–500.

49. Quartuccio N, Fox J, Kuk D, et al. Pediatric bone sarcoma: diagnostic performance of [18]F-FDG PET/CT versus conventional imaging for initial staging and follow-up. Am J Roentgenol 2015;204:153–60.

50. Guimarães JB, Rigo L, Lewin F, et al. The importance of PET/CT in the evaluation of patients with Ewing tumors. Radiol Bras 2015;48:175–80.

51. Costelloe CM, Macapinlac HA, Madewell JE, et al. 18F-FDG PET/CT as an indicator of progression-free and overall survival in osteosarcoma. J Nucl Med 2009;50:340–7.

52. Hawkins DS, Conrad EU, Butrynski JE, et al. [F-18]-fluorodeoxy-D-glucose-positron emission tomography response is associated with outcome for extremity osteosarcoma in children and young adults. Cancer 2009;115:3519–25.

53. Hoh CK, Hawkins RA, Dahlbom M, et al. Whole body skeletal imaging with [18F] fluoride ion and PET. J Comput Assist Tomogr 1993;17:34–41.

54. Hawkins DS, Schuetze SM, Butrynski JE, et al. [[18]F] Fluorodeoxyglucose positron emission tomography predicts outcome for ewing sarcoma family of tumors. J Clin Oncol 2005;23:8828–34.

55. Byun BH, Kong CB, Lim I, et al. Early response monitoring to neoadjuvant chemotherapy in osteosarcoma using sequential 18F-FDG PET/CT and MRI. Eur J Nucl Med Mol Imaging 2014;41: 1553–62.

56. Hoh C, Hawkins RA, Glaspy JA, et al. Cancer detection with whole-body PET using 2-[18F]Fluoro-2-Deoxy-D-Glucose. J Comput Assist Tomogr 1977; 17(4):582–9. Raven Press.

57. Brenner W, Bohuslavizki KH, Eary JF. PET imaging of osteosarcoma. J Nucl Med 2003;44:930–42.

58. Arvanitis C, Bendapudi PK, Tseng JR, et al. (18)F and (18)FDG PET imaging of osteosarcoma to non-invasively monitor in situ changes in cellular proliferation and bone differentiation upon MYC inactivation. Cancer Biol Ther 2008;7:1947–51.

59. Chou YH, Ko KY, Cheng MF, et al. 18F-NaF PET/CT images of cardiac metastasis from osteosarcoma. Clin Nucl Med 2016;41:708–9.

60. Brunkhorst T, Boerner AR, Bergh S, et al. Pretherapeutic assessment of tumour metabolism using a dual tracer PET technique. Eur J Nucl Med Mol Imaging 2002;29:1416.

61. Mosci C, Iagaru A, Sathekge M, et al. 18F NaF PET/CT in the assessment of malignant bone disease. PET Clin 2012;7:263–74.

# Skeletal Metastasis Evaluation

## Value and Impact of PET/Computed Tomography on Diagnosis, Management and Prognosis

Stephen M. Broski, MD[a], Jason R. Young, MD[a],
Ayse T. Kendi, MD[a],
Rathan M. Subramaniam, MD, PhD, MPH[b],*

### KEYWORDS

- Skeletal metastasis • PET/CT • FDG • NaF • Fluciclovine • Choline

### KEY POINTS

- A variety of benign processes, including inflammatory arthritis, osteoarthritis, osteomyelitis, fractures, fibrous dysplasia, and Paget's disease may show intense $^{18}$F-NaF uptake.
- In general, untreated lytic lesions tend to have a greater degree of $^{18}$F-FDG, $^{18}$F-fluciclovine, and $^{11}$C-choline activity compared to sclerotic metastases.
- Increased extent and degree of sclerosis within a metastasis on restaging PET/CT can indicate response to treatment or disease progression; correlation with changes in PET radiotracer activity in the lesion is necessary to make this distinction.
- $^{18}$F-fluciclovine and $^{11}$C-choline uptake has been described in several other malignancies in addition to prostate cancer, and also a variety of benign osseous lesions.
- Prostate cancer metastases can begin as intramedullary or osteolytic lesions, and become more sclerotic and less choline avid as response to therapy and healing occur.

## INTRODUCTION

The skeleton is one of the most frequent sites of metastatic disease. Breast and prostate cancers are the most common primary tumors to spread to bone, followed by thyroid, renal, and lung malignancies.[1] Development of bone metastases results in dramatically reduced patient survival[1] and has serious implications for therapy, especially given the rapidly expanding list of treatment options for oligometastatic disease.[2] Therefore, early and accurate detection of skeletal metastases is paramount.

The true mechanism of bone metastasis formation has not been fully elucidated, but the vicious-cycle hypothesis posits that tumor cells in bone first stimulate osteoclastic bone resorption

Disclosure: R.M. Subramaniam is a consultant to the Blue Earth Diagnostics. S.M. Broski is a consultant to Vyriad. The other authors have no commercial or financial conflicts of interest.
[a] Division of Nuclear Medicine, Department of Radiology, Mayo Clinic, 200 1st Street, SW Rochester, MN 55905, USA; [b] Division of Nuclear Medicine, Department of Radiology, Harold Simmons Comprehensive Cancer Center, University of Texas Southwestern Medical Center, 5323 Harry Hines Boulevard, Dallas, TX 75390-8896, USA
* Corresponding author.
E-mail address: rathan.subramaniam@UTsouthwestern.edu

PET Clin 14 (2019) 103–120
https://doi.org/10.1016/j.cpet.2018.08.006

through upregulation of receptor activator of nuclear factor kappa-B ligand (RANKL) among other factors, causing release of growth factors from the bone matrix, which then stimulate growth of tumor cells.[3] Some tumors, particularly prostate cancer, also produce osteoblast-stimulating factors that induce bone formation. Chemokines and cytokines produced by osteoblasts subsequently enhance tumor development. Thus, through a complex interaction of osteoclastic and osteoblastic factors, tumor deposits become established in bone, and osteolytic, osteoblastic, or mixed osteolytic/osteoblastic lesion morphology depends on the relative proportion of lytic or blastic processes unique to each tumor type.[3,4]

[99m]Tc-methyldiphosphonate bone scan is the most widely used molecular imaging technique to detect osseous metastases. It offers whole-body assessment, is widely available, cost-effective, and highly sensitive, showing sites of skeletal disease months before radiographs.[5] Because detection relies on bone formation, it has particular utility in prostate and breast cancer osseous metastases, which most commonly are osteoblastic or mixed osteolytic/osteoblastic. In contrast, diagnosis of small metastases, intramedullary metastases without reactive bone formation, and purely osteolytic lesions may be more limited. Although bone scan is very sensitive, its specificity suffers from a variety of benign conditions, including arthritis, inflammation, and trauma, which may elicit osteogenic bone formation and produce false-positive results.[5]

Recent years have seen unprecedented advances in PET technology, more widespread availability, and continued development of novel radiotracers that may be used in the evaluation of osseous metastatic disease. This article focuses on some of the most common PET imaging agents used for skeletal metastasis assessment, highlighting relative strengths and weaknesses.

## [18]F-FLUORIDE PET

[18]F-NaF was recognized as a useful radiotracer for skeletal imaging well before the advent of [99m]Tc-methylene diphosphonate (MDP), and was first introduced into clinical practice as early as 1962, receiving United States Food and Drug Administration (FDA) approval in 1972.[6] However, its imaging performance was limited with conventional gamma cameras owing to its high-energy 511-keV photons, and it was eventually supplanted by [99m]Tc-MDP. During the last 2 decades, widespread adoption of PET/computed tomography (CT) systems has led to renewed interest in this radiotracer.

[18]F-NaF shows high bone uptake, rapid blood pool and soft tissue clearance via bone deposition and renal excretion, and minimal serum protein binding, resulting in excellent target/background ratio and the ability to image less than 1 hour after injection.[7] The mechanism of [18]F-NaF osseous uptake is based on hydroxyl ion exchange on the surface of hydroxyapatite, forming fluorapatite. Uptake of [18]F-NaF is a function of both blood flow and osseous remodeling, similar to [99m]Tc-MDP. Pathologic processes that increase bone surface area exposure and result in more binding sites show increased uptake compared with background. Although uptake is greater in areas of osteoblastic activity, both osteolytic and osteoblastic processes may be shown.[7]

Recent data from the National Oncologic PET Registry (NOPR) examined the influence of 2839 [18]F-NaF-PET scans on the intended management of 2217 patients with osseous metastases (68% prostate, 17% breast, 6% lung, and 8% other cancers). In this cohort, [18]F-NaF-PET produced an intended change in therapeutic plan in 40.3% of overall patients.[8] Another recent NOPR study evaluating the concordance between the intended patient management after NaF-PET and inferred management on analysis of Medicare claims included 9898 NaF-PET scans.[9] There was claims agreement for planned surgery in 76.0% (19 of 25) lung, 75.4% (98 of 130) other cancers, and 58.9% (298 of 506) prostate cancer. Claims confirmed chemotherapy plans after NaF-PET done for initial staging or first osseous metastasis (FOM) in 81.0% and 73.5% for lung cancer (n = 148 and 136) and 69.4% and 67.5% for other cancers (n = 111 and 228). For radiotherapy plans, agreement ranged from 80.0% to 84.4% after initial staging and 68.4% to 74.0% for suspected FOM. Concordance of post–NaF-PET plans and claims was substantial and higher overall for initial staging than for FOM. These same investigators examined the association between NaF-PET results, Medicare hospice claims within 180 days, and 1-year survival in 21,167 NOPR examinations. In patients with evidence of new or progressing osseous metastasis compared with those without, there was a 2.0 to 7.5 times higher relative risk of hospice claims (all $P<.008$) and decreased 6-month survival (1.8–5.1 times greater risk of death, all $P<.0001$), depending on cancer type (prostate, breast, lung, or other). Thus, this study showed the impact of NaF-PET scan results on prognosis and patient management, particularly in difficult end-of-life treatment decisions.[10]

A recent meta-analysis by Shen and colleagues[11] in 2015 evaluating the diagnostic accuracy of [18]F-NaF-PET or PET/CT, [99m]Tc-MDP bone scintigraphy, and 2-deoxy-2-[$^{18}$F]-fluoro-D-glucose ($^{18}$F-flurodeoxyglucose [FDG])-PET/CT included 20 articles discussing 1170 patients. Compared with $^{99m}$Tc-MDP bone scintigraphy, $^{18}$F-NaF-PET or PET/CT showed both higher sensitivity (96% vs 88%, $P = .002$) and higher specificity (91% vs 80%, $P = .001$). Compared with FDG-PET/CT, $^{18}$F-fluoride PET/CT showed higher sensitivity (94% vs 73%, $P = .003$), whereas no significant difference was observed in specificity (88% vs 98%, $P = .06$).

Two-fold higher bone uptake, better target/background ratio, faster patient throughput, and improved spatial resolution are all potential advantages of $^{18}$F-NaF compared with $^{99m}$Tc-MDP. This finding has been borne out in numerous studies. A prospective study by Iagaru and colleagues[12] compared the performances of $^{99m}$Tc-MDP bone scintigraphy, $^{18}$F-NaF-PET/CT, and FDG-PET/CT to detect skeletal metastases in 52 patients with pathologically proven malignancies, including sarcomas, prostate cancers, and various other tumor types. They found 96% sensitivity and 93% specificity of $^{18}$F-NaF-PET/CT for detecting osseous metastases, compared with 67% and 96% for FDG-PET/CT, and 88% and 93% for planar $^{99m}$Tc-MDP scintigraphy. $^{18}$F-NaF-PET/CT also had the highest overall accuracy at 94%. They commented that combined FDG (for soft tissue metastases) and $^{18}$F-NaF (for bone metastases) PET/CT might be an optimal test to evaluate for metastatic disease, and later showed the usefulness of combined $^{18}$F-NaF/FDG-PET/CT in detecting osseous metastases versus CT,[13] $^{99m}$Tc-MDP scintigraphy, and whole-body magnetic resonance (MR) imaging.[14] Even-Sapir and colleagues[15] compared the utility of $^{18}$F-NaF-PET, $^{18}$F-NaF-PET/CT, $^{99m}$Tc-MDP single-photon emission CT (SPECT), and $^{99m}$Tc-MDP planar scintigraphy in patients with high risk prostate cancer. They found 100% sensitivity and 100% specificity of $^{18}$F-NaF-PET/CT for detecting osseous metastases, compared with 100% and 62% for $^{18}$F-NaF-PET, 70% and 57% for planar $^{99m}$Tc-MDP scintigraphy, and 92% and 82% for $^{99m}$Tc-MDP SPECT. In this study, 34 out of 156 osseous metastases revealed by $^{18}$F-NaF-PET/CT were not identified by planar bone scintigraphy. Similarly, greater sensitivity and specificity of $^{18}$F-NaF-PET/CT compared with $^{99m}$Tc-MDP SPECT and $^{99m}$Tc-MDP planar scintigraphy has been shown in skeletal metastasis evaluation in patients with urinary bladder carcinoma.[16] A 2015 prospective study examined 37 oncology patients with multiple different cancer types (most commonly breast, lung, prostate, and gastric cancer), and compared the performance of $^{18}$F-NaF-PET/CT and $^{99m}$Tc-MDP planar whole-body bone scintigraphy. In 33 out of 37 (89%) patients, $^{18}$F-NaF-PET/CT showed a greater number of skeletal metastases than bone scan, which the investigators attributed to the ability of $^{18}$F-NaF-PET/CT to show both lytic and blastic metastases, small lesions, and intramedullary metastases.[17] Corroborative findings were reported by Withofs and colleagues,[18] who showed superior accuracy of $^{18}$F-NaF-PET/CT compared with $^{99m}$Tc-MDP SPECT in detecting lumbar spine and pelvic lesions in patients with breast and prostate cancer.

Normally, $^{18}$F-NaF distributes evenly throughout the skeleton, with slightly greater uptake in the axial than appendicular skeleton. Increased uptake is present at sites of increased osseous turnover and remodeling, and most metastases show uptake, whether they are osteolytic, osteoblastic, or mixed.[7,15] Osteolytic metastases often manifest as centrally photopenic lesions with a peripheral rim of tracer activity. Because of its very high sensitivity, careful review of the CT fusion images and correlation with other imaging modalities is critical when interpreting these examinations. Multiple benign lesions, including osteophytes, degenerative endplate changes, and areas of subchondral sclerosis in osteoarthritic joints show uptake. Although there is significant overlap in standardized uptake values (SUVs) between benign and malignant osseous lesions,[7,19,20] some studies have shown that lesions with maximum SUV (SUV$_{max}$) greater than 45[21] or 50[22] are always malignant, whereas those with SUV$_{max}$ less than 12 are always degenerative.[22] Further study on the role of semiquantitative analysis in $^{18}$F-NaF-PET is warranted. In addition to degree, the pattern of uptake can be helpful. For instance, the linear uptake along a vertebral body endplate is usually caused by degenerative change, and can be used to exclude metastatic disease with high confidence.[7]

It is important to keep in mind that a variety of benign nonneoplastic processes, including inflammatory arthritis, osteoarthritis, osteomyelitis, fractures, fibrous dysplasia, and Paget disease, may also show variable, and sometimes intense, $^{18}$F-NaF uptake,[7] again underscoring the importance of PET/CT fusion and comparison with prior studies and other imaging modalities.

## $^{18}$F-FLURODEOXYGLUCOSE PET

FDG is a glucose analogue and the most widely used oncologic PET agent. It is taken up into cells via a family of glucose transporter proteins (primarily GLUT-1), and once in the cell is irreversibly phosphorylated by hexokinase and trapped.

A 110-minute physical half-life and short positron range make FDG a practical choice for imaging neoplastic processes, which show relative increased glucose use.

The time required for bone remodeling in response to metastatic disease often results in a lag period in which viable tumor may be present in the medullary space with little to no anatomic change. Often, it is only after treatment and subsequent bone healing that anatomic changes become evident. Therefore, there is opportunity to detect osseous metastatic disease on FDG-PET before it is apparent on conventional imaging. It is important to note differences between prototypical osteolytic and osteoblastic lesions. In general, untreated lytic lesions tend to have greater FDG avidity compared with sclerotic lesions, likely because of greater cellular displacement and attenuation of radiotracer emission by thickened bony trabeculae in sclerotic lesions compared with lytic ones.

Breast cancer bone metastases can be osteolytic, osteoblastic, or mixed. A recent study by Dashevsky and colleagues[23] showed that, on average, ductal carcinoma bone metastases are more FDG avid than lobular carcinoma (median $SUV_{max}$ of 6.6 vs 3.4, respectively). Further, they found that untreated lobular carcinoma metastases can appear as sclerotic, non–FDG-avid lesions (**Fig. 1**), and so knowledge of the histologic subtype is critical when interpreting FDG-PET/CT for breast cancer. Several studies have shown a higher sensitivity and specificity of FDG-PET/CT than bone scan in the detection of bone metastases in breast cancer.[24,25] Findings worrisome for progression of sclerotic lesions include increasing FDG avidity and/or enlarging volume of sclerosis (**Fig. 2**). This pattern is in contrast with lytic lesions, which often become sclerotic or mixed with decreasing FDG avidity in response to successful treatment[26] (**Fig. 3**).

Prostate cancer is a heterogeneous malignancy that can evolve through the course of disease. Although FDG has utility in detection and management of soft tissue prostate metastasis (particularly neuroendocrine subtypes) and has been shown to be valuable in detecting and assessing response of high-grade, castration-resistant prostate cancer,[27] there is little evidence to support utility regarding osseous metastasis.[28–30] However, in our practice, FDG-PET has an emerging role in evaluating osseous prostate metastases with neuroendocrine features, which can be FDG avid, while showing little or no choline uptake

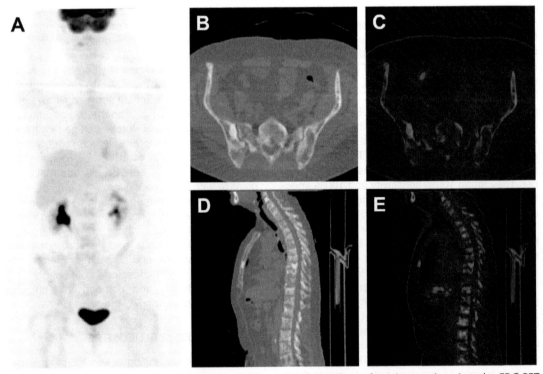

**Fig. 1.** A 71-year-old woman with lobular breast carcinoma and anemia, undergoing staging. Anterior FDG-PET maximum intensity projection (MIP) image (*A*) shows relatively normal FDG biodistribution. Axial CT (*B*) and fused PET/CT (*C*) images of the pelvis and sagittal CT (*D*) and fused PET/CT (*E*) images of the spine show diffuse non–FDG-avid osteoblastic skeletal metastases.

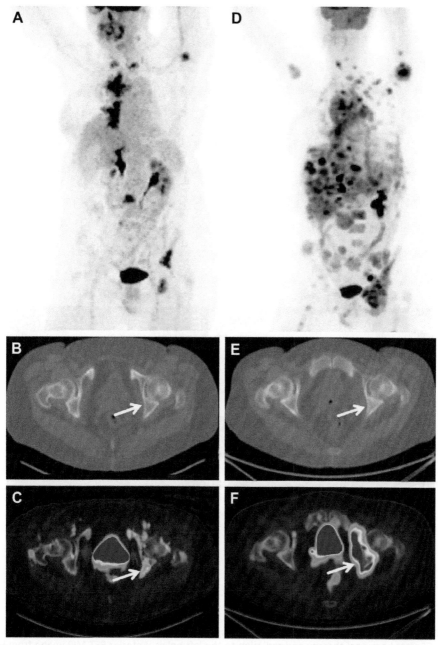

**Fig. 2.** A 59-year-old woman with invasive ductal breast carcinoma, following bilateral mastectomy undergoing restaging PET/CT after experiencing a pathologic sternal fracture. Pretreatment FDG-PET/CT shows an FDG-avid metastasis in the posterior left acetabulum (*arrow, C*) with little morphologic change on CT (*arrow, B*). Restaging FDG-PET/CT shows new sclerosis in the left acetabulum (*arrow, E*), increased size and FDG activity of the left acetabular metastasis, and new extraosseous extension (*arrow, F*) consistent with progression. Anterior MIP PET images *(A, D)* from the 2 examinations show marked overall disease progression, including diffuse osseous, nodal, and hepatic metastatic disease.

(Fig. 4). Neuroendocrine differentiation may be indicated by increased levels of serum markers (chromogranin A, lactate dehydrogenase, carcinoembryonic antigen) or clinical/imaging evidence of progressive disease with stable prostate-specific antigen (PSA) levels, and, in these patients, FDG-PET should be considered.

FDG-PET-CT is an excellent modality in detection of bone metastasis from both small cell and non–small cell lung cancer types, with several

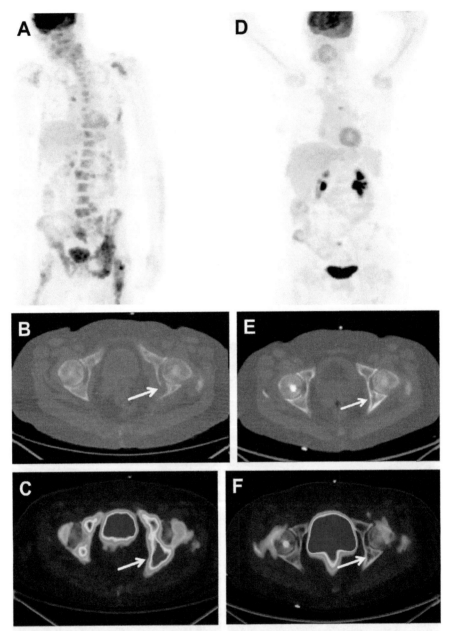

**Fig. 3.** A 62-year-old woman with invasive lobular breast carcinoma undergoing staging (*A–C*) and restaging (*D–F*) FDG-PET/CT after hormonal therapy and radiation to the left pelvis. Anterior PET MIP image from her staging PET/CT (*A*) shows diffuse hypermetabolic FDG-avid skeletal metastatic disease. Axial CT (*B*) and fused PET/CT (*C*) images of the pelvis show an intensely FDG-avid left acetabular metastasis with associated osteolysis and a pathologic fracture (*arrows*). Corresponding posttreatment anterior PET MIP (*D*), axial CT (*E*), and fused PET/CT (*F*) images show sclerosis, fracture healing, and normalized FDG activity in the left acetabulum consistent with positive treatment response (*arrows*).

studies showing superior diagnostic accuracy to both MR imaging and skeletal scintigraphy.[31–33] A recent meta-analysis showed pooled sensitivity and specificity for detection of bone metastasis in lung cancer of FDG-PET/CT of 92% and 98%, which was higher than FDG-PET, MR imaging, and bone scan.[34] Lung cancer bone metastases are commonly lytic, with a lesser proportion being mixed or osteoblastic. Viable osseous lung metastases are generally osteolytic and FDG avid (**Fig. 5**).

Bone is the second most common site of metastasis in renal cell carcinoma (RCC), and the most

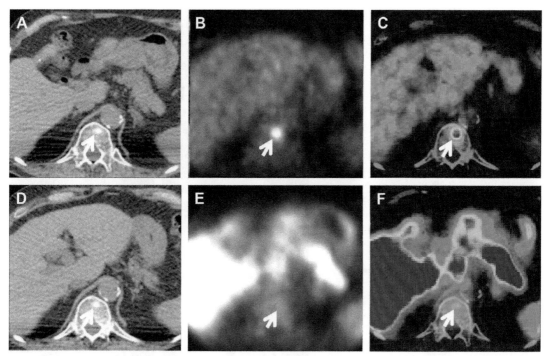

**Fig. 4.** An 85-year-old man with metastatic castrate-resistant prostate cancer. Axial CT (*A*), FDG-PET (*B*), and fused FDG-PET/CT (*C*) images show an FDG-avid sclerotic metastasis in the T10 vertebral body (*arrow*). Corresponding axial CT (*D*), ¹¹C-choline PET (*E*), and fused ¹¹C-choline PET/CT (*F*) images show no significant choline activity within the lesion. The patient's chromogranin A level was 572 ng/mL (normal, <93 ng/mL), and biopsy confirmed metastatic prostate cancer with neuroendocrine differentiation.

frequent locations of bony involvement are the pelvis and ribs (48%), followed by the spine (42%), and then long bones and skull.[35] Although detection of the primary lesion is limited because of intrinsically low RCC FDG uptake and physiologic uptake by the kidney, FDG-PET-CT clearly outperforms whole-body bone scans in evaluating osseous metastatic disease.[36] The major value of FDG-PET-CT seems to be in the postnephrectomy point of care, particularly for papillary RCC.[37] With RCC, low-level metabolism is expected and the threshold for determining abnormal activity should

be lowered. Although RCC osseous metastatic lesions may not be evident initially, growth to a certain size threshold may result in their detection, presenting the opportunity for monitoring disease and determining treatment response (**Fig. 6**).

Thyroid bone metastases appear similar to RCC: lytic and sometimes expansile with varying degrees of FDG avidity (**Fig. 7**). Several studies have shown whole-body iodine scintigraphy has greater sensitivity compared with FDG-PET/CT in detecting differentiated thyroid cancer (DTC) bone metastases.[38] However, the primary role of

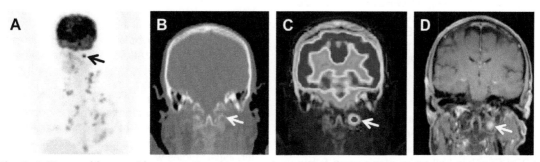

**Fig. 5.** A 65-year-old man with metastatic pulmonary adenocarcinoma. FDG-PET MIP (*A*), coronal CT (*B*), fused PET/CT (*C*), and gadolinium-enhanced fat-saturated coronal MR imaging images (*D*) show an osteolytic, FDG-avid, solidly enhancing metastasis within the left lateral mass of C1 (*arrows*).

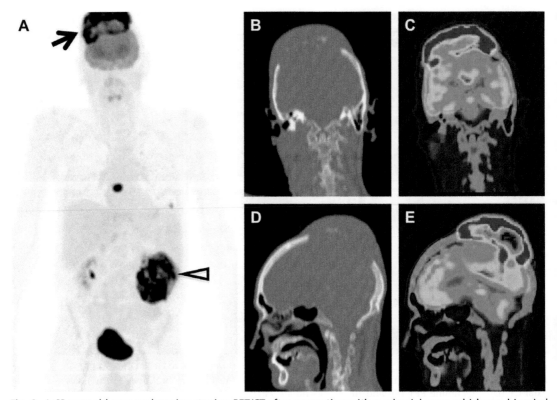

**Fig. 6.** A 63-year-old man undergoing staging PET/CT after presenting with a calvarial mass, which was biopsied and shown to be a poorly differentiated carcinoma. An anterior FDG-PET MIP (*A*) image shows a large, intensely FDG-avid left renal mass (*arrowhead*) and multiple metastases, including a large calvarial lesion (*arrow*). Coronal and sagittal CT (*B, D*) and fused PET/CT (*C, E*) images show a large, destructive, osteolytic, FDG-avid calvarial metastasis with central necrosis.

FDG-PET/CT in managing DTC is in the posttreatment setting (thyroidectomy/I-131 ablation) with increased serum thyroglobulin and negative whole-body iodine scan. These scenarios are suspicious for dedifferentiation of the thyroid carcinoma with impaired cellular iodine uptake and greater glucose metabolism (**Figs. 8** and **9**). In this setting, FDG-PET/CT has 89% sensitivity and 85% specificity.[39] FDG-PET/CT findings can also help predict overall survival in DTC. In a study by Qiu and colleagues[38] comparing FDG-PET/CT, bone scan, and I-131 SPECT/CT in 80 patients with DTC bone metastases, only FDG-PET/CT–positive bone disease was an independent prognosticator, with overall survival of 93% in the PET-negative group versus 69% in the PET-positive group. Anaplastic thyroid cancer (ATC) is a rare but aggressive type of thyroid carcinoma. FDG-PET-CT is well suited for evaluation of ATC, in part because of increased GLUT-1 cellular expression. The American Thyroid Association has a strong recommendation for use of FDG-PET-CT in both initial staging and follow-up of ATC, with particular mention of its helpfulness in identifying osseous metastasis.[40]

## 18F-FLUCICLOVINE PET

Anti-1-amino-3-[18]F-fluorocyclobutanecarboxylic acid ([18]F-fluciclovine) is an amino acid PET tracer that has been recently approved by the FDA for localization of recurrent prostate cancer in patients with increased PSA level.[41] It has been used to diagnose prostate cancer, breast cancer, and glioma.[41–43] Many amino acid transporters are upregulated in prostate cancer. The most common upregulated transporters are large neutral amino acid transporters (LATs: LAT1, LAT3, LAT4) and alanine-serine-cysteine transporters (ASCTs: ASCT1, ASCT2). Fluciclovine is predominantly transported by LAT1 and ASCT2, which are known to be associated with more aggressive tumor behavior.[41–43] The main advantage of [18]F-fluciclovine is low uptake by macrophages, reducing false-positives caused by inflammatory processes.[42]

Although assessment of skeletal metastases is essential in tumor staging, including prostate cancer, initial studies with [18]F-fluciclovine focused on detection of local recurrence in the prostate/prostatectomy bed and nodal disease.[41] Hence, there

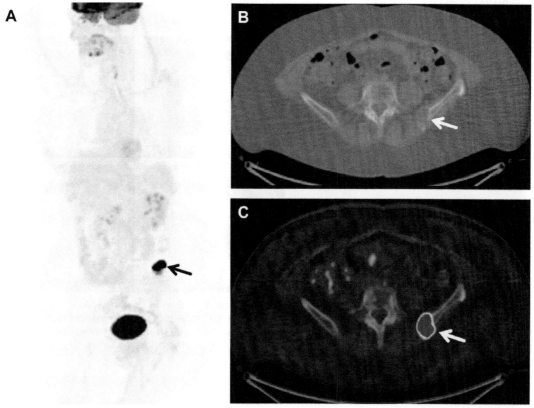

**Fig. 7.** A 68-year-old woman with papillary thyroid carcinoma, following subtotal thyroidectomy and radioactive iodine therapy. An increasing thyroglobulin level with negative conventional imaging prompted FDG-PET/CT. Anterior PET MIP (*A*), axial pelvic CT (*B*), and fused PET/CT (*C*) images show a solitary, FDG-avid, expansile, lytic lesion within the medial left iliac crest (*arrows*).

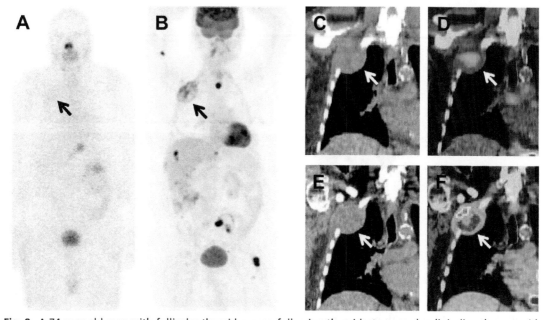

**Fig. 8.** A 74-year-old man with follicular thyroid cancer, following thyroidectomy and radioiodine therapy with increasing thyroglobulin level. Anterior planar (*A*), coronal CT (*C*), and fused SPECT/CT (*D*) images from an I-123 total-body iodide scan show only minimal iodine uptake within a large destructive right second rib metastasis (*arrows*). Corresponding PET MIP (*B*), CT (*E*), and fused PET/CT (*F*) images from an FDG-PET/CT examination show peripheral FDG activity (*arrows*) within the centrally necrotic mass, and multiple additional FDG-avid metastases that are not iodine avid.

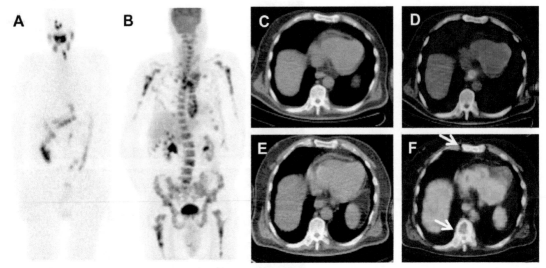

**Fig. 9.** A 62-year-old man with widely metastatic poorly differentiated thyroid carcinoma. Anterior planar (*A*), axial CT (*C*), and fused SPECT/CT (*D*) images from an I-123 total-body iodide scan show normal iodine distribution. Corresponding PET MIP (*B*), CT (*E*), and fused PET/CT (*F*) images from an FDG-PET/CT examination show widespread FDG-avid osseous metastatic disease, including the sternum and thoracic spine (*arrows, F*).

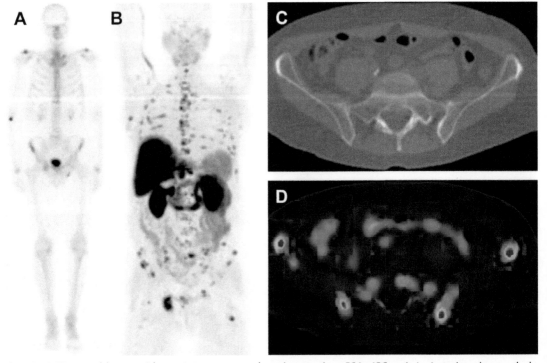

**Fig. 10.** A 72-year-old man with prostate cancer undergoing staging; PSA, 136 ng/mL. Anterior planar whole-body bone scan image (*A*) shows likely metastases in the medial left clavicle, several bilateral ribs, and the anterior right iliac crest. Anterior $^{11}$C-choline PET MIP image obtained the following day (*B*) shows innumerable choline-avid osseous metastases throughout the axial and appendicular skeleton. Axial CT (*C*) and fused $^{11}$C-choline PET/CT (*D*) images show multiple choline-avid intramedullary metastases in the pelvis, without corresponding abnormality on CT.

are fewer data regarding accuracy of detection of bone metastases with [18]F-fluciclovine. Nanni and colleagues[44] reported 7 out of 89 patients with prostate cancer with bone lesions, among whom 5 were positive with fluciclovine. This study showed that [18]F-fluciclovine has higher detection rates for local, lymph nodal, and bone metastasis compared with [11]C-choline. Fluciclovine also showed better tumor/background ratio compared with [11]C-choline. Other advantages of fluciclovine noted by the investigators included longer half-life (110 minutes), proven stability over time in vitro, easy production, and delayed renal clearance.[44] Schuster and colleagues[45] reported 3 out of 93 patients who had positive bone metastases on [18]F-fluciclovine PET with negative whole-body bone scans. Inoue and colleagues[46] reported 7 out of 10 patients with bone metastases that showed abnormal uptake on [18]F-fluciclovine.

[18]F-fluciclovine shows intense uptake in lytic bone lesions and moderate uptake in mixed lytic/sclerotic bone lesions. However, it has been observed that densely sclerotic bone lesions may show little or no [18]F-fluciclovine uptake,[41] perhaps /because of fewer malignant cells. Recently, Oka and colleagues[42] studied a rat model to identify accumulation of [18]F-fluciclovine in breast and prostate carcinoma bone metastases, and compared [18]F-fluciclovine uptake with FDG, [11]C/[18]F-choline, and [99m]Tc-MDP. These investigators showed accumulation of fluciclovine in both osteolytic and osteoblastic bone metastases, noting increased uptake in early-stage osteoblastic lesions with abundant cellular components. They also noted that fluciclovine revealed osteoblastic bone metastasis more clearly than FDG and choline. Hence, these investigators endorsed the combined use of bone scan (for densely sclerotic lesions) and fluciclovine (for osteolytic and early osteoblastic lesions) for evaluation of osseous metastatic disease in patients with prostate cancer.[42] Given the available evidence, [18]F-fluciclovine should not replace bone scan or [18]F NaF-PET/CT in clinical management of patients with prostate cancer.

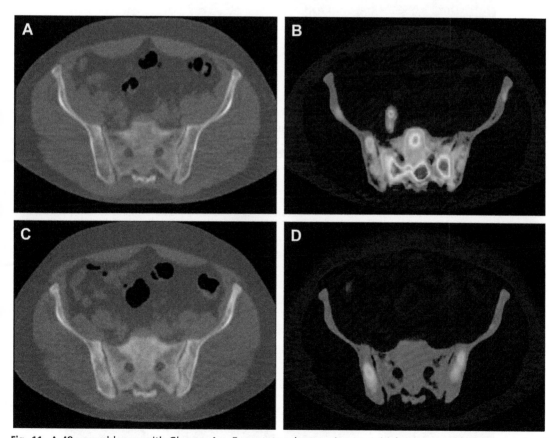

**Fig. 11.** A 48-year-old-man with Gleason 4 + 5 prostate adenocarcinoma. Initial staging axial CT (*A*) and fused [11]C-choline PET/CT (*B*) images show extensive choline-avid pelvic osseous metastases, with faint sclerosis. His initial PSA level was 1002 ng/mL. Follow-up axial CT (*C*) and fused [11]C-choline PET/CT (*D*) images after chemohormonal therapy show diffusely increased sclerosis with normalized choline activity consistent with response to treatment. Posttreatment PSA level was 2.8 ng/mL.

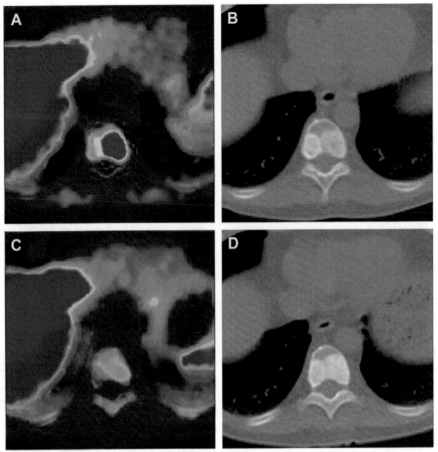

**Fig. 12.** A 56-year-old-man with Gleason 4 + 5 prostate adenocarcinoma following prostatectomy with biochemical recurrence. Axial CT (*A*) and fused $^{11}$C-choline PET/CT (*B*) images show 2 sclerotic, choline-avid metastases in the T10 vertebral body. Follow-up axial CT (*C*) and fused $^{11}$C-choline PET/CT (*D*) images after chemohormonal therapy show increased sclerosis and decreased choline activity consistent with response to treatment.

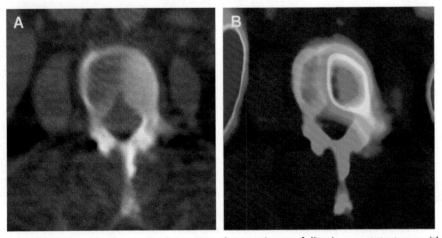

**Fig. 13.** A 62-year-old-man with Gleason 4 + 3 prostate adenocarcinoma, following prostatectomy with biochemical recurrence. Axial CT (*A*) and fused $^{11}$C-choline PET/CT (*B*) images through the L3 vertebral body show a sclerotic metastasis with intense choline activity.

Knowledge of normal physiologic distribution of fluciclovine, variants, and typical pattern of tumor uptake is important.[41,43] For bone lesions to be diagnosed as metastases, focal uptake should be visualized on maximum intensity projection (MIP) images. Uptake may occur with other malignancies such as squamous cell carcinoma of scalp, multiple myeloma, primary or metastatic tumors of brain, colon cancer, and lymphoma.[43] Uptake with benign conditions such as infection/inflammation should also be kept in mind during image interpretation. Normal heterogeneous bone marrow uptake may also compromise assessment of bone metastasis.[43] Fewer false-positives caused by inflammation have been reported with fluciclovine compared with FDG-PET/CT because of lower uptake of fluciclovine by inflammatory cells compared with FDG.[42] Degenerative uptake is also uncommon with fluciclovine, which is an advantage compared with FDG and [18]F-NaF-PET. Metabolically active bone lesions such as osteoid osteoma have been reported to have fluciclovine uptake as well.[41,43]

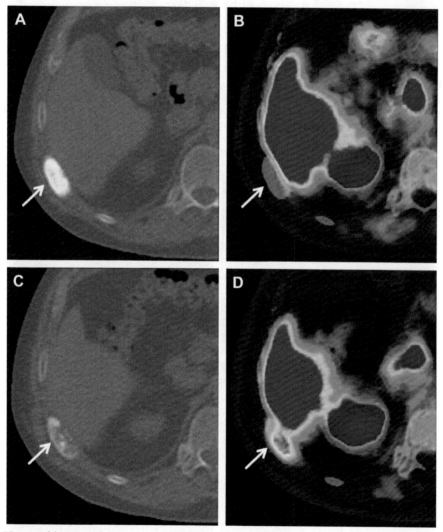

**Fig. 14.** A 72-year-old-man with prostate cancer following prostatectomy, salvage radiation therapy, chemohormonal therapy, and radiation to a right 10th rib metastasis. Increasing PSA level, currently 4.2 ng/mL. Axial CT (*A*) and fused [11]C-choline PET/CT (*B*) images show a densely sclerotic lesion without choline activity in the posterolateral right 10th rib consistent with a treated metastasis (*arrows*). Follow-up axial CT (*C*) and fused [11]C-choline PET/CT (*D*) images after PSA levels increased show new osteolysis and increased choline activity in the posterolateral right 10th rib consistent with reactivation of metastatic disease in a previously treated metastasis (*arrows*). The patient went on to cryoablation.

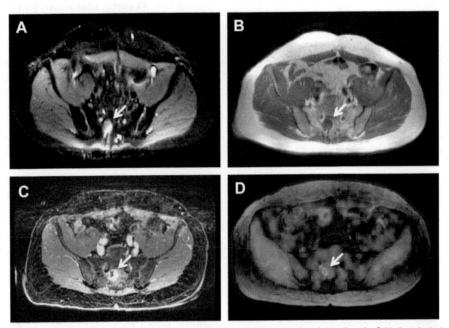

**Fig. 15.** A 63-year-old man with Gleason 5 + 4 prostate adenocarcinoma and PSA level of 62.5 ng/mL. Initial staging axial diffusion-weighted (*A*), T1-weighted (*B*), fat-saturated T1-weighted postgadolinium (*C*), and fused [11]C-choline PET/T1-weighted MR (*D*) images show an enhancing, marrow-replacing lesion with restricted diffusion and choline avidity in the S2 sacral segment consistent with an osseous metastasis (*arrows*).

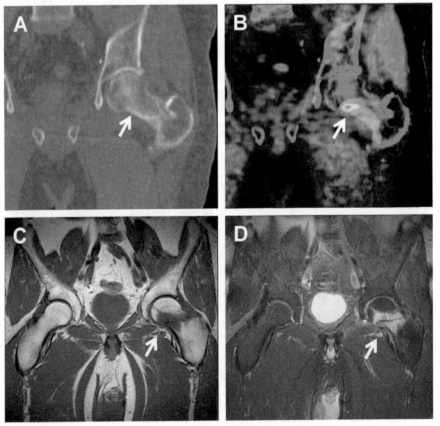

**Fig. 16.** A 64-year-old man with biochemically recurrent prostate cancer; PSA level, 9.1 ng/mL. Coronal CT (*A*) and fused [11]C-choline PET/CT (*B*) images show focal choline activity in the medial left femoral neck (*arrows*). Coronal T1-weighted (*C*) and T2-weighted fat-saturated (*D*) images from MR imaging performed 3 days later show a completed subcapital stress fracture with reactive bone marrow edema (*arrows*).

# ¹¹C-CHOLINE PET

¹¹C-choline PET/CT has emerged in recent years as a useful tool in the detection of biochemically recurrent prostate cancer, and was approved by the FDA for this purpose in 2012.[47] Choline is an essential component of cell membrane phospholipids, and various neoplasms have upregulated choline transport and phosphorylation, among them, prostate cancer. ¹¹C-choline is taken up by tumor cells and phosphorylated by choline kinase to form phosphorylated ¹¹C-choline, which is essentially trapped in tumor cells. ¹¹C-choline (half-life 20.4 minutes) rapidly clears from the circulation, with high clearance by the liver and kidneys. Its short half-life necessitates on-site cyclotron production, limiting widespread availability. Organs with the highest normal uptake include renal cortex, liver, pancreas, salivary glands, bowel, adrenal glands, and pituitary gland.

The traditional mainstays for imaging osseous metastatic disease in patients with prostate cancer are skeletal scintigraphy and CT, both of which exploit the tendency of prostate cancer metastases to be osteoblastic. However, ¹¹C-choline

PET/CT has been shown to be much more sensitive than skeletal scintigraphy in several studies.[48–50] It has also been shown that bone resorption precedes bone production in prostate cancer, and patients with prostate cancer may present with osteolytic, osteoblastic, and intramedullary mestastases.[51–53] Given this, ¹¹C-choline PET/CT has been shown to be superior to bone scan and conventional imaging given the ability to show nonsclerotic and CT occult bone metastases (**Fig. 10**).

Some studies have shown correlation between ¹¹C-choline PET SUVs and morphologic CT features of osseous metastases. Ceci and colleagues[51] showed an average $SUV_{max}$ of 7.84 for osteolytic metastases, versus 6.98 for intramedullary lesions, and 5.71 for osteoblastic metastases ($P = .001$). These investigators also found faster PSA doubling time ($P = .01$) and higher PSA velocity ($P = .01$) in osteolytic metastases versus osteoblastic ones. Similarly, Tuncel and colleagues[54] observed an average $SUV_{max}$ of 6.0 and attenuation of 458 Hounsfield units (HU) for lesions reported as positive on ¹¹C-choline PET/CT compared with $SUV_{max}$ of 2.5 and mean of 787

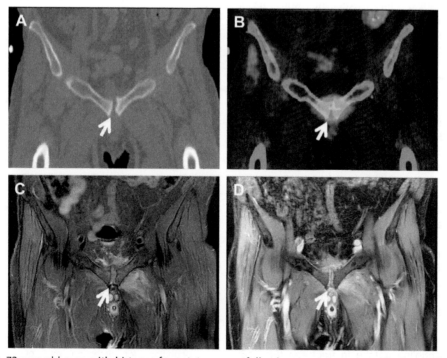

**Fig. 17.** A 72-year-old man with history of prostate cancer following prostatectomy, radiation, and androgen deprivation therapy with biochemical recurrence. Coronal CT (*A*) and fused ¹¹C-choline PET/CT (*B*) images show subtle erosive changes, periarticular sclerosis, and moderate choline activity about the pubic symphysis (*arrows*). Coronal T2-weighted (*C*) and fat-saturated postgadolinium spoiled gradient recalled (*D*) MR images show bone marrow edema and enhancement about the pubic symphysis without evidence of osseous metastasis (*arrows*). The clinical and radiologic findings were consistent with osteitis pubis.

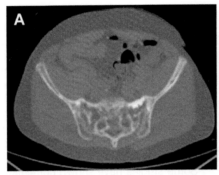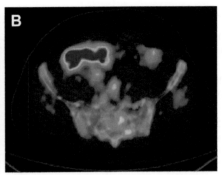

Fig. 18. A 68-year-old man with history of recurrent metastatic prostate cancer following prostatectomy and androgen deprivation therapy. Axial CT (*A*) and fused [11]C-choline PET/CT (*B*) images show changes of Paget disease in the sacrum and both iliac bones with moderate choline activity.

HU for lesions reported as negative. Therefore, it seems that many prostate cancer metastases initially begin as intramedullary or osteolytic and become more sclerotic and less choline avid as responses to therapy and healing occur (**Figs. 11** and **12**), although densely sclerotic lesions may still show intense choline activity (**Fig. 13**). Locally recurrent disease manifesting as a new choline-avid osteolytic lesion occurring within a sclerotic non–choline-avid treated metastasis has also been recognized (**Fig. 14**).

MR imaging has excellent soft tissue contrast and the capability to show intramedullary metastases before cortical destruction occurs or osteoblastic activity ensues, thereby having many of the same advantages as [11]C-choline PET/CT. In a recent meta-analysis, MR imaging was shown to have a 95% sensitivity and 96% specificity for detecting skeletal metastases in patients with prostate cancer on a per-patient basis, compared with 87% and 97%, respectively, for choline PET/CT[50]; there were insufficient data to extrapolate per-lesion data. [11]C-choline PET/MR imaging may therefore be useful in patients with prostate cancer, given the combination of excellent osseous anatomic depiction, superior soft tissue contrast, and functional information such as restricted diffusion on MR imaging combined with the metabolic information afforded by PET/CT (**Fig. 15**).

However, choline is also important for methyl-metabolism, cholinergic neurotransmission, transmembrane signaling, and lipid transport and metabolism, and focal uptake in bone is not 100% specific for prostate cancer metastases. Increased choline uptake in fractures (**Fig. 16**), inflammatory and degenerative lesions (**Fig. 17**), and benign neoplastic lesions such as fibrous dysplasia[55] and Paget disease of bone[56] (**Fig. 18**) has been seen, and so careful scrutiny of the CT portion of PET/CT examinations is critical.

## SUMMARY

Recent years have seen unprecedented advances in PET technology and the introduction of several new PET radiopharmaceuticals that may be useful for assessment of skeletal metastatic disease. These new PET agents have significant advantages compared with [99m]Tc-MDP scintigraphy, including superior diagnostic accuracy, higher spatial resolution, and shorter imaging times, often with the ability to show soft tissue local recurrence and metastasis in the same examination. Although these agents have excellent diagnostic utility, they are not 100% specific for skeletal metastasis, and so normal patterns of biodistribution, benign osseous lesions that may show radiotracer uptake, and the significance of morphologic changes on CT such as osteolysis or osteosclerosis must be kept in mind to ensure accurate interpretation.

## REFERENCES

1. Siegel RL, Miller KD, Jemal A. Cancer statistics, 2017. CA Cancer J Clin 2017;67(1):7–30.
2. Van Poppel H, De Meerleer G, Joniau S. Oligometastatic prostate cancer: metastases-directed therapy? Arab J Urol 2016;14(3):179–82.
3. Mundy GR. Metastasis to bone: causes, consequences and therapeutic opportunities. Nat Rev Cancer 2002;2(8):584–93.
4. David Roodman G, Silbermann R. Mechanisms of osteolytic and osteoblastic skeletal lesions. Bonekey Rep 2015;4:753.
5. Bombardieri E, Setti L, Kirienko M, et al. Which metabolic imaging, besides bone scan with 99mTc-phosphonates, for detecting and evaluating bone metastases in prostatic cancer patients? An open discussion. Q J Nucl Med Mol Imaging 2015;59(4):381–99.
6. Blau M, Ganatra R, Bender MA. 18 F-fluoride for bone imaging. Semin Nucl Med 1972;2(1):31–7.

7. Bastawrous S, Bhargava P, Behnia F, et al. Newer PET application with an old tracer: role of 18F-NaF skeletal PET/CT in oncologic practice. Radiographics 2014;34(5):1295–316.

8. Hillner BE, Siegel BA, Hanna L, et al. Impact of (18) F-fluoride PET on intended management of patients with cancers other than prostate cancer: results from the national ONCOLOGIC PET registry. J Nucl Med 2014;55(7):1054–61.

9. Hillner BE, Hanna L, Makineni R, et al. Intended versus inferred treatment after 18F-fluoride PET performed for evaluation of osseous metastatic disease in the national oncologic PET registry. J Nucl Med 2018;59(3):421–6.

10. Gareen IF, Hillner BE, Hanna L, et al. Hospice admission and survival after 18F-fluoride PET performed for evaluation of osseous metastatic disease in the national oncologic PET registry. J Nucl Med 2018;59(3):427–33.

11. Shen CT, Qiu ZL, Han TT, et al. Performance of 18F-fluoride PET or PET/CT for the detection of bone metastases: a meta-analysis. Clin Nucl Med 2015; 40(2):103–10.

12. Iagaru A, Mittra E, Dick DW, et al. Prospective evaluation of (99m)Tc MDP scintigraphy, (18)F NaF PET/CT, and (18)F FDG PET/CT for detection of skeletal metastases. Mol Imaging Biol 2012; 14(2):252–9.

13. Sampath SC, Sampath SC, Mosci C, et al. Detection of osseous metastasis by 18F-NaF/18F-FDG PET/CT versus CT alone. Clin Nucl Med 2015;40(3):e173–7.

14. Minamimoto R, Loening A, Jamali M, et al. Prospective comparison of 99mTc-MDP scintigraphy, combined 18F-NaF and 18F-FDG PET/CT, and whole-body MRI in patients with breast and prostate cancer. J Nucl Med 2015;56(12):1862–8.

15. Even-Sapir E, Metser U, Mishani E, et al. The detection of bone metastases in patients with high-risk prostate cancer: 99mTc-MDP planar bone scintigraphy, single- and multi-field-of-view SPECT, 18F-fluoride PET, and 18F-fluoride PET/CT. J Nucl Med 2006;47(2):287–97.

16. Chakraborty D, Bhattacharya A, Mete UK, et al. Comparison of 18F fluoride PET/CT and 99mTc-MDP bone scan in the detection of skeletal metastases in urinary bladder carcinoma. Clin Nucl Med 2013;38(8):616–21.

17. Araz M, Aras G, Kucuk ON. The role of 18F-NaF PET/CT in metastatic bone disease. J Bone Oncol 2015;4(3):92–7.

18. Withofs N, Grayet B, Tancredi T, et al. 1)(8)F-fluoride PET/CT for assessing bone involvement in prostate and breast cancers. Nucl Med Commun 2011; 32(3):168–76.

19. Schirrmeister H. Detection of bone metastases in breast cancer by positron emission tomography. Radiol Clin North Am 2007;45(4):669–76, vi.

20. Segall G, Delbeke D, Stabin MG, et al. SNM practice guideline for sodium 18F-fluoride PET/CT bone scans 1.0. J Nucl Med 2010;51(11):1813–20.

21. Beheshti M, Vali R, Waldenberger P, et al. Detection of bone metastases in patients with prostate cancer by F-18 fluorocholine and F-18 fluoride PET-CT: a comparative study. Eur J Nucl Med Mol Imaging 2008;35(10):1766–74.

22. Muzahir S, Jeraj R, Liu G, et al. Differentiation of metastatic vs degenerative joint disease using semi-quantitative analysis with (18)F-NaF PET/CT in castrate resistant prostate cancer patients. Am J Nucl Med Mol Imaging 2015;5(2):162–8.

23. Dashevsky BZ, Goldman DA, Parsons M, et al. Appearance of untreated bone metastases from breast cancer on FDG PET/CT: importance of histologic subtype. Eur J Nucl Med Mol Imaging 2015; 42(11):1666–73.

24. Hahn S, Heusner T, Kummel S, et al. Comparison of FDG-PET/CT and bone scintigraphy for detection of bone metastases in breast cancer. Acta Radiol 2011;52(9):1009–14.

25. Morris PG, Lynch C, Feeney JN, et al. Integrated positron emission tomography/computed tomography may render bone scintigraphy unnecessary to investigate suspected metastatic breast cancer. J Clin Oncol 2010;28(19):3154–9.

26. Al-Muqbel KM, Yaghan RJ, Al-Omari MH, et al. Clinical relevance of 18F-FDG-negative osteoblastic metastatic bone lesions noted on PET/CT in breast cancer patients. Nucl Med Commun 2016;37(6):593–601.

27. Jadvar H. Is there use for FDG-PET in prostate cancer? Semin Nucl Med 2016;46(6):502–6.

28. Spratt DE, Gavane S, Tarlinton L, et al. Utility of FDG-PET in clinical neuroendocrine prostate cancer. Prostate 2014;74(11):1153–9.

29. Kitajima K, Murphy RC, Nathan MA, et al. Update on positron emission tomography for imaging of prostate cancer. Int J Urol 2014;21(1):12–23.

30. Jadvar H. Molecular imaging of prostate cancer: PET radiotracers. AJR Am J Roentgenol 2012; 199(2):278–91.

31. Wu Y, Li P, Zhang H, et al. Diagnostic value of fluorine 18 fluorodeoxyglucose positron emission tomography/computed tomography for the detection of metastases in non-small-cell lung cancer patients. Int J Cancer 2013;132(2):E37–47.

32. Liu T, Xu JY, Xu W, et al. Fluorine-18 deoxyglucose positron emission tomography, magnetic resonance imaging and bone scintigraphy for the diagnosis of bone metastases in patients with lung cancer: which one is the best?–a meta-analysis. Clin Oncol (R Coll Radiol) 2011;23(5):350–8.

33. Lee JW, Lee SM, Lee HS, et al. Comparison of diagnostic ability between (99m)Tc-MDP bone scan and (18)F-FDG PET/CT for bone metastasis in patients

with small cell lung cancer. Ann Nucl Med 2012; 26(8):627–33.

34. Qu X, Huang X, Yan W, et al. A meta-analysis of (1)(8)FDG-PET-CT, (1)(8)FDG-PET, MRI and bone scintigraphy for diagnosis of bone metastases in patients with lung cancer. Eur J Radiol 2012;81(5): 1007–15.

35. Zekri J, Ahmed N, Coleman RE, et al. The skeletal metastatic complications of renal cell carcinoma. Int J Oncol 2001;19(2):379–82.

36. Wu HC, Yen RF, Shen YY, et al. Comparing whole body 18F-2-deoxyglucose positron emission tomography and technetium-99m methylene diphosphate bone scan to detect bone metastases in patients with renal cell carcinomas - a preliminary report. J Cancer Res Clin Oncol 2002;128(9):503–6.

37. Nakatani K, Nakamoto Y, Saga T, et al. The potential clinical value of FDG-PET for recurrent renal cell carcinoma. Eur J Radiol 2011;79(1):29–35.

38. Qiu ZL, Xue YL, Song HJ, et al. Comparison of the diagnostic and prognostic values of 99mTc-MDP-planar bone scintigraphy, 131I-SPECT/CT and 18F-FDG-PET/CT for the detection of bone metastases from differentiated thyroid cancer. Nucl Med Commun 2012;33(12):1232–42.

39. Dong MJ, Liu ZF, Zhao K, et al. Value of 18F-FDG-PET/PET-CT in differentiated thyroid carcinoma with radioiodine-negative whole-body scan: a meta-analysis. Nucl Med Commun 2009;30(8):639–50.

40. Smallridge RC, Ain KB, Asa SL, et al. American Thyroid Association guidelines for management of patients with anaplastic thyroid cancer. Thyroid 2012; 22(11):1104–39.

41. Savir-Baruch B, Zanoni L, Schuster DM. Imaging of prostate cancer using fluciclovine. PET Clin 2017; 12(2):145–57.

42. Oka S, Kanagawa M, Doi Y, et al. PET tracer 18F-fluciclovine can detect histologically proven bone metastatic lesions: a preclinical study in rat osteolytic and osteoblastic bone metastasis models. Theranostics 2017;7(7):2048–64.

43. Schuster DM, Nanni C, Fanti S, et al. Anti-1-amino-3-18F-fluorocyclobutane-1-carboxylic acid: physiologic uptake patterns, incidental findings, and variants that may simulate disease. J Nucl Med 2014;55(12): 1986–92.

44. Nanni C, Schiavina R, Brunocilla E, et al. 18F-Fluciclovine PET/CT for the detection of prostate cancer relapse: a comparison to 11C-Choline PET/CT. Clin Nucl Med 2015;40(8):e386–91.

45. Schuster DM, Nieh PT, Jani AB, et al. Anti-3-[(18)F]FACBC positron emission tomography-computerized tomography and (111)In-capromab pendetide single photon emission computerized tomography-computerized tomography for recurrent prostate carcinoma: results of a prospective clinical trial. J Urol 2014;191(5):1446–53.

46. Inoue Y, Asano Y, Satoh T, et al. Phase IIa clinical trial of trans-1-amino-3-(18)F-fluoro-cyclobutane carboxylic acid in metastatic prostate cancer. Asia Ocean J Nucl Med Biol 2014;2(2):87–94.

47. FDA approves 11C-choline for PET in prostate cancer. J Nucl Med 2012;53(12):11N.

48. Fuccio C, Castellucci P, Schiavina R, et al. Role of 11C-choline PET/CT in the re-staging of prostate cancer patients with biochemical relapse and negative results at bone scintigraphy. Eur J Radiol 2012; 81(8):e893–6.

49. Picchio M, Spinapolice EG, Fallanca F, et al. [11C] Choline PET/CT detection of bone metastases in patients with PSA progression after primary treatment for prostate cancer: comparison with bone scintigraphy. Eur J Nucl Med Mol Imaging 2012;39(1):13–26.

50. Shen GH, Deng HF, Hu S, et al. Comparison of choline-PET/CT, MRI, SPECT, and bone scintigraphy in the diagnosis of bone metastases in patients with prostate cancer: a meta-analysis. Skeletal Radiol 2014;43(11):1503–13.

51. Ceci F, Castellucci P, Graziani T, et al. 11C-choline PET/CT identifies osteoblastic and osteolytic lesions in patients with metastatic prostate cancer. Clin Nucl Med 2015;40(5):e265–70.

52. Keller ET, Brown J. Prostate cancer bone metastases promote both osteolytic and osteoblastic activity. J Cell Biochem 2004;91(4):718–29.

53. Murphy RC, Kawashima A, Peller PJ. The utility of 11C-choline PET/CT for imaging prostate cancer: a pictorial guide. AJR Am J Roentgenol 2011;196(6): 1390–8.

54. Tuncel M, Souvatzoglou M, Herrmann K, et al. [(11)C]Choline positron emission tomography/computed tomography for staging and restaging of patients with advanced prostate cancer. Nucl Med Biol 2008;35(6):689–95.

55. Gu CN, Hunt CH, Lehman VT, et al. Benign fibrous dysplasia on [(11)C]choline PET: a potential mimicker of disease in patients with biochemical recurrence of prostate cancer. Ann Nucl Med 2012; 26(7):599–602.

56. Leitch CE, Goenka AH, Howe BM, et al. Imaging features of Paget's disease on 11C choline PET/CT. Am J Nucl Med Mol Imaging 2017;7(3):105–10.

# Hybrid Imaging (PET-Computed Tomography/ PET-MR Imaging) of Bone Metastases

Christian Schmidkonz, MD[a],*, Stephan Ellmann, MD[b],
Philipp Ritt, PhD[a], Frank W. Roemer, MD[b],
Ali Guermazi, MD, PhD[c], Michael Uder, MD[b],
Torsten Kuwert, MD[a], Tobias Bäuerle, MD[b]

## KEYWORDS

- Hybrid imaging • PET/computed tomography (CT) • PET/MR imaging • Bone metastases

## KEY POINTS

- PET/computed tomography (CT) and PET/MR imaging imply great potential for characterization of unclear bone lesions.
- PET/CT and PET/MR imaging enable assessment of the entire skeleton in 1 imaging session.
- PET/CT and PET/MR imaging show superior performance for the detection and follow-up of bone metastases compared with conventional imaging methods.
- Although PET/CT has an established role in the staging and treatment assessment of bone metastases, the potential value of PET/MR imaging in the clinical needs to be further explored.

## INTRODUCTION

Bone metastases occur much more frequently than primary bone tumors.[1] Metastases to the skeleton are observed in up to 70% of all cancer patients,[2] with the skeleton being among the 3 most commonly affected metastatic sites together with lung and liver.[3,4] Breast and prostate tumors are most likely to metastasize to the bone followed by lung, thyroid, and kidney tumors.[5] The presence of bone metastases in cancer patients has a considerable effect on mortality and morbidity including complications like pain, pathologic fractures, impaired mobility, hypercalcemia, spinal cord or nerve root compression, and bone marrow infiltration.[6] Early detection of bone metastases is

therefore pivotal for accurate staging, choice of optimal treatment strategies, and therapeutic monitoring.

Established localized treatment strategies include surgical excision or radiation beam therapy.[7,8] Systemic treatment is a crucial component for disseminated disease. Besides chemotherapy, bisphosphonates are frequently used to reduce the rate of complications, bone pain, and to improve the quality of life.[9] Recently, denosumab, a human monoclonal antibody against the receptor activator of nuclear factor-kappa B ligand (RANKL) as the main driver of osteoclast formation, function, and survival in bone metastases, was integrated in systemic therapy approaches (eg, in patients with prostate cancer), showing a reduced rate of

Conflicts of Interest Statement: The authors have no conflict of interest.
[a] Department of Nuclear Medicine, University Medical Center Erlangen, Ulmenweg 18, Erlangen 91054, Germany; [b] Department of Radiology, University Medical Center Erlangen, Ulmenweg 18, Erlangen 91054, Germany; [c] Department of Radiology, Quantitative Imaging Center, Boston University School of Medicine, Boston, 72 East Concord Street, Boston, MA 02118, USA
* Corresponding author. Clinic of Nuclear Medicine, University of Erlangen-Nuremberg, Ulmenweg 18, Erlangen 91054, Germany.
E-mail address: christian.schmidkonz@uk-erlangen.de

PET Clin 14 (2019) 121–133
https://doi.org/10.1016/j.cpet.2018.08.003

skeletal related events compared with intravenous zoledronic acid.[10] Additionally, radium-223 dichloride (Xofigo), a targeted α-emitter, improved overall survival and reduced the rate of skeletal-related events in patients with castration-resistant prostate cancer and symptomatic bone metastases,[11] and thus was approved by the US Food and Drug Administration (FDA).[12] The mechanisms responsible for metastatic tumor growth in the skeleton are complex and involve the stimulation of osteoclasts and osteoblasts by tumor cells expressing factors like parathyroid hormone-related protein (PTHrP).[13] The resulting imbalance between resorption and production of bone matrix subsequently leads to osteoclastic, osteoblastic, or mixed metastatic disease.[14] The release of bone-derived factors such as transforming growth factor-β (TGF-β) consequently stimulates tumor cells to express PTHrP in a positive feedback mechanism. To break this vicious cycle,[15] imaging of bone metastases is of utmost importance for the detection and follow-up of metastatic disease, especially in monitoring treatment response upon local or systemic therapy.

Although serum markers like alkaline phosphatase give valuable information on bone turnover,[16] imaging is indispensable to acquire information on the anatomic localization, size, and metabolism of osseous lesions. Widely used modalities for diagnosing and staging of bone metastases include morphologic imaging techniques such as conventional radiographs, computed tomography (CT), and MR imaging.[17] In addition, nuclear medicine imaging techniques including planar scintigraphy, single photon emission CT (SPECT), and PET enable the assessment of metabolic parameters.[18] In recent years, the implementation of hybrid imaging techniques including SPECT/CT, PET/CT, and PET/MR imaging, which combine the strengths of morphologic and metabolic imaging techniques, opened a new perspective on detection and therapeutic monitoring of skeletal disease, and bone metastases in particular.[19–23]

## BONE SCINTIGRAPHY AND SINGLE PHOTON EMISSION COMPUTED TOMOGRAPHY/COMPUTED TOMOGRAPHY

Several reports emphasize the high sensitivity of bone scintigraphy in the diagnosis of osseous metastases.[19,24] However, specificity is limited, because tracer accumulation in bone scintigraphy reflects the metabolic reaction of bone to several disease processes including neoplasia, trauma, or inflammation.[25] A particular problem results from enhanced diphosphonate uptake in degenerative processes. In most cases, this enhancement affects the vertebral column and the pelvis. Especially in planar scintigraphy, the differentiation of deforming spondylosis and spondylarthrosis from metastases and the exact localization of the respective lesions is hampered.[26] The use of SPECT/CT reduces the rate of equivocal lesions compared with planar bone scan because of better anatomic localization of lesions and higher lesion-to-background contrast, providing increased diagnostic accuracy over planar bone scintigraphy or SPECT alone.[24,27] For detection of bone metastases in patients with prostate cancer, direct comparison between [18]F-Fluoride PET/CT and SPECT/CT using [99m]Tc-MDP showed higher sensitivity and specificity for PET/CT.[18] A recent study prospectively evaluated and compared the performance of [99m]Tc-HDP planar bone scan, [99m]Tc-HDP SPECT/CT, [18]F-fluoride PET/CT, and [18]F-fluoride PET/MR imaging for diagnosing bone metastases.[28] In contrast to previous work, this study found that [18]F-fluoride PET/CT and PET/MR imaging did not significantly improve sensitivity and specificity for detecting osseous metastases over SPECT/CT on a per patient basis. Yet the authors noted that PET/CT and PET/MR imaging revealed a higher number of lesions compared with SPECT/CT, which could potentially result in significant differences in sensitivity for larger patient populations.

For neuroendocrine tumors, van Binnebeek and colleagues[29] reported superiority of [68]Ga-DOTA-TOC-PET/CT over [111]In-pentetreotide SPECT/CT for detection of metastatic lesions in 53 patients. In a lesion-by-lesion and organ-by-organ analysis, PET/CT showed a twofold higher sensitivity than SPEC/CT predominantly for metastatic lesions in the skeleton and in the liver.

Recently several [99m]Tc-labeled SPECT-compatible small molecule inhibitors, targeting the prostate-specific membrane antigen (PSMA), were developed.[30] So far only 2 studies evaluated the role of [99m]Tc-labeled MIP-1404, one of these novel PSMA ligands, in patients with biochemical recurrence of prostate cancer for the detection of PSMA-positive lesions.[31,32] SPECT/CT with [99m]Tc-labeled MIP-1404 proved a high probability of detecting PSMA-positive lesions in patients with PSA values of at least 2 ng/mL, with detection rates comparable to those of [68]Ga-PSMA PET/CT.[33] However, the results indicated that at lower PSA-levels [68]Ga-PSMA PET/CT might be preferable.

Generally, differences in detection rates between SPECT/CT and PET/CT might be due to PET's higher spatial resolution compared with SPECT, which becomes especially important when evaluating small lesions. However, the broader availability and lower costs of SPECT compared with PET still make it a highly valuable tool for diagnostic imaging.

## PET/COMPUTED TOMOGRAPHY

The introduction of [18]F-fluorodeoxyglucose (FDG) PET had marked impact on patient management.[34,35] Increase in size, detection of an abnormal mass, change in tissue attenuation, and abnormal contrast media uptake are the main criteria for a diagnosis of malignancy using purely morphologic imaging approaches.[36] However, these criteria may be misleading, especially after treatment.[37] A metabolic technique like [18]F-FDG PET is inferior to conventional imaging in terms of spatial resolution and localization of abnormalities,[38] but coregistration of PET with CT images allows the combination of detailed anatomic localization with metabolic data and thus improves diagnostic performance over each modality used as a stand-alone.[39] In the past, time-consuming coregistration of separate imaging procedures was performed manually or by using complicated fusion models, hampered by changes in patient position and organ location between the 2 procedures.[40] The development of an integrated hybrid PET/CT scanner for the simultaneous acquisition of morphologic (CT) and metabolic (PET) data made image fusion applicable in the clinical routine and enabled PET/CT to position itself as a standard imaging instrument for oncologic evaluation.[41]

For imaging of bone metastases, [18]F-fluoride and [18]F-FDG are the most frequently used radiopharmaceuticals.[42] The use of these radiotracers allows retrieving information from the bone and the soft tissue components of bone metastases. Application of [18]F-fluoride and [18]F-FDG reflects areas of enhanced bone remodeling and tumor cell glucose metabolism, respectively.[6] [18]F-fluoride is an analogue of the hydroxyl group found in the hydroxyapatite bone crystals and shows high and rapid bone uptake and fast blood clearance resulting in high target-to-background ratios while being deposited in the bone compartment.[43] The accumulation of [18]F-FDG because of metabolic trapping is related to the amount of viable tumor cells and the glucose metabolism of skeletal lesions and therefore primarily represents the hypercellular soft tissue compartment of bone metastases.[44] [18]F-FDG PET/CT features superior diagnostic performance for the detection of distant metastases of lung, breast, and head and neck cancer compared with conventional imaging methods.[45–47]

### Diagnostic Performance of [18]F-Fluorodeoxyglucose PET/Computed Tomography

For the detection of bone metastases, [18]F-FDG PET/CT demonstrated higher sensitivity and specificity in patients with lung- and breast cancer compared with bone scintigraphy.[48,49] A meta-analysis of 2940 patients with lung cancer compared [18]F-FDG PET/CT, [18]F-FDG PET, MR imaging, and bone scintigraphy for the diagnosis of bone metastases in patients with lung cancer.[50] [18]F-FDG PET/CT showed the highest pooled sensitivity with 92%, compared with 87% for [18]F-FDG PET, 77% for MR imaging, and 86% for bone scintigraphy. The pooled specificity of [18]F-FDG PET/CT, [18]F-FDG PET, MR imaging, and bone scintigraphy yielded values of 98%, 94%, 92%, and 88%, respectively, with [18]F-FDG PET/CT again showing the best performance. A large meta-analysis including 145 studies compared [18]F-FDG PET/CT, CT, MR imaging, and bone scintigraphy for the detection of bone metastases.[51] The results indicated an equivalent sensitivity on a per-patient basis of PET and MR imaging of 90%, higher than for CT and bone scintigraphy alone, with 73% and 86%, respectively. The pooled specificity for PET, MR imaging, CT, and bone scan were 97%, 95%, 95%, and 81%, respectively. On a per-lesion basis, the pooled sensitivity was higher for PET and MR imaging, with 87% and 90% compared with CT and bone scintigraphy, with 77% and 75%, respectively. The pooled specificity on per-lesion basis again was higher for PET and MR imaging, with 97% and 96%, compared with CT and bone scintigraphy with 83% and 94%, respectively.[51] Although [18]F-FDG PET/CT was reported to show higher sensitivity for the detection of osteolytic metastases, sensitivity for the detection of osteoblastic metastases is reduced.[52] The reason for this might be the different uptake mechanism in osteolytic and osteoblastic bone metastases. Osteoblast activity and proliferation in sclerotic metastases result in an increase of bone matrix and a relative decrease in cell density, leading to lower FDG accumulation, because FDG uptake in tissue represents the underlying glucose metabolism and thus cell density.[53] The proper interpretation of [18]F-FDG PET/CT requires knowledge of the physiologic distribution and its variations to avoid misinterpretations. [18]F-FDG uptake is not tumor specific and can also be seen in healthy tissue or benign disease (eg, in inflammation or post-traumatic repair that could be mistaken for cancer).[54]

In patients with lymphoma, [18]F-FDG PET/CT has been used successfully for primary staging and therapeutic response evaluation.[55] Upstaging in a relevant proportion of patients with bone marrow involvement is reported when [18]F-FDG PET/CT is compared with staging based on conventional CT.[56] However, in patients with chemotherapy followed by stimulants such as granulocyte colony-stimulating factors, the bone marrow shows diffuse increased FDG accumulation mimicking progressive disease.[57] Interestingly, in patients with breast cancer under antiestrogen therapy, the so-called flare phenomenon seen on bone scan in patients with response to treatment was also found in [18]F-FDG PET/CT.[58]

## Diagnostic Performance of [18]F-fluoride PET/Computed Tomography

Besides [18]F-FDG and [99m]Tc-MDP for primary staging of bone metastases, [18]F-fluoride is frequently used in bone imaging. Before the introduction of [99m]Tc-based agents for bone scintigraphy, [18]F-fluoride was initially used as a planar scintigraphy tracer despite the fact that the emitted 511-keV photons are suboptimal for conventional nuclear medicine scanners.[59] With the widespread availability of PET scanners and the improved logistics for the delivery of [18]F radiopharmaceuticals, [18]F-fluoride experienced a resurgence.[60] Bone uptake of [18]F-fluoride is twofold higher than that of [99m]Tc-MDP; the capillary permeability of [18]F-F is higher, and its faster blood clearance results in better target-to-background ratios.[61] Several studies compared [18]F-fluoride PET/CT to other nuclear medicine and hybrid imaging modalities. In 44 patients with high-risk prostate cancer, Even-Sapir and colleagues[18] reported higher specificity for [18]F-fluoride PET/CT than for [18]F-fluoride PET alone and higher sensitivity and specificity than for bone scan and SPECT/CT using [99m]Tc-MDP. The comparison of [18]F-fluoride PET/CT, [18]F-FDG PET/CT, and [99m]Tc-MDP in patients with lung, prostate, and breast cancers yielded the highest sensitivity and negative predictive value for [18]F-fluoride PET/CT in all 3 malignancies.[62] In patients with lung cancer, [18]F-fluoride PET/CT demonstrated superior image quality and evaluation of skeletal disease extent over [18]F-FDG PET/CT and [99m]Tc-MDP, whereas [18]F-FDG PET/CT allows superior detection of extraskeletal disease, which can change patient management.[43] Accounting for the different tracer accumulations, the combination of [18]F-FDG PET/CT and [18]F-fluoride PET/CT was proposed and evaluated in a pilot study with 14 patients,[63] showing feasibility of this novel approach. Thereafter, an international multicenter trial in 115 patients was conducted, demonstrating the superiority of combined [18]F-Fluoride/[18]F-FDG PET/CT for detection of bone metastases, while providing accurate detection of tracer uptake outside the skeleton when compared to [18]F-FDG PET/CT alone.[44] These promising results need further evaluation to identify the most suitable scenarios for routine clinical use.

## Radiotracers for Neuroendocrine Tumors

Although [18]F-fluoride and [18]F-FDG are the most commonly used radiopharmaceuticals in clinical routine, [68]Ga-Dotatoc/Dotatate is preferred for the detection of neuroendocrine tumors (NETs).[64] This tumor entity originates from neuroendocrine cells within several different organs.[65] They are characterized by the overexpression of somatostatin receptors (SSRs) on the cell surface, with $SSR_2$ and $SSR_5$ expressed in high density in 70% to 100% of GEP-NETs.[66] These receptors are an ideal target for diagnostic and therapeutic radiopharmaceuticals such as the SPECT-compatible [111]In-pentreotide and the PET-compatible [68]Ga-Dotatoc/Dotatate/Dotanoc. Van Binnebeek and colleagues[29] compared both substances in patients with metastatic neuroendocrine tumors. The use of [68]Ga-Dotatoc-PET/CT resulted in the detection of a significantly higher number of tumor lesions, especially in the skeleton and in the liver. These results go in line with the findings of Buchmann and colleagues,[67] who demonstrated the superiority of [68]Ga-Dotatoc-PET/CT over [111]In-pentreotide for the detection of metastases in the lung and skeleton. Compared with conventional CT imaging for the detection of bone metastases, Ambrosini and colleagues[64] found higher sensitivity, specificity, and positive and negative predictive values for [68]Ga-Dotanoc-PET/CT.

## Radiotracers for Prostate Cancer

In patients with prostate cancer, prognosis is strongly associated with the presence or absence of metastases. The skeletal system is the location most frequently involved in metastatic spread as demonstrated in large autopsy studies.[68] Current guidelines recommend CT and MR imaging for the detection of lymphatic and visceral spread, while bone scintigraphy is the modality of choice for exclusion of bone metastases.[69] Although CT and MR imaging have limited diagnostic accuracy for the diagnosis of malignant foci (eg, lymph node involvement is primarily diagnosed by the size of lymph nodes),[70,71] the diagnostic sensitivity of bone scintigraphy is reduced by relatively low tumor-to-normal ratios of metastases.

The development of [68]Ga- and [18]F-labelled PSMA PET ligands targeting the extracellular domain of the PSMA receptor, which is expressed up to 100- to 1000-fold higher on prostate cancer cells, was a major breakthrough.[30] [68]Ga-labeled PSMA is the most widely used PET tracer for the work-up of prostate cancer and increasingly replaces the previously used

[18]F-choline PET, which lacks sensitivity, especially in patients with low PSA levels.[72,73] [68]Ga-PSMA PET/CT has proven to be an excellent imaging technique for staging of patients with primary prostate cancer[74–76] and with biochemical recurrence after primary therapy,[77,78] providing 1-stop shop imaging for evaluation of soft tissue and bone metastases (**Fig. 1**). Afshar-Oromieh and colleagues[77] performed a retrospective analysis of 319 patients who underwent [68]Ga-PSMA PET/CT for staging of recurrent prostate cancer. In 83% of all patients at least 1 PSMA-positive lesion indicative of prostate cancer was detected. Bone metastases were the most frequently detected lesion type, with a total of 359 metastases, followed by 328 lymph node metastases. Regarding tracer uptake, lymph node metastases showed highest contrast, followed by bone metastases. Comparison of [18]F-choline PET/CT with [68]Ga-PSMA PET/CT in 37 patients with biochemical relapse of prostate cancer yielded higher overall detection rates of [68]Ga-PSMA PET/CT with higher $SUV_{max}$ of lesions and lower uptake of background tissue, resulting in higher tumor-to-background ratios for [68]Ga-PSMA PET/CT. Concerning both $SUV_{max}$ of lesions and their tumor-to-background ratio, the most

significant differences between the 2 imaging techniques were observed in lymph node metastases followed by bone metastases, showing higher detection rates of bone metastases for the [68]Ga labeled PET tracer compared with the [18]F-choline labeled compound.[73] Direct comparison between [68]Ga-PSMA PET and planar [99m]Tc-DPD bone scan in skeletal staging of prostate cancer patients showed higher sensitivity and specificity for overall bone involvement and for the region-based analysis.[79] The additional value of morphologic information of low-dose CT in [68]Ga-PSMA PET and [99m]Tc-DPD-SPECT was evaluated by Janssen and colleagues.[80] [68]Ga-PSMA PET outperformed [99m]Tc-DPD SPECT in detecting bone metastases, while the additional information of low-dose CT resulted in a significant reduction of equivocal lesions in both modalities.

For assessment of treatment response and follow-up of osteoblastic lesions, CT is often inconclusive. Therefore, [68]Ga-PSMA PET/CT, with PSMA-uptake in the sclerotic lesion representing the presence of vital tumor cells, might become an important method to determine response or progression of skeletal disease in patients with prostate cancer (**Fig. 2**).

**08/15**

**04/16**

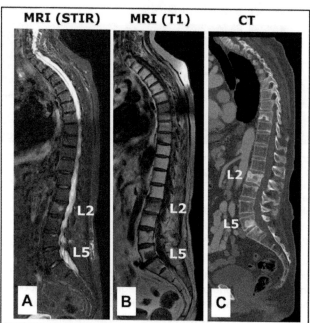
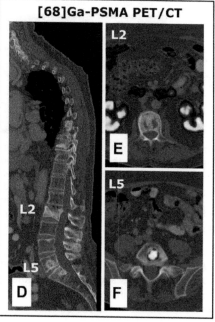

**Fig. 1.** 79-year-old patient with prostate cancer bone metastases. Bone lesions were diagnosed in 08/15 in lumbar vertebral body (LVB) #2 and #5 with MR imaging (*A, B*) and CT (*C*). Beginning bone compression was observed in LVB #2 in 08/15 and progressed in 04/16 as shown in (*D*). CT information alone is not conclusive to discriminate between compression (osteoporotic) and pathologic fracture (tumor infiltration of bone marrow). The [68]Ga-PSMA PET/CT, however, indicates the absence of tumor in LVB #2 (*E*) but presence of metastatic infiltration in LVB #5 (*F*).

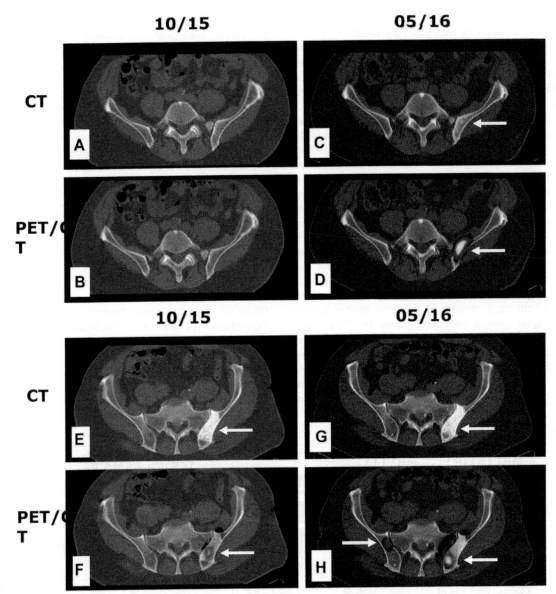

**10/15**                    **05/16**

CT

A        C

PET/C
T

B        D

**10/15**                    **05/16**

CT

E        G

PET/C
T

F        H

**Fig. 2.** 66-year-old patient with prostate cancer bone metastases under chemotherapy. Although CT indicates minimal sclerosis in the proximal left iliac bone as indicator of progressive disease in 05/16 compared with 10/15 (CT, *A*, *C*, *White arrow*), new PSMA-uptake is clearly visible in this localization in 05/16 as ($^{68}$Ga-PSMA PET/CT *D*) while still absent in 10/15 (*B*). In the distal left iliac bone, a sclerotic lesion is already present at baseline (*E*, 10/15, *White arrows*), and, based on CT-morphology, almost unchanged after therapy (*G*, 05/16, *White arrow*). In $^{68}$Ga-PSMA PET/CT, however, there is an increase of radiotracer-uptake over time in the left iliac bone and a novel lesion in the right iliac bone without CT-morphologic changes (*arrows*; *F*, 10/15 and *H*, 05/16).

As evidenced by the previously mentioned studies, PET/CT is superior to the other conventional and hybrid imaging modalities in detecting bone metastases in various cancers.

**PET/MR IMAGING**

With regard to soft tissue contrast, MR imaging is clearly superior to CT. Therefore, MR imaging is the imaging modality of choice for accurate morphologic tumor staging in many oncologic diseases. Especially in imaging of the brain, parenchymal abdominal organs, and the bone marrow, the use of MR imaging may be advantageous. Although T1- and T2-weighted sequences form the basis of MR morphologic imaging, functional information is provided by a variety of MR imaging techniques.[81,82] Among these, diffusion-weighted MR imaging provides a quantifiable imaging biomarker (apparent diffusion coefficient, ADC) through measurement of the diffusion properties of water within tissues.[83,84] ADC changes result from shifts of water molecules from the extracellular to the intracellular space, increased cellular density, and disruption of cellular membrane depolarization commonly associated with malignancies.[85–87] MR spectroscopy determines the concentration of various metabolites such as amino acids in a specific region of interest, being most widely used in the evaluation of brain tumors or prostate cancer.[88,89] These functional and molecular imaging techniques represent only a selection of the available applications to approach oncologic diseases in MR imaging. With regard to bone metastases, the excellent soft tissue contrast of MR imaging enables capture of early stages of malignant bone marrow infiltration.[90,91] Tumor proliferation in the bone marrow results in hypointense T1 and hyperintense T2 signal, as well as relatively strong contrast media uptake, regularly seen in osteolytic disease. In contrast to these findings, the described signal changes might be less pronounced or even absent in osteoblastic metastases because of the lower tumor cellularity.[6] For evaluation of structures adjacent to bone when the intramedullary tumor has penetrated cortical bone and infiltrates nerves or the spinal cord, MR imaging is capable of reliably determining tumor expansion[92,93] (Fig. 3). The use of morphologic and functional MR imaging techniques enables the assessment of complementary data in bone metastases and increases the accurate assignment of PET-positive findings to anatomic structures.[94]

Although the initial development of PET/MR imaging scanners was in the experimental field, prototype systems have rapidly progressed to systems that are now clinically available and used for oncologic patients routinely at some centers. Initial designs included systems in which MR imaging and PET scanners were placed side by side connected by a moving table on which the patient underwent PET and MR imaging consecutively.[82,95] This type of PET/MR imaging contains conventional photomultipliers that show a high sensitivity to magnetic fields. The replacement of these with avalanche photodiodes, which are unaffected by magnetic fields, led to the development of new hybrid scanner designs that include photon detectors in the main magnetic field.[96,97] Thereby whole-body tumor staging in 1 session has become feasible.

## PET/Computed Tomography Versus PET/MR Imaging

Several studies comparing PET/MR imaging with PET/CT and conventional imaging modalities in radiology and nuclear medicine have been conducted so far. Eiber and colleagues[98] compared the performance of whole-body integrated [18]F-FDG PET/MR imaging with [18]F-FDG PET/CT for the evaluation of malignant bone lesions. The overall performance of PET/MR imaging and PET/CT in patients who underwent both scans sequentially using [18]F-FDG was equivalent for detection and characterization of bone lesions. However, lesion delineation and allocation of PET-positive findings were superior in PET/MR imaging including diagnostic T1-weighted TSE or T1-weighted Dixon in-phase sequences compared with PET/CT. This finding might be of clinical relevance, especially in early bone marrow infiltration and bone lesions with low uptake on PET. The implementation of T1-weighted TSE sequences for oncologic PET/MR imaging to screen for suspicious skeletal lesions might be advantageous.

Samarin and colleagues[99] compared the performance of PET/CT and PET/MR imaging for the detection of bone metastases in 24 patients with malignant tumors who underwent both imaging modalities for staging or restaging under therapy and suspicion of bone metastases. As demonstrated by Eiber and colleagues,[98] the overall detection rate showed no significant difference; however, PET/MR imaging provided higher reader confidence and improved conspicuity compared with PET/CT. Beiderwellen and colleagues[100] enrolled 67 patients who suffered from different primary tumors, including malignant melanoma, breast cancer, nonsmall cell lung cancer, colorectal cancer, and others. A total of 75 bone lesions were present in 10 patients, of which 48 lesions were metastases, and 27 lesions were benign. PET/MR imaging allowed identification of all bone metastases, while PET/CT identified 45 of 48 bone metastases correctly (94%). In benign lesions, PET/CT outperformed PET/MR imaging by correctly identifying 96% bone lesions compared with 67% in PET/MR imaging. The benign lesions missed by PET/MR imaging consisted of PET-negative osteosclerotic lesions. The lower specificity of MR imaging, especially for osteosclerotic lesions is well known, since especially cortical bone yields only very low signal intensities in MR imaging.[20] Although the overall conspicuity of malignant lesions was excellent in both imaging modalities, PET/MR imaging exhibited significantly higher values in the subgroup of bone metastases

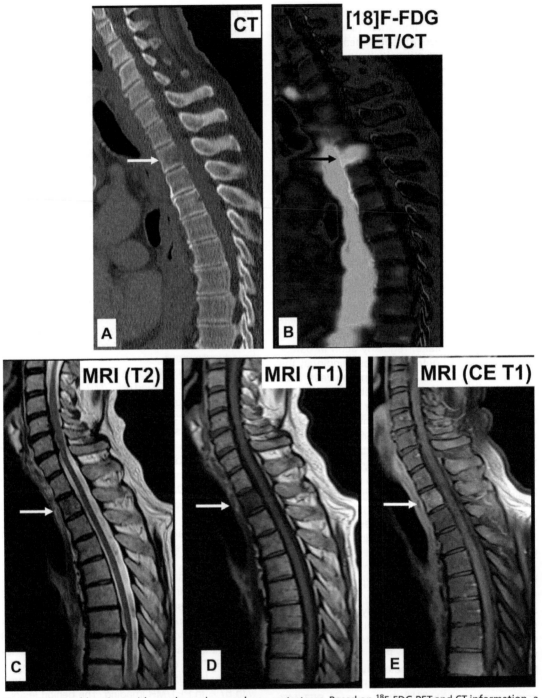

**Fig. 3.** 60-year-old patient with esophageal cancer bone metastases. Based on [18]F-FDG PET and CT information, a lytic bone metastasis can be diagnosed with disruption of the dorsal cortical bone of thoracic vertebral body #2 (*arrows* in *A, B*). However, an infiltration of the myelon could not be ruled out with PET/CT alone. On MR imaging (*C*, T2; *D*, T1; *E*, contrast-enhanced T1, *white arrows*), no signs of tumor growth into the spinal canal or the myelon were seen.

less than 5 mm in size. Regarding $SUV_{max}$ values of PET-positive lesions, both imaging modalities showed good correlation, but lower $SUV_{max}$ values were found for PET/MR imaging, with a mean

difference of −3.5%. This might be explained by the challenging attenuation correction of PET data based on MR images.[101] In PET/CT, the CT transmission data are routinely used for

**Table 1**
**Advantages and disadvantages of PET/CT and PET/MR imaging in the assessment of bone metastases**

|  | PET/CT | PET/MR Imaging |
|---|---|---|
| Advantages | Faster imaging protocols<br>Easier attenuation correction<br>Assessment of bone and bone structure (cortical and cancellous bone) to define phenotype of metastasis (lytic or blastic) and to determine bone stability/fracture risk | Higher soft tissue contrast<br>No additional radiation exposure<br>Additional functional techniques available (diffusion weighted imaging, dynamic contrast-enhanced MR imaging) |
| Disadvantages | Limited soft tissue contrast: Bone marrow infiltration without bone destruction may not be visible on CT component<br>Additional radiation exposure | Cost intensive, available only in dedicated medical centers<br>Longer image acquisition times<br>Implants for example, pacemaker are contraindicated<br>Limited information on bone structure |

attenuation correction.[102] In PET/MR imaging, however, intensity values do not reflect the X-ray density of tissue; thus image processing of MR imaging data is required in order to generate attenuation correction maps.[103,104] Proposed approaches to MR imaging-based attenuation correction include tissue segmentation, the use of atlases or templates, and pattern recognition techniques.[105–107] In many of these approaches, tissue segmentation is performed with substitution of bone by soft tissue, causing an underestimation of tracer in osseous and soft tissue lesions adjacent to bones of almost 16%.[103] The errors depend substantially on lesion composition, with the largest error being seen in sclerotic lesions.[103] Therefore, to accurately quantify uptake values in whole-body PET/MR imaging for bony structures, appropriate attenuation correction maps are necessary, especially when comparing data obtained from PET/MR imaging and PET/CT.

In prostate cancer imaging, hybrid PET/MR imaging was mainly performed using choline tracers such as $^{18}$F-choline and $^{11}$C-choline.[108,109] As described for $^{18}$F-FDG, the diagnostic performance of $^{18}$F-choline PET/CT and PET/MR imaging was comparable, with better anatomic allocation of lesions in PET/MR imaging. The introduction of the more specific PSMA ligands in PET/CT will most probably result in application also in PET/MR imaging. In the study by Freitag and colleagues,[94] 26 patients underwent PET/CT and PET/MR imaging for the evaluation of lymph node and bone metastases. Comparison of the PET components yielded no discordant findings in the 28 depicted bone lesions, while 2 PET-positive bone metastases could not be confirmed morphologically using low-dose CT but were

assessable on MR imaging. Again, the overall conspicuity was higher on MR imaging compared with CT.

In summary, the available data suggest that bone metastases can be accurately and reliably be depicted by PET/MR imaging with a similar overall detection rate compared with PET/CT, but higher reader confidence and conspicuity for anatomic allocation of PET-positive findings. **Table 1** summarizes the advantages and disadvantages of PET/CT and PET/MR imaging.

## SUMMARY

For detection and evaluation of treatment response in bone metastases, imaging modalities like CT or MR imaging and metabolic imaging approaches like SPECT and PET justifiably play a significant role. The combination of metabolic and morphologic imaging represented by PET/CT and PET/MR imaging bares great potential for improved characterization and follow-up of bone metastases, enabling whole-body oncologic imaging in 1 session. Although PET/CT is already commonly used in the clinical practice supported by a large number of representative studies, the so far available data of PET/MR imaging for this purpose look promising but have to be clarified in further clinical validation studies.

## REFERENCES

1. Bussard KM, Gay CV, Mastro AM. The bone microenvironment in metastasis; what is special about bone? Cancer Metastasis Rev 2008;27:41–55.

2. Coleman R. Metastatic bone disease: clinical features, pathophysiology and treatment strategies. Cancer Treat Rev 2001;27:165–76.

3. Vassiliou V, Andreopoulos D, Frangos S, et al. Bone metastases: assessment of therapeutic response through radiological and nuclear medicine imaging modalities. Clin Oncol 2011;23:632–45.

4. Yu H, Tsai Y-Y, Hoffe SE. Overview of diagnosis and management of metastatic disease to bone. Cancer Control 2012;19:84–91.

5. Rubens RD. Bone metastases: incidence and complications. Cancer and the skeleton. London: Martin Dunitz; 2000. p. 33–42.

6. Bäuerle T, Semmler W. Imaging response to systemic therapy for bone metastases. Eur Radiol 2009;19:2495–507.

7. Nielsen OS, Munro A, Tannock I. Bone metastases: pathophysiology and management policy. J Clin Oncol 1991;9:509–24.

8. Arcangeli G, Micheli A, Arcangeli G, et al. The responsiveness of bone metastases to radiotherapy: the effect of site, histology and radiation dose on pain relief. Radiother Oncol 1989;14:95–101.

9. Ross J, Saunders Y, Edmonds P, et al. A systematic review of the role of bisphosphonates in metastatic disease. Health Technol Assess 2004;8(4):1–176.

10. Fizazi K, Carducci M, Smith M, et al. Denosumab versus zoledronic acid for treatment of bone metastases in men with castration-resistant prostate cancer: a randomised, double-blind study. Lancet 2011;377:813–22.

11. Sartor O, Coleman R, Nilsson S, et al. Effect of radium-223 dichloride on symptomatic skeletal events in patients with castration-resistant prostate cancer and bone metastases: results from a phase 3, double-blind, randomised trial. Lancet Oncol 2014;15:738–46.

12. Kluetz PG, Pierce W, Maher VE, et al. Radium Ra 223 dichloride injection: US Food and Drug Administration drug approval summary. Clin Cancer Res 2014;20:9–14.

13. Mundy GR. Metastasis: metastasis to bone: causes, consequences and therapeutic opportunities. Nat Rev Cancer 2002;2:584.

14. Guise TA, Mohammad KS, Clines G, et al. Basic mechanisms responsible for osteolytic and osteoblastic bone metastases. Clin Cancer Res 2006; 12:6213s–6s.

15. Guise T. The vicious cycle of bone metastases. J Musculoskelet Neuronal Interact 2002;2:570–2.

16. Leung K, Fung K, Sher A, et al. Plasma bone-specific alkaline phosphatase as an indicator of osteoblastic activity. J Bone Joint Surg Br 1993; 75:288–92.

17. O'Sullivan GJ, Carty FL, Cronin CG. Imaging of bone metastasis: an update. World J Radiol 2015; 7:202.

18. Even-Sapir E, Metser U, Mishani E, et al. The detection of bone metastases in patients with high-risk prostate cancer: 99mTc-MDP planar bone scintigraphy, single-and multi-field-of-view SPECT, 18F-fluoride PET, and 18F-fluoride PET/CT. J Nucl Med 2006;47:287–97.

19. Römer W, Nömayr A, Uder M, et al. SPECT-guided CT for evaluating foci of increased bone metabolism classified as indeterminate on SPECT in cancer patients. J Nucl Med 2006;47:1102–6.

20. Schmidt GP, Schoenberg SO, Schmid R, et al. Screening for bone metastases: whole-body MRI using a 32-channel system versus dual-modality PET-CT. Eur Radiol 2007;17:939–49.

21. Pichler BJ, Kolb A, Nägele T, et al. PET/MRI: paving the way for the next generation of clinical multimodality imaging applications. J Nucl Med 2010;51: 333–6.

22. Wiesmüller M, Quick HH, Navalpakkam B, et al. Comparison of lesion detection and quantitation of tracer uptake between PET from a simultaneously acquiring whole-body PET/MR hybrid scanner and PET from PET/CT. Eur J Nucl Med Mol Imaging 2013;40:12–21.

23. Kuwert T, Ritt P. PET/MRI and PET/CT: is there room for both at the top of the food chain? Eur J Nucl Med Mol Imaging 2016;43:209–11.

24. Utsunomiya D, Shiraishi S, Imuta M, et al. Added value of SPECT/CT fusion in assessing suspected bone metastasis: comparison with scintigraphy alone and nonfused scintigraphy and CT. Radiology 2006;238:264–71.

25. Hamaoka T, Madewell JE, Podoloff DA, et al. Bone imaging in metastatic breast cancer. J Clin Oncol 2004;22:2942–53.

26. Love C, Din AS, Tomas MB, et al. Radionuclide bone imaging: an illustrative review. Radiographics 2003;23:341–58.

27. Schillaci O, Danieli R, Manni C, et al. Is SPECT/CT with a hybrid camera useful to improve scintigraphic imaging interpretation? Nucl Med Commun 2004;25:705–10.

28. Löfgren J, Mortensen J, Rasmussen SH, et al. A prospective study comparing 99mTc-hydroxy-ethylene-diphosphonate planar bone scintigraphy and whole-body SPECT/CT with 18F-fluoride PET/CT and 18F-fluoride PET/MRI for diagnosing bone metastases. J Nucl Med 2017;58:1778–85.

29. Van Binnebeek S, Vanbilloen B, Baete K, et al. Comparison of diagnostic accuracy of 111In-pentetreotide SPECT and 68Ga-DOTATOC PET/CT: a lesion-by-lesion analysis in patients with metastatic neuroendocrine tumours. Eur Radiol 2016;26: 900–9.

30. Afshar-Oromieh A, Babich JW, Kratochwil C, et al. The rise of PSMA ligands for diagnosis and therapy of prostate cancer. J Nucl Med 2016;57:79S–89S.

31. Reinfelder J, Kuwert T, Beck M, et al. First experience with SPECT/CT using a 99mTc-labeled inhibitor for prostate-specific membrane antigen in patients with biochemical recurrence of prostate cancer. Clin Nucl Med 2017;42:26–33.

32. Schmidkonz C, Hollweg C, Beck M, et al. 99m Tc-MIP-1404-SPECT/CT for the detection of PSMA-positive lesions in 225 patients with biochemical recurrence of prostate cancer. Prostate 2018; 78(1):54–63.

33. Perera M, Papa N, Christidis D, et al. Sensitivity, specificity, and predictors of positive 68 Ga–prostate-specific membrane antigen positron emission tomography in advanced prostate cancer: a systematic review and meta-analysis. Eur Urol 2016; 70:926–37.

34. Rigo P, Paulus P, Kaschten B, et al. Oncological applications of positron emission tomography with fluorine-18 fluorodeoxyglucose. Eur J Nucl Med 1996;23:1641–74.

35. Cohade C, Wahl RL. PET scanning and measuring the impact of treatment. Cancer J 2002;8:119–34.

36. Israel O, Mor M, Gaitini D, et al. Combined functional and structural evaluation of cancer patients with a hybrid camera-based PET/CT system using 18F-FDG. J Nucl Med 2002;43:1129–36.

37. Hutchings M, Barrington SF. PET/CT for therapy response assessment in lymphoma. J Nucl Med 2009;50:21S–30S.

38. Bar-Shalom R, Yefremov N, Guralnik L, et al. Clinical performance of PET/CT in evaluation of cancer: additional value for diagnostic imaging and patient management. J Nucl Med 2003;44:1200–9.

39. Townsend DW, Cherry SR. Combining anatomy and function: the path to true image fusion. Eur Radiol 2001;11(10):1968–74.

40. Israel O, Keidar Z, Iosilevsky G, et al. The fusion of anatomic and physiologic imaging in the management of patients with cancer. Semin Nucl Med 2001;31:191–205.

41. Beyer T, Townsend DW, Brun T, et al. A combined PET/CT scanner for clinical oncology. J Nucl Med 2000;41:1369.

42. Choi J, Raghavan M. Diagnostic imaging and image-guided therapy of skeletal metastases. Cancer Control 2012;19:102–12.

43. Iagaru A, Mittra E, Dick DW, et al. Prospective evaluation of 99mTc MDP scintigraphy, 18F NaF PET/CT, and 18F FDG PET/CT for detection of skeletal metastases. Mol Imaging Biol 2012;14:252–9.

44. Iagaru A, Mittra E, Mosci C, et al. Combined 18F-fluoride and 18F-FDG PET/CT scanning for evaluation of malignancy: results of an international multicenter trial. J Nucl Med 2013;54:176–83.

45. De Wever W, Ceyssens S, Mortelmans L, et al. Additional value of PET-CT in the staging of lung cancer: comparison with CT alone, PET alone and visual correlation of PET and CT. Eur Radiol 2007; 17:23–32.

46. Du Y, Cullum I, Illidge TM, et al. Fusion of metabolic function and morphology: sequential [18F] fluorodeoxyglucose positron-emission tomography/computed tomography studies yield new insights into the natural history of bone metastases in breast cancer. J Clin Oncol 2007; 25:3440–7.

47. Yoon DY, Hwang HS, Chang SK, et al. CT, MR, US, 18F-FDG PET/CT, and their combined use for the assessment of cervical lymph node metastases in squamous cell carcinoma of the head and neck. Eur Radiol 2009;19:634–42.

48. Krüger S, Buck AK, Mottaghy FM, et al. Detection of bone metastases in patients with lung cancer: 99mTc-MDP planar bone scintigraphy, 18F-fluoride PET or 18F-FDG PET/CT. Eur J Nucl Med Mol Imaging 2009;36:1807.

49. Hahn S, Heusner T, Kümmel S, et al. Comparison of FDG-PET/CT and bone scintigraphy for detection of bone metastases in breast cancer. Acta Radiol 2011;52:1009–14.

50. Qu X, Huang X, Yan W, et al. A meta-analysis of 18 FDG-PET–CT, 18 FDG-PET, MRI and bone scintigraphy for diagnosis of bone metastases in patients with lung cancer. Eur J Radiol 2012; 81:1007–15.

51. Yang H-L, Liu T, Wang X-M, et al. Diagnosis of bone metastases: a meta-analysis comparing 18FDG PET, CT, MRI and bone scintigraphy. Eur Radiol 2011;21:2604–17.

52. Huyge V, Garcia C, Vanderstappen A, et al. Progressive osteoblastic bone metastases in breast cancer negative on FDG-PET. Clin Nucl Med 2009;34:417–20.

53. Nakai T, Okuyama C, Kubota T, et al. Pitfalls of FDG-PET for the diagnosis of osteoblastic bone metastases in patients with breast cancer. Eur J Nucl Med Mol Imaging 2005;32:1253–8.

54. Rosenbaum SJ, Lind T, Antoch G, et al. False-positive FDG PET uptake– the role of PET/CT. Eur Radiol 2006;16:1054–65.

55. Kostakoglu L, Cheson BD. Current role of FDG PET/CT in lymphoma. Eur J Nucl Med Mol Imaging 2014;41:1004–27.

56. Schaefer NG, Strobel K, Taverna C, et al. Bone involvement in patients with lymphoma: the role of FDG-PET/CT. Eur J Nucl Med Mol Imaging 2007; 34:60–7.

57. Chiang SB, Rebenstock A, Guan L, et al. Diffuse bone marrow involvement of Hodgkin lymphoma mimics hematopoietic cytokine-mediated FDG uptake on FDG PET imaging. Clin Nucl Med 2003; 28:674–6.

58. Dehdashti F, Flanagan FL, Mortimer JE, et al. Positron emission tomographic assessment

of" metabolic flare" to predict response of metastatic breast cancer to antiestrogen therapy. Eur J Nucl Med 1999;26:51–6.

59. Shirazi PH, Rayudu GV, Fordham EW. Review of solitary 18F bone scan lesions. Radiology 1974; 112:369–72.

60. Grant FD, Fahey FH, Packard AB, et al. Skeletal PET with 18F-fluoride: applying new technology to an old tracer. J Nucl Med 2008;49:68–78.

61. Even-Sapir E. Imaging of malignant bone involvement by morphologic, scintigraphic, and hybrid modalities. J Nucl Med 2005;46:1356–67.

62. Damle NA, Bal C, Bandopadhyaya G, et al. The role of 18F-fluoride PET-CT in the detection of bone metastases in patients with breast, lung and prostate carcinoma: a comparison with FDG PET/CT and 99mTc-MDP bone scan. Jpn J Radiol 2013;31:262–9.

63. Iagaru A, Mittra E, Yaghoubi SS, et al. Novel strategy for a cocktail 18F-fluoride and 18F-FDG PET/CT scan for evaluation of malignancy: results of the pilot-phase study. J Nucl Med 2009;50:501–5.

64. Ambrosini V, Nanni C, Zompatori M, et al. 68Ga-DOTA-NOC PET/CT in comparison with CT for the detection of bone metastasis in patients with neuroendocrine tumours. Eur J Nucl Med Mol Imaging 2010;37:722–7.

65. Modlin IM, Oberg K, Chung DC, et al. Gastroenteropancreatic neuroendocrine tumours. Lancet Oncol 2008;9:61–72.

66. Reubi JC, Waser B. Concomitant expression of several peptide receptors in neuroendocrine tumours: molecular basis for in vivo multireceptor tumour targeting. Eur J Nucl Med Mol Imaging 2003;30:781–93.

67. Buchmann I, Henze M, Engelbrecht S, et al. Comparison of 68Ga-DOTATOC PET and 111In-DTPAOC (Octreoscan) SPECT in patients with neuroendocrine tumours. Eur J Nucl Med Mol Imaging 2007;34:1617–26.

68. Bubendorf L, Schöpfer A, Wagner U, et al. Metastatic patterns of prostate cancer: an autopsy study of 1,589 patients. Hum Pathol 2000;31: 578–83.

69. Heidenreich A, Bastian PJ, Bellmunt J, et al. EAU guidelines on prostate cancer. Part 1: screening, diagnosis, and local treatment with curative intent—update 2013. Eur Urol 2014;65:124–37.

70. Hövels A, Heesakkers R, Adang E, et al. The diagnostic accuracy of CT and MRI in the staging of pelvic lymph nodes in patients with prostate cancer: a meta-analysis. Clin Radiol 2008;63: 387–95.

71. Eiber M, Beer AJ, Holzapfel K, et al. Preliminary results for characterization of pelvic lymph nodes in patients with prostate cancer by diffusion-weighted MR-imaging. Invest Radiol 2010;45: 15–23.

72. Pfister D, Porres D, Heidenreich A, et al. Detection of recurrent prostate cancer lesions before salvage lymphadenectomy is more accurate with 68Ga-PSMA-HBED-CC than with 18F-fluoroethylcholine PET/CT. Eur J Nucl Med Mol Imaging 2016;43: 1410–7.

73. Afshar-Oromieh A, Zechmann CM, Malcher A, et al. Comparison of PET imaging with a 68Ga-labelled PSMA ligand and 18F-choline-based PET/CT for the diagnosis of recurrent prostate cancer. Eur J Nucl Med Mol Imaging 2014;41:11–20.

74. Fendler WP, Schmidt DF, Wenter V, et al. 68Ga-PSMA PET/CT detects the location and extent of primary prostate cancer. J Nucl Med 2016;57: 1720–5.

75. Herlemann A, Wenter V, Kretschmer A, et al. 68 Ga-PSMA positron emission tomography/computed tomography provides accurate staging of lymph node regions prior to lymph node dissection in patients with prostate cancer. Eur Urol 2016;70: 553–7.

76. Maurer T, Gschwend JE, Rauscher I, et al. Diagnostic efficacy of 68 gallium-PSMA positron emission tomography compared to conventional imaging for lymph node staging of 130 consecutive patients with intermediate to high risk prostate cancer. J Urol 2016;195:1436–43.

77. Afshar-Oromieh A, Avtzi E, Giesel FL, et al. The diagnostic value of PET/CT imaging with the 68Ga-labelled PSMA ligand HBED-CC in the diagnosis of recurrent prostate cancer. Eur J Nucl Med Mol Imaging 2015;42:197–209.

78. Eiber M, Maurer T, Souvatzoglou M, et al. Evaluation of hybrid 68Ga-PSMA ligand PET/CT in 248 patients with biochemical recurrence after radical prostatectomy. J Nucl Med 2015;56:668–74.

79. Pyka T, Okamoto S, Dahlbender M, et al. Comparison of bone scintigraphy and 68Ga-PSMA PET for skeletal staging in prostate cancer. Eur J Nucl Med Mol Imaging 2016;43:2114–21.

80. Janssen J-C, Meißner S, Woythal N, et al. Comparison of hybrid 68Ga-PSMA-PET/CT and 99mTc-DPD-SPECT/CT for the detection of bone metastases in prostate cancer patients: additional value of morphologic information from low dose CT. Eur Radiol 2018;28(2):610–9.

81. Buchbender C, Heusner TA, Lauenstein TC, et al. Oncologic PET/MRI, part 1: tumors of the brain, head and neck, chest, abdomen, and pelvis. J Nucl Med 2012;53:928–38.

82. Drzezga A, Souvatzoglou M, Eiber M, et al. First clinical experience with integrated whole-body PET/MR: comparison to PET/CT in patients with oncologic diagnoses. J Nucl Med 2012;53: 845–55.

83. Charles-Edwards EM. Diffusion-weighted magnetic resonance imaging and its application to cancer. Cancer Imaging 2006;6:135.

84. Mori S, Barker PB. Diffusion magnetic resonance imaging: its principle and applications. Anat Rec 1999;257:102–9.

85. Malayeri AA, El Khouli RH, Zaheer A, et al. Principles and applications of diffusion-weighted imaging in cancer detection, staging, and treatment follow-up. Radiographics 2011;31:1773–91.

86. Desouza N, Reinsberg S, Scurr E, et al. Magnetic resonance imaging in prostate cancer: the value of apparent diffusion coefficients for identifying malignant nodules. Br J Radiol 2007;80:90–5.

87. Partridge SC, Mullins CD, Kurland BF, et al. Apparent diffusion coefficient values for discriminating benign and malignant breast MRI lesions: effects of lesion type and size. AJR Am J Roentgenol 2010;194:1664–73.

88. Gujar SK, Maheshwari S, Björkman-Burtscher I, et al. Magnetic resonance spectroscopy. J Neuroophthalmol 2005;25:217–26.

89. Fütterer JJ, Briganti A, De Visschere P, et al. Can clinically significant prostate cancer be detected with multiparametric magnetic resonance imaging? A systematic review of the literature. Eur Urol 2015;68:1045–53.

90. Imamura F, Kuriyama K, Seto T, et al. Detection of bone marrow metastases of small cell lung cancer with magnetic resonance imaging: early diagnosis before destruction of osseous structure and implications for staging. Lung Cancer 2000;27:189–97.

91. Steinborn MM, Heuck AF, Tiling R, et al. Whole-body bone marrow MRI in patients with metastatic disease to the skeletal system. J Comput Assist Tomogr 1999;23:123–9.

92. Godersky JC, Smoker WR, Knutzon R. Use of magnetic resonance imaging in the evaluation of metastatic spinal disease. Neurosurgery 1987;21:676–80.

93. Buhmann S, Becker C, Duerr HR, et al. Detection of osseous metastases of the spine: comparison of high resolution multi-detector-CT with MRI. Eur J Radiol 2009;69:567–73.

94. Freitag MT, Radtke JP, Hadaschik BA, et al. Comparison of hybrid 68Ga-PSMA PET/MRI and 68Ga-PSMA PET/CT in the evaluation of lymph node and bone metastases of prostate cancer. Eur J Nucl Med Mol Imaging 2016;43:70–83.

95. Zaidi H, Ojha N, Morich M, et al. Design and performance evaluation of a whole-body Ingenuity TF PET–MRI system. Phys Med Biol 2011;56:3091.

96. Disselhorst JA, Bezrukov I, Kolb A, et al. Principles of PET/MR imaging. J Nucl Med 2014;55:2S–10S.

97. Pichler BJ, Judenhofer MS, Catana C, et al. Performance test of an LSO-APD detector in a 7-T MRI scanner for simultaneous PET/MRI. J Nucl Med 2006;47:639–47.

98. Eiber M, Takei T, Souvatzoglou M, et al. Performance of whole-body integrated 18F-FDG PET/MR in comparison to PET/CT for evaluation of malignant bone lesions. J Nucl Med 2014;55:191–7.

99. Samarin A, Hüllner M, Queiroz MA, et al. 18F-FDG-PET/MR increases diagnostic confidence in detection of bone metastases compared with 18F-FDG-PET/CT. Nucl Med Commun 2015;36:1165–73.

100. Beiderwellen K, Huebner M, Heusch P, et al. Whole-body [18F] FDG PET/MRI vs. PET/CT in the assessment of bone lesions in oncological patients: initial results. Eur Radiol 2014;24:2023–30.

101. Hofmann M, Pichler B, Schölkopf B, et al. Towards quantitative PET/MRI: a review of MR-based attenuation correction techniques. Eur J Nucl Med Mol Imaging 2009;36:93–104.

102. Kinahan PE, Hasegawa BH, Beyer T. X-ray-based attenuation correction for positron emission tomography/computed tomography scanners. Semin Nucl Med 2003;33:166–79.

103. Samarin A, Burger C, Wollenweber SD, et al. PET/MR imaging of bone lesions–implications for PET quantification from imperfect attenuation correction. Eur J Nucl Med Mol Imaging 2012;39:1154–60.

104. Burger C, Goerres G, Schoenes S, et al. PET attenuation coefficients from CT images: experimental evaluation of the transformation of CT into PET 511-keV attenuation coefficients. Eur J Nucl Med Mol Imaging 2002;29:922–7.

105. Martinez-Möller A, Souvatzoglou M, Delso G, et al. Tissue classification as a potential approach for attenuation correction in whole-body PET/MRI: evaluation with PET/CT data. J Nucl Med 2009;50:520–6.

106. Schulz V, Torres-Espallardo I, Renisch S, et al. Automatic, three-segment, MR-based attenuation correction for whole-body PET/MR data. Eur J Nucl Med Mol Imaging 2011;38:138–52.

107. Hofmann M, Bezrukov I, Mantlik F, et al. MRI-based attenuation correction for whole-body PET/MRI: quantitative evaluation of segmentation-and atlas-based methods. J Nucl Med 2011;52:1392–9.

108. Arce-Calisaya P, Souvatzoglou M, Eiber M, et al. Sensitivity of PET/MRI to detect recurrence of prostate cancer. Eur J Nucl Med Mol Imaging 2013;40:799.

109. Lord M, Ratib O, Vallée J-P. 18F-fluorocholine integrated PET/MRI for the initial staging of prostate cancer. Eur J Nucl Med Mol Imaging 2011;38:2288.

# Metastatic Seeding Attacks Bone Marrow, Not Bone
## Rectifying Ongoing Misconceptions

William Y. Raynor, BS[a,b], Abdullah Al-Zaghal, MD[a],
Mahdi Zirakchian Zadeh, MD, MHM[c],
Siavash Mehdizadeh Seraj, MD[a],
Abass Alavi, MD, MD (Hon), PhD (Hon), DSc (Hon)[a,*]

**KEYWORDS**

• Skeletal metastasis • Bone marrow • Cancer • Bone scintigraphy • FDG • NaF • PET-CT

**KEY POINTS**

- Although bone scintigraphy and fluorine-18 ([18]F)-sodium fluoride PET–computed tomography (CT) portray osteoblastic reaction to malignant activity, [18]F-fluorodeoxyglucose (FDG) PET-CT can detect abnormal metabolism in cancer cells directly.
- FDG PET-CT and tumor-specific tracers are powerful modalities for detecting skeletal metastases that have not yet caused osseous manifestations.
- FDG PET-CT can be particularly useful for assessing the response of malignant cells to treatment.

## INTRODUCTION

Skeletal metastases often arise from hematogenous spread to the red marrow, which later causes bone remodeling at the site of the metastasis.[1] Seeding of tumor emboli can occur through the bloodstream, as well as by retrograde venous flow or direct extension. Circulating tumor stem cells adhere to the endothelial lining of blood vessels, extravasate into the bone marrow (BM) space, and degrade bone matrix by secreting proteolytic enzymes.[2] Starting at birth until the second decade of life, when most BM is hematopoietic red marrow, conversion of red marrow to fatty yellow marrow eventually results in the concentration of hematopoietic BM in the axial skeleton and proximal humerus and femur in adults (**Fig. 1**).[3] As a result, the axial skeleton is commonly involved in early metastatic disease,

whereas the extremities are typically spared.[4] After malignant cells have been seeded in the red marrow, osteoblasts and osteoclasts are involved in the remodeling of the surrounding bone and can result in a sclerotic, lytic, or mixed lesion visible with bone scintigraphy or radiographic studies (**Fig. 2**). However, local bone remodeling constitutes indirect evidence for tumor activity, and small intramedullary lesions are unlikely to be visualized. Therefore, molecular imaging modalities that directly characterize the metabolic activity of tumor cells can detect metastases earlier and assess response to therapy with greater sensitivity, justifying them as more appropriate in this setting.

In general, imaging modalities for skeletal metastases can be classified as detecting either disease in BM or subsequent bone reaction. Of the modalities that assess BM, MR imaging and BM

[a] Department of Radiology, University of Pennsylvania, 3400 Spruce Street, Philadelphia, PA 19104, USA;
[b] Department of Radiology, Drexel University College of Medicine, 230 N Broad Street, Philadelphia, PA 19102, USA; [c] Department of Radiology, Children's Hospital of Philadelphia, 3401 Civic Center Boulevard, Philadelphia, PA 19104, USA
* Corresponding author.
*E-mail address:* abass.alavi@uphs.upenn.edu

PET Clin 14 (2019) 135–144
https://doi.org/10.1016/j.cpet.2018.08.005

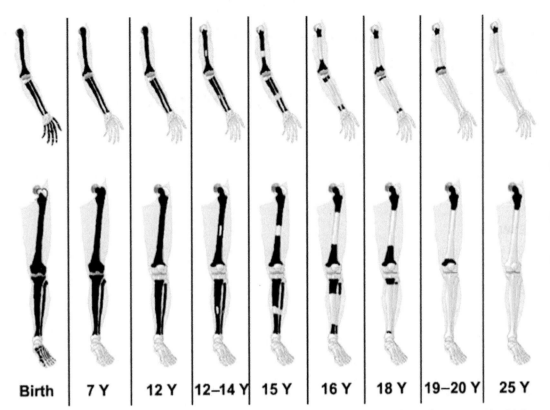

**Fig. 1.** The amount and distribution of red marrow in tubular bones from birth until 25 years. The highest amount of red marrow (*black*) is found at birth and it is converted to yellow marrow with age. These images clarify the lack of metastatic lesions in the extremities of adult population. In other words, lack of BM after the second decade of life in the distal part of the upper and lower extremities protects it from malignant invasion. (*From* Blebea JS, Houseni M, Torigian DA, et al, Structural and functional imaging of normal bone marrow and evaluation of its age-related changes. Semin Nucl Med 2007;37(3):186; with permission.)

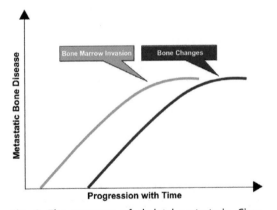

**Fig. 2.** The sequence of skeletal metastasis. Circulating tumor cells invade the highly vascularized BM as metastatic seeds, followed by a lag phase of unknown length comprising a dormant phase. Then, dysregulation of osteoclast-mediated bone resorption and osteoblast-mediated bone deposition by tumor cells leads to either osteoblastic or osteolytic phenotypes.

scintigraphy (BMS) visualize changes in the BM compartment, whereas PET combined with fluorine-18 ($^{18}$F)-fluorodeoxyglucose (FDG) or other specific tracers directly characterizes malignant tissue activity. Computed tomography (CT) is able to visualize cortical destruction and reactive bone formation, and bone scintigraphy and PET with $^{18}$F-sodium fluoride (NaF) portray osteoblastic lesions. The availability of these various modalities has led to controversy regarding the relative clinical utility of structural imaging modalities (CT and MR imaging), functional imaging modalities that assess abnormal activity in BM (FDG PET and others), and functional imaging modalities that assess osseous abnormalities (bone scintigraphy and NaF PET). Over the last 5 decades, bone scintigraphy was used in the initial screening for metastatic bone disease because it was low cost, widely available, and considered highly sensitive. However, the principles behind indirect assessment of skeletal metastases with bone scintigraphy, NaF PET, and CT have been called into question in favor of modalities that target the malignant activity in the BM.[5–8] This article discusses the strengths and limitations of both new and established functional modalities in the assessment of skeletal metastases.

## IMAGING OSSEOUS ABNORMALITIES AS INDIRECT EVIDENCE FOR TUMOR ACTIVITY

Conventional bone scintigraphy with tracers, such as technetium-99m ($^{99m}$Tc)-methylene diphosphonate (MDP), is commonly used to detect osteoblastic activity in response to bone destruction by cancer cells.[9–11] False-positive findings on bone scan can be due to fractures, osteoarthritis, or degenerative changes. Bone scintigraphy combined with CT has been shown to increase diagnostic accuracy.[12] In addition to studies with $^{99m}$Tc-MDP, functional imaging of bone can performed with NaF PET. Advantages of NaF as a tracer include higher plasma clearance and minimal serum protein binding, increasing the contrast in uptake between bone and soft tissue.[13] Furthermore, the use of PET rather than planar scintigraphy allows for increased resolution and sensitivity. Hydroxide ($OH^-$) ions on the surface of hydroxyapatite bone matrix exchange with the $^{18}F^-$ ion, occurring preferentially at sites of active mineralization.[14,15] NaF PET has been used to diagnose and assess metastases in breast cancer,[16–18] prostate cancer,[19–24] and non-small cell lung cancer.[24–26]

In a comparison between NaF PET-CT and NaF PET alone, 44 subjects with cancer with a variety of primary tumors were imaged with a hybrid PET-CT scanner.[27] Of the 111 malignant lesions identified by NaF PET, 94 were confirmed with lytic or sclerotic pattern on CT. Regarding the remaining lesions, 16 appeared normal on CT and 1 was falsely characterized as benign by PET-CT. Diagnosis of lesions was confirmed by histopathology, imaging, and clinical follow-up, or diagnostic CT or MR imaging. Combining NaF PET with CT increased specificity from 72% to 97% and sensitivity from 72% to 85%. In a similar study that compared findings of planar bone scintigraphy, single-photon emission CT (SPECT), NaF PET, and NaF PET-CT in 44 subjects with prostate cancer, NaF PET and NaF PET-CT were found to be more sensitive than SPECT, which was more sensitive than bone scintigraphy.[19] In 3 subjects with newly diagnosed disease, the presence of metastases was detected with NaF PET-CT that had been missed with bone scintigraphy, informing the alteration of patient management from local therapy to systemic therapy.

Several studies have used NaF PET to assess treatment response in metastatic prostate cancer with conflicting results regarding its utility.[23,28–30] A study in 60 subjects with prostate cancer undergoing primary definitive therapy and various antineoplastic therapies found significant associations between changes in NaF uptake and clinical impression, as well as overall survival.[23] Lesion response to radium-223 ($^{223}$Ra)-dichloride was assessed with NaF PET-CT in 10 metastatic castration-resistant prostate cancers.[28] Each subject underwent 6 treatment cycles, and imaging was performed before the first cycle, after the first cycle, and after the sixth cycle. Although response to therapy was evident by NaF PET-CT after the sixth cycle, the investigators determined that imaging after the first cycle was not informative about the treatment outcome. These findings were corroborated by a similar study in which 14 subjects were imaged at baseline, after 3 cycles of $^{223}$Ra, and after 6 cycles of $^{223}$Ra.[30] No significant association was found between skeletal disease burden after 3 cycles and after 6 cycles, suggesting that interim imaging is not useful in predicting treatment outcome.

Although longitudinal studies in larger patient settings would be of interest to explore the utility of NaF PET in assessing response to therapy, the shortcomings of indirectly imaging malignant skeletal involvement cannot be ignored. The role of these modalities must be reassessed while considering the advantages of FDG PET and the use of specific tracers that target cancer cell markers.

## ROLE OF FLUORINE-18-FLUORODEOXYGLUCOSE IN ASSESSING TUMOR CELL ACTIVITY

Increased glucose transport and utilization results in a high rate of glycolysis in tumor cells, which can be detected by FDG PET. By contrast, BMS visualizes normal BM without direct evidence of disease activity, which appears as a negative defect. FDG PET also has the advantages of increased spatial and contrast resolution, precise localization, and accurate quantification compared with BMS (**Fig. 3**).[31–35] Studies have shown that FDG PET is an effective modality for the detection of skeletal metastases.[34,36–39] The relative utilities of bone scintigraphy and FDG PET in detecting skeletal metastases have been compared, with controversial results.[10,40–43] The use of both imaging modalities may provide complementary information, and some studies suggest that bone scintigraphy may better detect sclerotic lesions whereas FDG PET is preferable for mixed and lytic lesions.[44–46] Other studies suggest that FDG PET-CT is more sensitive and specific

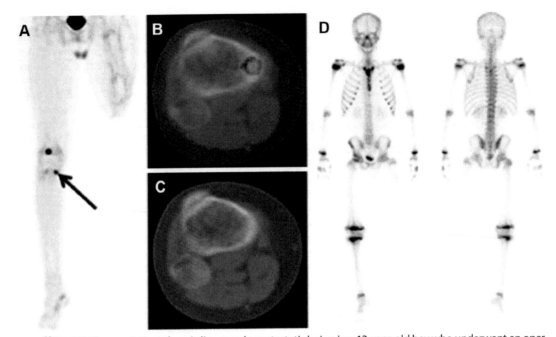

**Fig. 3.** $^{99m}$Tc-MDP bone scintigraphy misdiagnosed a metastatic lesion in a 13-year-old boy who underwent an operation for left femoral osteosarcoma 16 months previously. (*A, B*) Maximal intensity projection and fused transaxial images of FDG PET-CT showed a focal hypermetabolic lesion with a maximum standard uptake value of 7.4 in the right tibia, suggesting bone metastasis (*arrow*). Another focal hypermetabolic lesion also suggesting bone metastasis was noted in the right femur. These 2 lesions were confirmed as bone metastases with clinical follow-up. (*C*) A transaxial CT image of FDG PET-CT showed no significant lesion in the right tibia. (*D*) $^{99m}$Tc-MDP bone scintigraphy showed no definite high uptake in the right tibia except age-related growth plate region uptake. (*Reprinted by permission from* Springer Nature. *From* Byun, BH, et al. Comparison of (18)F-FDG PET/CT and (99 m)Tc-MDP bone scintigraphy for detection of bone metastasis in osteosarcoma. Skeletal Radiol, 2013. 42(12): p. 1678.)

compared with bone scintigraphy for detecting bone metastases.[47–50] Furthermore, FDG PET may be useful in selecting biopsy sites, assessing response to therapy, and improving staging.[36–38] Changes in FDG uptake with treatment of breast cancer were found to be significantly associated with changes in clinical assessment of response, tumor marker value, time to progression, and time to a skeletal-related event.[51,52]

A study comparing MR imaging, FDG PET, and bone scintigraphy imaged 21 pediatric subjects with a variety of malignancies and found that the sensitivity of FDG PET (90%) for detecting skeletal metastases was significantly higher compared with either of the other 2 modalities (82% for MR imaging, 71% for bone scintigraphy).[53] Another comparison between FDG PET and bone scintigraphy assessed metastases in 257 subjects with lung cancer and concluded that FDG PET was more accurate, sensitive, and specific.[34] Although NaF PET-CT is more sensitive in identifying osseous abnormalities, FDG PET-CT can better detect metastases to BM and small lytic lesions, allowing for superior prognostication in patients with breast cancer.[16]

A limitation of FDG PET in this setting is the effect of cytokine therapy, which increases FDG uptake in BM for up to 4 weeks and can mask or mimic lesions caused by skeletal metastasis.[54–56] Therefore, patients having completed cytokine therapy should delay imaging by FDG PET for at least 2 weeks. Additionally, FDG PET has been reported as having lower sensitivity for detecting sclerotic lesions, possibly due to the presence of fewer tumor cells or lower glycolytic activity.[57–60] The effectiveness of FDG PET in detecting skeletal metastases may be affected by tumor type and tumor biology, warranting future studies into discrepant results between studies. Despite these shortcomings, FDG PET has been shown to have many strengths in the application of skeletal metastases and can additionally provide information about the primary tumor, lymph node involvement, and metastases to other organs.

## PROSTATE-SPECIFIC MEMBRANE ANTIGEN

Prostate cancer is among the most frequently diagnosed malignancies in men older than the age of 50 years. With the introduction of modern quantitative techniques and advancements of imaging technology, it is now possible to identify previously undetectable metastatic lesions. This will result in a shift in the definition of disease assessment and improved outcomes. Skeletal bone is not uncommonly involved, and skeletal metastasis is seen in about 30% of the patients with predominant osteoblastic nature.[61] Over the last few decades, conventional imaging modalities, such as radiograph, CT, and bone scanning, were used to evaluate bone metastasis.

Over the last few years, radiolabeled gallium-68 ([68]Ga)–prostate-specific membrane antigen (PSMA) has been introduced as a novel radiopharmaceutical and powerful PET probe for the imaging of prostate cancer. Since then, the management of prostate cancer has changed dramatically (**Fig. 4**).[62–64] PSMA PET has a higher detection rate than standard bone scintigraphy regarding lesion number.[65] It is now commonly used to assess soft tissue metastatic and lymph node disease, in particular. However, there are a limited number of studies assessing the utility of this promising tracer in detecting bone lesions.[66] PSMA PET-CT scans show diagnostic potential but likely will not be available for widespread use in the United States for several years.

## CARBON-11 CHOLINE

Choline is an essential component of the phospholipids forming the cellular membrane. Prostate cancer cells have an increase in the proliferative level, as well as the activity, of the enzyme choline kinase, in turn, increasing the levels of choline.[67] Recent developments of new PET tracers, such as carbon-11 ([11]C)-choline and [18]F-choline, have shown promising results for the evaluation of bone metastasis in prostate cancer. A study by Picchio and colleagues,[68] which included 78 subjects with relapsing prostate cancer, found that [11]C-choline had a lower sensitivity (89% vs 100%) but significantly higher specificity (98% vs 75%) than bone scans. Fuccio and colleagues[69] studied 123 subjects with prostate cancer and reported a high sensitivity and specificity of [11]C-choline (86% and 100%, respectively) in the detection of bone metastatic lesions.

## EVOLVING ROLE OF DUAL-TIME-POINT IMAGING IN HEMATOLOGICAL MALIGNANCIES

It has been shown that FDG uptake in malignant tumors increases from 1-hour to 4-hour scans,

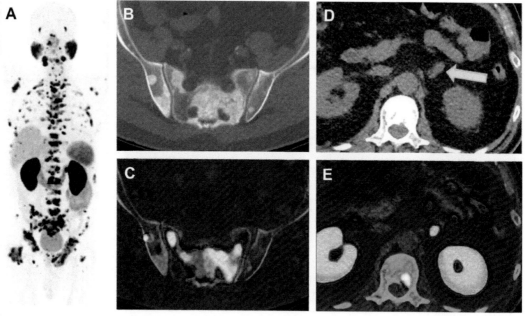

**Fig. 4.** A 75-year-old man with prostate cancer and known lymph node and bone metastases undergoing restaging with PSMA PET because of a rising prostate-specific antigen (252 ng/mL). On coronal (*A*) maximum intensity projection, disseminated intense uptake in the entire skeleton is visible. Axial CT images show the extensive sclerosis (*B*), corresponding to increased uptake on the fused PSMA PET-CT (*C*). A minimally enlarged suprarenal gland on the left would probably not have been reported as a suspicious lesion on CT (*yellow arrow*) (*D*); however, the intense PSMA accumulation suggested suprarenal gland metastasis (*E*). (*Reprinted by permission from Springer Nature. From Fankhauser, CD, et al. Current and potential future role of PSMA-PET in patients with castration-resistant prostate cancer. World J Urol, 2018 Jul 20. https://doi.org/10.1007/s00345-018-2408-2.*)

whereas benign and normal tissue show a decline in uptake 60 to 90 minutes after the administration of FDG. This allows optimal detection of malignant lesions on delayed scans.[70–72] Previous early and delayed imaging (or dual-time-point imaging [DTPI]) studies have demonstrated a promising role in distinguishing normal and inflammatory tissue from malignant lesions.[72,73] Percent increase or retention index could be useful in distinguishing malignant from benign activity in the BM because they have the same pattern of increasing FDG uptake with DTPI. Researchers had also correlated DTPI analysis with treatment response and disease outcome. For instance, Taghvaei and colleagues[74] determined the dynamics of FDG uptake in focal lesions in subjects with multiple myeloma between 1-hour and 3-hour scans with a novel method of FDG PET quantification (ROVER; ABX, Radeberg, Germany) (**Figs. 5** and **6**). This research was designed to demonstrate that change in FDG uptake over time could predict prognosis and disease outcomes in this population. The investigators noted that the increase in mean standardized uptake value ($SUV_{mean}$) and partial volume corrected $SUV_{mean}$ was significantly higher in lesions with a partial response compared with lesions with a complete response. Therefore, they concluded that percentage increase in FDG uptake from early to delayed scans could predict the degree of aggressiveness and response to chemotherapy.

## THE NECESSITY OF GLOBAL DISEASE ASSESSMENT IN OPTIMAL MANAGEMENT OF PATIENTS WITH CANCER

Currently, most PET images are assessed by assigning small regions of interest to several sites of abnormal uptake of FDG or other tracers to measure the degree of disease activity at baseline and following interventions. This approach is suboptimal due to a variety of technical factors and may provide misleading results. Small regions of interest lead to generating values that are substantially underestimated (partial volume effect) and, therefore, do not reflect the true levels of metabolic activity of the disease sites at various stages of management of patients with cancer.[75] Also, these measurements are nonreproducible because no clear-cut rules for assigning these regions have been established at this time. Furthermore, the results conveyed to the attending physicians are confusing because this approach provides an overload of standardized uptake values for multiple lesions and may not accurately guide physicians to adopt the appropriate course for managing their patients. Therefore, over the years, attempts have been made to correct for partial volume effect in each lesion and subsequently determine global disease activity for each abnormality and the entire disease sites based on their volume and corrected metabolic activity.[76,77] This logical

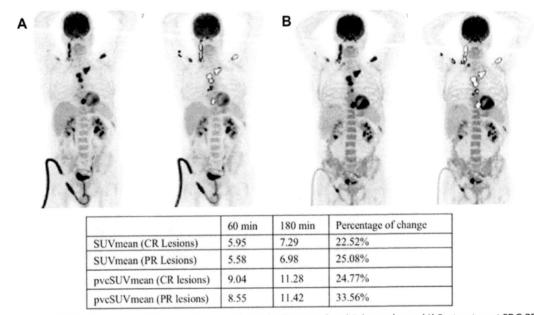

| | 60 min | 180 min | Percentage of change |
|---|---|---|---|
| SUVmean (CR Lesions) | 5.95 | 7.29 | 22.52% |
| SUVmean (PR Lesions) | 5.58 | 6.98 | 25.08% |
| pvcSUVmean (CR lesions) | 9.04 | 11.28 | 24.77% |
| pvcSUVmean (PR lesions) | 8.55 | 11.42 | 33.56% |

**Fig. 5.** FDG PET-CT scans of a 60-year-old man with newly diagnosed multiple myeloma. (*A*) Pretreatment FDG PET scan 1 hour after administration of FDG tracer. (*B*) Pretreatment FDG PET scan 3 hours after administration of FDG tracer (ROVER; ABX, Radeberg, Germany). The table shows the percentage of change in the $SUV_{mean}$ and $pvcSUV_{mean}$ of the CR and PR lesions in the patient from 1-hour to 3-hour scans. CR, complete response; PR, partial response; pvc, partial volume correction; $SUV_{mean}$, mean standardized uptake value.

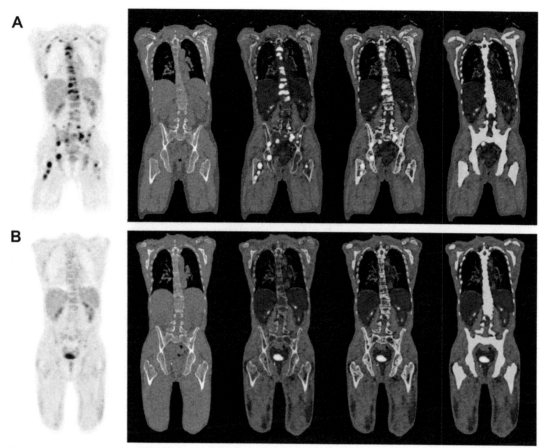

**Fig. 6.** Whole body FDG PET and fused FDG PET-CT images of a 60-year-old man diagnosed with multiple myeloma. Iterative threshold algorithm based on Hounsfield units, allowing the segmentation of the entire skeleton by a smoothing and closing algorithm (OsiriX software; Pixmeo SARL; Bernex, Switzerland), which provides global SUV$_{mean}$ (GSUV$_{mean}$) that represents whole BM involvement in multiple myeloma patients. (*A*) GSUV$_{mean}$ before initiating treatment was 2.02, whereas (*B*) after finishing the course of treatment the GSUV$_{mean}$ dropped to 1.10.

approach results in generating substantially robust numbers that are statistically reliable for making an informed decision. The authors believe global assessment is of great importance in assessing primary tumors, as well as metastatic sites, including lesions that are located in the skeletal system.

## SUMMARY

Although different tracers and modalities may provide complementary information regarding tumor biology, certain modalities are more accurate than others, depending on tumor type and tumor characteristics. FDG PET-CT and tumor-specific tracers have the potential to play an important role in detecting skeletal metastases that have not yet caused osseous manifestations, as well as the assessment of therapy. New radiopharmaceuticals are becoming available that may provide

additional methods that directly assess cancer cell metabolism, decreasing the usefulness of modalities that only provide information regarding osteoblastic reaction. FDG PET-CT should be the leading imaging modality in the evaluation of most malignant BM metastases, and the use of bone scintigraphy (conventional or PET-based) should be abandoned in the near future.

## REFERENCES

1. Morgan-Parkes JH. Metastases: mechanisms, pathways, and cascades. AJR Am J Roentgenol 1995; 164(5):1075–82.
2. Roodman GD. Mechanisms of bone metastasis. N Engl J Med 2004;350(16):1655–64.
3. Blebea JS, Houseni M, Torigian DA, et al. Structural and functional imaging of normal bone marrow and evaluation of its age-related changes. Semin Nucl Med 2007;37(3):185–94.

4. Kamby C, Guldhammer B, Vejborg I, et al. The presence of tumor cells in bone marrow at the time of first recurrence of breast cancer. Cancer 1987;60(6): 1306–12.

5. Lucignani G. Bone and marrow imaging: do we know what we see and do we see what we want to know? Eur J Nucl Med Mol Imaging 2007;34(7): 1123–6.

6. Basu S, Alavi A. Bone marrow and not bone is the primary site for skeletal metastasis: critical role of [18F]fluorodeoxyglucose positron emission tomography in this setting. J Clin Oncol 2007;25(10): 1297 [author reply: 1297–9].

7. Basu S, Torigian D, Alavi A. Evolving concept of imaging bone marrow metastasis in the twenty-first century: critical role of FDG-PET. Eur J Nucl Med Mol Imaging 2008;35(3):465–71.

8. Caglar M, Kupik O, Karabulut E, et al. Detection of bone metastases in breast cancer patients in the PET/CT era: do we still need the bone scan? Rev Esp Med Nucl Imagen Mol 2016;35(1):3–11.

9. Hamaoka T, Madewell JE, Podoloff DA, et al. Bone imaging in metastatic breast cancer. J Clin Oncol 2004;22(14):2942–53.

10. Shie P, Cardarelli R, Brandon D, et al. Meta-analysis: comparison of F-18 Fluorodeoxyglucose-positron emission tomography and bone scintigraphy in the detection of bone metastases in patients with breast cancer. Clin Nucl Med 2008;33(2):97–101.

11. Roberts CC, Daffner RH, Weissman BN, et al. ACR appropriateness criteria on metastatic bone disease. J Am Coll Radiol 2010;7(6):400–9.

12. Even-Sapir E. Imaging of malignant bone involvement by morphologic, scintigraphic, and hybrid modalities. J Nucl Med 2005;46(8):1356–67.

13. Blake GM, Fogelman I, Bone radionuclide imaging, quantitation and bone densitometry. In: McCready R, Gnanasegaran G, Bomanji JB, editors. A history of radionuclide studies in the UK: 50th Anniversary of the British Nuclear Medicine Society. Cham (CH): Springer; 2016. p. 111–20.

14. Bang S, Baud CA. Topographical distribution of fluoride in iliac bone of a fluoride-treated osteoporotic patient. J Bone Miner Res 1990;5(Suppl 1):S87–9.

15. Narita N, Kato K, Nakagaki H, et al. Distribution of fluoride concentration in the rat's bone. Calcif Tissue Int 1990;46(3):200–4.

16. Piccardo A, Puntoni M, Morbelli S, et al. 18F-FDG PET/CT is a prognostic biomarker in patients affected by bone metastases from breast cancer in comparison with 18F-NaF PET/CT. Nuklearmedizin 2015;54(4):163–72.

17. Abikhzer G, Srour S, Fried G, et al. Prospective comparison of whole-body bone SPECT and sodium 18F-fluoride PET in the detection of bone metastases from breast cancer. Nucl Med Commun 2016; 37(11):1160–8.

18. Brito AE, Santos A, Sasse AD, et al. 18F-Fluoride PET/CT tumor burden quantification predicts survival in breast cancer. Oncotarget 2017;8(22): 36001–11.

19. Even-Sapir E, Metser U, Mishani E, et al. The detection of bone metastases in patients with high-risk prostate cancer: 99mTc-MDP Planar bone scintigraphy, single- and multi-field-of-view SPECT, 18F-fluoride PET, and 18F-fluoride PET/CT. J Nucl Med 2006;47(2):287–97.

20. Minamimoto R, Loening A, Jamali M, et al. Prospective comparison of 99mTc-MDP scintigraphy, combined 18F-NaF and 18F-FDG PET/CT, and whole-body MRI in patients with breast and prostate cancer. J Nucl Med 2015;56(12):1862–8.

21. Etchebehere EC, Araujo JC, Fox PS, et al. Prognostic factors in patients treated with 223Ra: the role of skeletal tumor burden on baseline 18F-Fluoride PET/CT in predicting overall survival. J Nucl Med 2015;56(8):1177–84.

22. Hillner BE, Siegel BA, Hanna L, et al. 18F-fluoride PET used for treatment monitoring of systemic cancer therapy: results from the National Oncologic PET Registry. J Nucl Med 2015;56(2):222–8.

23. Apolo AB, Lindenberg L, Shih JH, et al. Prospective study evaluating Na18F PET/CT in predicting clinical outcomes and survival in advanced prostate cancer. J Nucl Med 2016;57(6):886–92.

24. Damle NA, Bal C, Bandopadhyaya GP, et al. The role of 18F-fluoride PET-CT in the detection of bone metastases in patients with breast, lung and prostate carcinoma: a comparison with FDG PET/CT and 99mTc-MDP bone scan. Jpn J Radiol 2013; 31(4):262–9.

25. Kruger S, Buck AK, Mottaghy FM, et al. Detection of bone metastases in patients with lung cancer: 99mTc-MDP planar bone scintigraphy, 18F-fluoride PET or 18F-FDG PET/CT. Eur J Nucl Med Mol Imaging 2009;36(11):1807–12.

26. Rao L, Zong Z, Chen Z, et al. 18F-Labeled NaF PET-CT in detection of bone metastases in patients with preoperative lung cancer. Medicine (Baltimore) 2016;95(16):e3490.

27. Even-Sapir E, Metser U, Flusser G, et al. Assessment of malignant skeletal disease: initial experience with 18F-fluoride PET/CT and comparison between 18F-fluoride PET and 18F-fluoride PET/CT. J Nucl Med 2004;45(2):272–8.

28. Kairemo K, Joensuu T. Radium-223-dichloride in castration resistant metastatic prostate cancer-preliminary results of the response evaluation using F-18-Fluoride PET/CT. Diagnostics (Basel) 2015; 5(4):413–27.

29. Murray I, Chittenden SJ, Denis-Bacelar AM, et al. The potential of (223)Ra and (18)F-fluoride imaging to predict bone lesion response to treatment with (223)Ra-dichloride in castration-resistant prostate

cancer. Eur J Nucl Med Mol Imaging 2017;44(11): 1832–44.

30. Kairemo K, Milton DR, Etchebehere E, et al. Final outcome of 223Ra-therapy and the role of 18F-fluoride-PET in response evaluation in metastatic castration resistant prostate cancer -a single institution experience. Curr Radiopharm 2018;11(2):147–52.

31. Basu S, Zaidi H, Houseni M, et al. Novel quantitative techniques for assessing regional and global function and structure based on modern imaging modalities: implications for normal variation, aging and diseased states. Semin Nucl Med 2007;37(3): 223–39.

32. Durski JM, Srinivas S, Segall G. Comparison of FDG-PET and bone scans for detecting skeletal metastases in patients with non-small cell lung cancer. Clin Positron Imaging 2000;3(3):97–105.

33. El-Haddad G, Zhuang H, Gupta N, et al. Evolving role of positron emission tomography in the management of patients with inflammatory and other benign disorders. Semin Nucl Med 2004;34(4): 313–29.

34. Cheran SK, Herndon JE 2nd, Patz EF Jr. Comparison of whole-body FDG-PET to bone scan for detection of bone metastases in patients with a new diagnosis of lung cancer. Lung Cancer 2004;44(3): 317–25.

35. Alavi A, Lakhani P, Mavi A, et al. PET: a revolution in medical imaging. Radiol Clin North Am 2004;42(6): 983–1001, vii.

36. Kumar R, Maillard I, Schuster SJ, et al. Utility of fluorodeoxyglucose-PET imaging in the management of patients with Hodgkin's and non-Hodgkin's lymphomas. Radiol Clin North Am 2004;42(6): 1083–100.

37. Kumar R, Chawla M, Basu S, et al. PET and PET-CT imaging in treatment monitoring of breast cancer. PET Clin 2009;4(4):359–69.

38. Moog F, Bangerter M, Kotzerke J, et al. 18-F-fluorodeoxyglucose-positron emission tomography as a new approach to detect lymphomatous bone marrow. J Clin Oncol 1998;16(2):603–9.

39. Mavi A, Lakhani P, Zhuang H, et al. Fluorodeoxyglucose-PET in characterizing solitary pulmonary nodules, assessing pleural diseases, and the initial staging, restaging, therapy planning, and monitoring response of lung cancer. Radiol Clin North Am 2005;43(1):1–21, ix.

40. Niikura N, Costelloe CM, Madewell JE, et al. FDG-PET/CT compared with conventional imaging in the detection of distant metastases of primary breast cancer. Oncologist 2011;16(8):1111–9.

41. Balci TA, Koc ZP, Komek H. Bone scan or (18)f-fluorodeoxyglucose positron emission tomography/computed tomography; which modality better shows bone metastases of breast cancer? Breast Care (Basel) 2012;7(5):389–93.

42. Schirrmeister H, Guhlmann A, Elsner K, et al. Sensitivity in detecting osseous lesions depends on anatomic localization: planar bone scintigraphy versus 18F PET. J Nucl Med 1999;40(10):1623–9.

43. Hong S, Li J, Wang S. 18FDG PET-CT for diagnosis of distant metastases in breast cancer patients. A meta-analysis. Surg Oncol 2013;22(2):139–43.

44. Hsu WK, Virk MS, Feeley BT, et al. Characterization of osteolytic, osteoblastic, and mixed lesions in a prostate cancer mouse model using 18F-FDG and 18F-fluoride PET/CT. J Nucl Med 2008;49(3):414–21.

45. Chua S, Gnanasegaran G, Cook GJ. Miscellaneous cancers (lung, thyroid, renal cancer, myeloma, and neuroendocrine tumors): role of SPECT and PET in imaging bone metastases. Semin Nucl Med 2009; 39(6):416–30.

46. Cook GJ, Houston S, Rubens R, et al. Detection of bone metastases in breast cancer by 18FDG PET: differing metabolic activity in osteoblastic and osteolytic lesions. J Clin Oncol 1998;16(10):3375–9.

47. Rong J, Wang S, Ding Q, et al. Comparison of 18 FDG PET-CT and bone scintigraphy for detection of bone metastases in breast cancer patients. A meta-analysis. Surg Oncol 2013;22(2):86–91.

48. Abe K, Sasaki M, Kuwabara Y, et al. Comparison of 18FDG-PET with 99mTc-HMDP scintigraphy for the detection of bone metastases in patients with breast cancer. Ann Nucl Med 2005;19(7):573–9.

49. Hahn S, Heusner T, Kümmel S, et al. Comparison of FDG-PET/CT and bone scintigraphy for detection of bone metastases in breast cancer. Acta Radiol 2011;52(9):1009–14.

50. Bury T, Barreto A, Daenen F, et al. Fluorine-18 deoxyglucose positron emission tomography for the detection of bone metastases in patients with non-small cell lung cancer. Eur J Nucl Med 1998;25(9): 1244–7.

51. Specht JM, Tam SL, Kurland BF, et al. Serial 2-[18F] fluoro-2-deoxy-D-glucose positron emission tomography (FDG-PET) to monitor treatment of bone-dominant metastatic breast cancer predicts time to progression (TTP). Breast Cancer Res Treat 2007; 105(1):87–94.

52. Stafford SE, Gralow JR, Schubert EK, et al. Use of serial FDG PET to measure the response of bone-dominant breast cancer to therapy. Acad Radiol 2002;9(8):913–21.

53. Daldrup-Link HE, Franzius C, Link TM, et al. Whole-body MR imaging for detection of bone metastases in children and young adults: comparison with skeletal scintigraphy and FDG PET. AJR Am J Roentgenol 2001;177(1):229–36.

54. Gundlapalli S, Ojha B, Mountz JM. Granulocyte colony-stimulating factor: confounding F-18 FDG uptake in outpatient positron emission tomographic facilities for patients receiving ongoing treatment of lymphoma. Clin Nucl Med 2002;27(2):140–1.

55. Hollinger EF, Alibazoglu H, Ali A, et al. Hematopoietic cytokine-mediated FDG uptake simulates the appearance of diffuse metastatic disease on whole-body PET imaging. Clin Nucl Med 1998; 23(2):93–8.

56. Sugawara Y, Fisher SJ, Zasadny KR, et al. Preclinical and clinical studies of bone marrow uptake of fluorine-1-fluorodeoxyglucose with or without granulocyte colony-stimulating factor during chemotherapy. J Clin Oncol 1998;16(1):173–80.

57. Shreve PD, Grossman HB, Gross MD, et al. Metastatic prostate cancer: initial findings of PET with 2-deoxy-2-[F-18]fluoro-D-glucose. Radiology 1996; 199(3):751–6.

58. Yeh SD, Imbriaco M, Larson SM, et al. Detection of bony metastases of androgen-independent prostate cancer by PET-FDG. Nucl Med Biol 1996;23(6):693–7.

59. Morris MJ, Akhurst T, Osman I, et al. Fluorinated deoxyglucose positron emission tomography imaging in progressive metastatic prostate cancer. Urology 2002;59(6):913–8.

60. Fogelman I, Cook G, Israel O, et al. Positron emission tomography and bone metastases. Semin Nucl Med 2005;35(2):135–42.

61. Bubendorf L, Schöpfer A, Wagner U, et al. Metastatic patterns of prostate cancer: an autopsy study of 1,589 patients. Hum Pathol 2000;31(5):578–83.

62. Afshar-Oromieh A, Malcher A, Eder M, et al. PET imaging with a [68Ga]gallium-labelled PSMA ligand for the diagnosis of prostate cancer: biodistribution in humans and first evaluation of tumour lesions. Eur J Nucl Med Mol Imaging 2013;40(4):486–95.

63. Afshar-Oromieh A, Haberkorn U, Eder M, et al. [68Ga]Gallium-labelled PSMA ligand as superior PET tracer for the diagnosis of prostate cancer: comparison with 18F-FECH. Eur J Nucl Med Mol Imaging 2012;39(6):1085–6.

64. Eder M, Schäfer M, Bauder-Wüst U, et al. 68Ga-complex lipophilicity and the targeting property of a urea-based PSMA inhibitor for PET imaging. Bioconjug Chem 2012;23(4):688–97.

65. Pyka T, Okamoto S, Dahlbender M, et al. Comparison of bone scintigraphy and (68)Ga-PSMA PET for skeletal staging in prostate cancer. Eur J Nucl Med Mol Imaging 2016;43(12):2114–21.

66. Fankhauser CD, Poyet C, Kroeze SGC, et al. Current and potential future role of PSMA-PET in patients with castration-resistant prostate cancer. World J Urol 2018. https://doi.org/10.1007/s00345-018-2408-2.

67. Richter JA, Rodríguez M, Rioja J, et al. Dual tracer 11C-choline and FDG-PET in the diagnosis of biochemical prostate cancer relapse after radical treatment. Mol Imaging Biol 2010;12(2):210–7.

68. Picchio M, Spinapolice EG, Fallanca F, et al. [11C] Choline PET/CT detection of bone metastases in patients with PSA progression after primary treatment for prostate cancer: comparison with bone scintigraphy. Eur J Nucl Med Mol Imaging 2012;39(1): 13–26.

69. Fuccio C, Castellucci P, Schiavina R, et al. Role of 11C-choline PET/CT in the re-staging of prostate cancer patients with biochemical relapse and negative results at bone scintigraphy. Eur J Radiol 2012; 81(8):e893–6.

70. Basu S, Kung J, Houseni M, et al. Temporal profile of fluorodeoxyglucose uptake in malignant lesions and normal organs over extended time periods in patients with lung carcinoma: implications for its utilization in assessing malignant lesions. Q J Nucl Med Mol Imaging 2009;53(1):9–19.

71. Boerner AR, Weckesser M, Herzog H, et al. Optimal scan time for fluorine-18 fluorodeoxyglucose positron emission tomography in breast cancer. Eur J Nucl Med 1999;26(3):226–30.

72. Houshmand S, Salavati A, Segtnan EA, et al. Dual-time-point imaging and delayed-time-point fluorodeoxyglucose-PET/computed tomography imaging in various clinical settings. PET Clin 2016;11(1): 65–84.

73. Kumar R, Loving VA, Chauhan A, et al. Potential of dual-time-point imaging to improve breast cancer diagnosis with (18)F-FDG PET. J Nucl Med 2005; 46(11):1819–24.

74. Taghvaei R, Oestergaard B, Zadeh MZ, et al. Correlation of dual time point FDG-PET with response to chemotherapy in multiple myeloma. J Nucl Med 2017;58(Suppl. 1).

75. Alavi A, Werner TJ, Høilund-Carlsen PF, et al. Correction for partial volume effect is a must, not a luxury, to fully exploit the potential of quantitative PET imaging in clinical oncology. Mol Imaging Biol 2018;20(1):1–3.

76. Basu S, Zaidi H, Salavati A, et al. FDG PET/CT methodology for evaluation of treatment response in lymphoma: from "graded visual analysis" and "semiquantitative SUVmax" to global disease burden assessment. Eur J Nucl Med Mol Imaging 2014; 41(11):2158–60.

77. Houshmand S, Salavati A, Hess S, et al. An update on novel quantitative techniques in the context of evolving whole-body PET imaging. PET Clin 2015; 10(1):45–58.

# Pediatric Musculoskeletal Imaging
## The Indications for and Applications of PET/ Computed Tomography

Hedieh Khalatbari, MD, MBA[a],*,
Marguerite T. Parisi, MD, MS[a,b], Neha Kwatra, MD[c],
Douglas J. Harrison, MD, MS[d], Barry L. Shulkin, MD, MBA[e]

## KEYWORDS

• PET/CT • FDG • 18F • Pediatric • Musculoskeletal

## KEY POINTS

- Fluorodeoxyglucose (FDG) PET/computed tomography (CT) is useful for pediatric patients with oncologic disorders.
- FDG PET/CT is useful for pediatric patients with inflammatory/infectious disorders.
- 18F sodium fluoride is an excellent bone imaging agent.

## INTRODUCTION

In PET/computed tomography (CT), the functional data provided by the use of a positron-emitting radiopharmaceutical is combined with the anatomic information, higher spatial resolution, and tissue characterization of CT. The most common indications for the performance of musculoskeletal PET/CT in children include the diagnosis, staging, and therapeutic response monitoring of malignancy primarily using fluorine-18 fluorodeoxyglucose ($^{18}$F-FDG) and, with the resurgence of interest in fluoride-18 sodium fluoride imaging ($^{18}$F-NaF), skeletal trauma. Unlike in adults, there is a limited role for $^{18}$F-FDG PET/CT in the evaluation of musculoskeletal infections in children, although the introduction of newer radiotracers such as Gallium-68 ($^{68}$Ga) may change that dynamic.

PET/magnetic resonance (MR) is a promising hybrid modality that combines the functional information provided by a positron-emitting radiopharmaceutical with MR rather than CT. The MR component is used not only for attenuation correction but to provide anatomic and, using diffusion-weighted imaging, another type of functional information. Compared with CT, MR has superior soft tissue contrast and its lack of ionizing radiation is of particular importance in the pediatric population, which is believed to be more sensitive to the effects of ionizing radiation than are adults. To date, the use of PET/MR has been hampered by equipment costs, difficulties with attenuation correction in lung and bone, and the long scanning times involved in imaging compared with PET/CT.[1,2] Despite the potential advantages

The authors have no conflicts of interest to report regarding this article.
[a] Department of Radiology, University of Washington School of Medicine, Seattle Children's Hospital, 4800 Sandpoint Way NE, Seattle, WA 98105, USA; [b] Department of Pediatrics, University of Washington School of Medicine, Seattle Children's Hospital, 4800 Sandpoint Way NE, Seattle, WA 98105, USA; [c] Division of Nuclear Medicine and Molecular Imaging, Department of Radiology, Boston Children's Hospital, Harvard Medical School, 300 Longwood Avenue, Boston, MA 02115, USA; [d] Department of Pediatrics, MD Anderson Cancer Center, 7600 Beechnut Street, Houston, TX 77074, USA; [e] Department of Diagnostic Imaging, St Jude Children's Research Hospital, 262 Danny Thomas Place, Memphis, TN 38105, USA
* Corresponding author. Department of Radiology, Seattle Children's Hospital, MA.7.220, 4800 Sandpoint Way Northeast, Seattle, WA 98105.
E-mail address: Hedieh.khalatbari@seattlechildrens.org

PET Clin 14 (2019) 145–174
https://doi.org/10.1016/j.cpet.2018.08.008
1556-8598/19/© 2018 Elsevier Inc. All rights reserved.

of PET-MR, a discussion of the pediatric musculo-skeletal applications of this technique is beyond the scope of this article.

## SPECIAL CONSIDERATIONS WHEN PERFORMING MUSCULOSKELETAL PET/COMPUTED TOMOGRAPHY IN CHILDREN

It is of utmost importance when performing PET/CT in children to be cognizant of the unique differences between children and adults. Children are not just small adults. There are age-related developmental and physiologic variants that can mimic pathology. Familiarity with these processes is often a key component to the proper interpretation of musculoskeletal PET/CT in children. For example, increased uptake may be a normal variant seen in the Waldeyer ring, the thymus, and activated brown adipose tissue. Physiologically increased uptake is present in the physes before adulthood.[3,4] Moreover, there are differences in the disease processes, their presentations, and patterns of involvement when encountered in children as opposed to adults.

Recently, there has been debate concerning the validity of the linear no-dose threshold theory as it relates to the health effects of the low-dose radiation exposure that occurs with diagnostic imaging.[5] Despite this controversy, there is evidence that the risk of adverse, radiation-induced health effects is greater in children than adults.[6,7] Not only are children said to be more sensitive to radiation than adults, they have a longer expected life span in which to manifest radiation-induced injury. Consequently, it is in the best interest of the pediatric patient not only to ensure that when requested, musculoskeletal PET-CT imaging is the right test, performed using the "right dose, for the right patient, at the right time," but that the imaging procedure is performed to the highest technical standards, using the lowest administered radiopharmaceutical dose that will result in obtaining appropriate diagnostic information.[8]

In an effort to reduce pediatric radiation exposures related to nuclear medicine procedures, 2 groups, one in North America and the second in Europe, developed guidelines for administered radiopharmaceutical activities in children.[9,10] These easily accessible consensus guidelines for pediatric-specific, weight-based radiopharmaceutical administered activities have since been harmonized[11] and recently updated.[12,13] These guidelines should be used when performing musculoskeletal PET/CT in children of all ages.

It should be recognized that performing PET-CT results in a higher radiation dose to the patient than performing PET alone.[14,15] The incremental increase in radiation dose depends on the type of CT performed. There are several options for the type of CT used in PET/CT imaging.[15]

These include diagnostic CT for attenuation correction and localization (2–10 mSV), low-dose CT for attenuation correction and localization (0.3–2.2 mSV radiation dose), selective (limited or bone localization) CT (0.2–1 mSV radiation dose), and ultralow-dose CT for attenuation correction only (0.06–0.3 mSV radiation dose).[14,15] When determining the imaging protocol, each case should be evaluated individually, using best practices to adjust CT parameters to a lower radiation dose while maintaining diagnostic utility. The recent review article by Parisi and colleagues[15] discusses various strategies to optimize the performance of pediatric PET-CT, including dose reduction strategies, as well as special considerations in patient preparation, image acquisition, and interpretation that are unique to children, including the need for whole-body imaging (**Fig. 1**).

## RADIOTRACERS FOR MUSCULOSKELETAL PET/COMPUTED TOMOGRAPHY
### *18F-Fluorodeoxyglucose*

18F-FDG, the most widely used of all PET radiotracers, is a glucose analog that is carried into cells by the glucose transport system. Once within the cell, 18F-FDG is converted to 18F-2'-FDG-6-phosphate, which unlike glucose is then trapped and accumulates at a rate proportionate to glucose utilization.[16] Both malignant and activated infectious or inflammatory cells use glucose as an energy source, resulting in high 18F-FDG accumulation at sites of malignancy, inflammation, and infection.

There are several advantages of performing 18F-FDG PET/CT for musculoskeletal imaging compared with the conventional nuclear medicine techniques such as technetium 99m-methylene diphosphonate bone scan ($^{99m}$Tc-MDP) or labeled white blood cell scans. These include high spatial and contrast resolution, high target to background ratios, short imaging times, precise localization of abnormalities, high sensitivity, high interobserver agreement, and, when optimized protocols are used, relatively low radiation dose compared with either $^{67}$Gallium ($^{67}$Ga) citrate or radiolabeled white blood cell imaging for tumors and/or infection.[17] Although disadvantages include somewhat limited availability, relatively high cost, and the need for sedation in young children, the most important limitation of 18F-FDG is the inability to use this radiotracer to reliably distinguish infection from noninfectious inflammation or malignancy.[18]

The most common indication for the performance of 18F-FDG PET/CT musculoskeletal

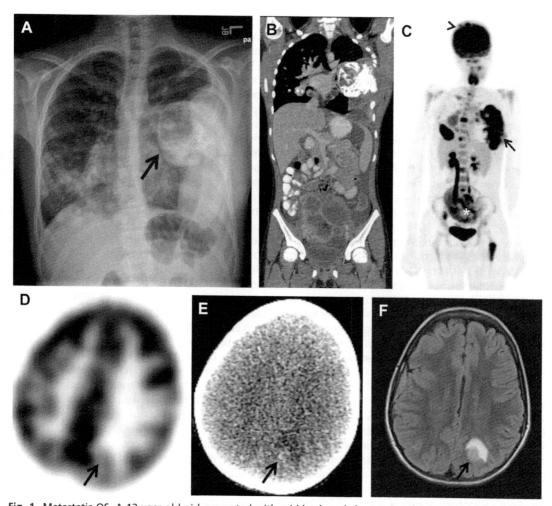

**Fig. 1.** Metastatic OS. A 13-year-old girl presented with mid-back and chest pain. Chest radiograph (*A*) demonstrated a partially calcified chest wall mass (*arrow*), left pleural effusion, and multiple bilateral pulmonary nodules. Coronal soft tissue image from a contrast-enhanced CT of the chest, abdomen, and pelvis (*B*) confirmed the findings identified on plain film imaging and, further, identified a second necrotic soft tissue mass (*asterisk*) in the pelvis in addition to several vertebral lytic bone metastases (not shown). Anterior maximal intensity projection (MIP) image (*C*) from a whole-body $^{18}$F-FDG PET/CT scan demonstrates not only the hypermetabolic (SUV$_{max}$ 13.6) primary left chest wall mass (*arrow*), multiple pulmonary nodules and the necrotic soft tissue mass in the pelvis (*asterisk*), but confirms the presence of multiple sites of osseous metastatic disease involving multilevel vertebral bodies, the right iliac bone, proximal left proximal femur, and the right calvarium (*arrowhead* in [*C*]). Close attention to the axial PET (*D*) and corresponding low-dose CT (*E*) images through the brain in this patient demonstrated an unsuspected, subtle left parietal lobe metastasis (*arrows* in [*D*] and [*E*]), confirmed on corresponding T2 fluid-attenuated inversion recovery (FLAIR) image (*F*) of the brain MR imaging (*arrow* in [*F*]). This case not only demonstrates the exquisite sensitivity of $^{18}$F-FDG PET/CT in the diagnosis and staging of osteosarcoma, but also illustrates the importance of obtaining whole-body PET/CT in children of all ages.

imaging in children is oncologic, including the diagnosis, staging, and therapeutic response monitoring of a variety of malignancies. The pediatric malignancies that are typically evaluated with $^{18}$F-FDG PET-CT include Hodgkin and non-Hodgkin lymphomas, primary and secondary bone as well as soft tissue sarcomas, and those neuroblastomas that are nonavid or poorly avid on $^{123}$Iodine ($^{123}$I) metaiodobenzylguanidine (mIBG) scanning. Less common oncologic applications include evaluation for potential malignant transformation of a plexiform neurofibroma in neurofibromatosis type 1 as well as detection of the primary site of disease in those with malignancy and an unknown primary.[19,20]

The use of $^{18}$F-FDG in the identification of and therapeutic response monitoring of those with infection continues to increase, particularly in adults. In children, [18]F-FDG use has been reported in a variety of infectious and inflammatory conditions,[21–23] most pertinent to this review, acute and chronic osteomyelitis.[24,25]

The recommended European Association of Nuclear Medicine (EANM) administered activity for a whole-body [18]F-FDG PET/CT study is calculated by multiplying the baseline activity of 25.9 Megabecquerel (MBq) by a multiple based on the patient's weight; this multiple ranges from 1 to 14 for patients weighing 1 to 68 kg, respectively, with a minimum administered activity of 26 MBq.[13] In the 1-year to 15-year age group, these doses will result in an effective dose range of 6.7 to 7.2 mSv.[26] In the 2016 version of the North American (NA) consensus guidelines, the proposed administered activity for [18]F-FDG is 3.6 to 5.2 MBq/kg (0.1–0.14 mCi/kg) with the recommendation that the low end of the range be used in smaller patients. It is also important to consider the imaging time per bed position as a factor in choosing the appropriate radiopharmaceutical administered dose, as longer bed position time may allow for decrease in administered [18]F-FDG dose.[12,27]

## [18]F-Sodium Fluoride

Blau and colleagues[28] first demonstrated the clinical utility of [18]F-NaF for bone scanning in 1962. This radiopharmaceutical was later approved for use by the US Food and Drug Administration (FDA) in 1972. Although [18]F-NaF proved to be an excellent radiopharmaceutical for bone imaging, there were important technical and logistic limitations to its use. These included the need to use rectilinear scanners with thick crystals because of high-energy 511 keV annihilation photons produced by the decay of [18]F, as well as the relatively short physical half-life of the radiotracer (110 minutes). With the wider availability of Molybdenum-99/Technetium-99m ([99]Mo/[99m]Tc) generators, increasing use of Anger-type gamma cameras, and the introduction of diphosphonates in the 1970s, there was a sharp decline in the use of [18]F-NaF. [99m]Tc-labeled diphosphonates, particularly [99m]Tc-MDP were accepted as, and still remain, the radiopharmaceutical agent of choice for skeletal scintigraphy.[29,30]

Beginning in the 1990s, there was a resurgence of interest in the use of [18]F-NaF for bone imaging. This was due to the concomitant development of clinical PET scanners and resultant robust commercial systems for production, use, and ready delivery of positron-emitting agents, including [18]F-FDG and [18]F-NaF. Currently, more widespread use of [18]F-NaF has been hindered by extensive past experience with [99m]Tc-MDP scintigraphy and reimbursement concerns at most sites, particularly in pediatrics.[31,32]

[18]F-NaF demonstrates a similar uptake pattern but has superior pharmacokinetic characteristics compared with [99m]Tc-MDP. Injected [18]F-NaF is rapidly cleared from the plasma in a biexponential manner.[33] All of the [18]F-NaF that is delivered to bone is retained initially on the surface of the hydroxyapatite matrix by chemisorption and subsequently incorporated in to the crystalline matrix.[34] There is minimal binding of the [18]F-NaF to serum proteins compared with 30% binding for MDP, which results in greater single-pass extraction by bone and rapid clearance of activity from blood, thereby allowing bone imaging in less than an hour after injection, compared with 3 to 4 hours with MDP.[19,35,36] The total uptake of [18]F-NaF by the bone is approximately twofold higher in comparison with a similar dose of MDP, improving sensitivity. The localization of [18]F-NaF in the skeleton is dependent on regional blood flow, as well as on new bone formation, and is cleared from the body by renal excretion similar to MDP.

Similar to [18]F-FDG PET/CT, advantages of [18]F-NaF PET/CT include high bone-to-background ratios and short imaging times. One limitation of [18]F-NaF is that its effective dose is approximately 70% higher than the effective dose of [99m]Tc-MDP. However, the high bone-to-background ratio of [18]F-NaF permits a 50% reduction in injected radiopharmaceutical administered activity without adverse effect on image quality. Using this approach, the effective doses of [18]F-NaF and [99m]Tc-MDP would be comparable.[37] In fact, the higher sensitivity, improved image quality, and shorter imaging times achieved with [18]F-NaF PET/CT have led some investigators to propose it be used as an alternative to [99m]Tc-MDP scintigraphy for musculoskeletal applications in children.[19,38]

The Society of Nuclear Medicine practice guidelines for the performance and interpretation of [18]F-NaF PET suggest that it might be appropriate for imaging a variety of benign and malignant skeletal conditions.[39] In the pediatric setting, the more common indications include assessment of back pain, sports-related bone injuries, nonaccidental trauma (NAT), and other benign tumors, with more limited experience with malignant bone tumors and detection of metastases.[38,40–43]

Although dose estimates may vary with the use of different models of [18]F-NaF and [99m]Tc-MDP biokinetics, the effective dose resulting from [18]F-NaF PET is largely similar to an appropriate weight-based administered activity of [99m]Tc-MDP.[36,43] The updated North American Consensus Guidelines recommend an [18]F-NaF dose of 2.2 MBq/kg (0.06 mCi/kg) with a minimum activity of 14 MBq (0.38 mCi).[12] The radiation exposure from low-dose CT performed for skeletal localization is similar for $^{18}$F-NaF PET/CT and $^{99m}$Tc-MDP single-photon emission CT (SPECT)/CT.

## Gallium-68

Newly added to the PET-CT armamentarium are a number of radiotracers labeled with $^{68}$Ga, a generator-derived positron-emitter, which can be used in the imaging of infection and inflammation in both preclinical and clinical settings[44] as well as in the identification, staging, and therapeutic response monitoring of somatostatin receptor tumors such as pheochromocytoma, carcinoid, and in children, neuroblastoma.[45]

$^{67}$Gallium citrate, the predecessor of $^{68}$Ga-citrate, has been used for infection imaging. The mechanism of uptake for both of these radiotracers includes both nonspecific and specific processes, including vasodilation, binding to transferrin in plasma, as well as binding to lactoferrin and siderophores.[46] $^{68}$Ga has advantages compared with $^{67}$Ga, including shorter half-life, improved and expanded labeling choices thereby allowing linkage to different compounds via chelators, shorter imaging times, and improved dosimetry. $^{68}$Ga-labeled PET/CT also enables much higher-quality images compared with $^{67}$Ga SPECT imaging.[44]

According to the 2016 NA consensus guidelines, the administered activity of $^{68}$GA-DOTATOC or $^{68}$Ga-DOTATATE is 2.7 MBq/kg (0.074 mCi/kg) with a minimum and maximum administered activity of 14 MBq (0.38 mCi) and 185 MBq (5 mCi), respectively.[12,47]

## INDICATIONS FOR IMAGING AND THE USE OF PET/COMPUTED TOMOGRAPHY PARAMETERS AS SURROGATE BIOMARKERS

The main indications for anatomic and functional imaging in malignancy include diagnosis, evaluation of the local extent of the primary site, tumor grading, staging, including the detection of metastases, evaluating response to treatment, and screening for recurrence. $^{18}$F-FDG PET/CT also has been used to determine the best site for tumor biopsy. Another, equally important role for PET/CT in tumor imaging is as a surrogate biomarker of response that can be used for prognostication, either at the time of initial diagnosis or after neoadjuvant chemotherapy. Prognostication is valuable, as it may guide treatment intensification (administering more therapy to achieve an excellent outcome) or deintensification (administering less

therapy to achieve an excellent outcome). Many of the studies investigating the role of $^{18}$F-FDG PET/CT for prognostication in bone sarcomas as well as other, nonmusculoskeletal malignancies suffer from small sample size, heterogeneity of sample, and retrospective nature.

The PET/CT parameters or radiotracer uptake metrics that have been used in prognostication, primarily although not exclusively with $^{18}$F-FDG, have included the following[48,49]:

- Maximum standardized uptake value ($SUV_{max}$) at diagnosis and after a variable number of cycles of chemotherapy (pretherapeutic and posttherapeutic; ie, SUV1 and SUV2, respectively), as well as change in $SUV_{max}$ between the 2 studies
- Total lesion glycolysis (TLG) which is defined as metabolic tumor volume (MTV) multiplied by mean SUV ($SUV_{mean}$)
  - MTV is defined as the volume of tumor with activity above a specified threshold[50]
  - $SUV_{mean}$ is defined as the average SUV in a region of interest and is less susceptible to noise than $SUV_{max}$
- Lean body mass corrected SUV peak ($SUL_{peak}$) is measured by placing a 1.2-cm-diameter region of interest (1 $cm^3$ volume sphere) in the most FDG-avid portion of the tumor and correcting the SUV for lean body mass[51]
  - $SUL_{peak}$ is a metric for the "Positron Emission Response Criteria in Solid Tumors" (PERCIST) 1.0 criteria[51]

Multiple investigators have tried to correlate these parameters with clinical outcomes such as progression-free survival, overall survival, and metastasis-free survival, as well as using them as a surrogate for processes such as tumor necrosis (percentage of necrotic tumor in the resected primary tumor after chemotherapy determined by pathology). Investigators have also tried to assess the role of dual-time-point $^{18}$F-FDG PET/CT in imaging bone sarcomas; that is, obtaining 2 sets of scans, the first after an uptake period of 60 minutes and the second after a longer uptake period, such as 120 or 150 minutes. The hypothesis is that the differential radiotracer uptake between these 2 time points may be helpful in both detection and the characterization of neoplasms.[48,49,52]

## MUSCULOSKELETAL INDICATIONS FOR PEDIATRIC PET/COMPUTED TOMOGRAPHY
### Tumor Imaging

Bone tumors, either benign or malignant, may present with pain, swelling, pathologic fracture, decreased use of a limb, or neurologic changes. Alternatively, they may be identified as an incidental finding on clinical examination or imaging. Typically, malignant bone tumors present with gradually worsening, nonmechanical pain. Swelling becomes apparent only once the tumor has broken through the cortex and starts growing beneath or outside the periosteum. In this clinical setting, the differential diagnosis includes malignant and benign bone tumors, infection, hematological disorder, and metastases. The prevalence of each of these diseases depends on the patient's age. The most common primary bone neoplasm in the diaphysis is Ewing sarcoma (ES), whereas in the metaphysis it is osteosarcoma.[53]

Imaging of bone tumors starts with radiographs, which determine the location and size of the tumor, its pattern of bone destruction, matrix type, the presence and type of periosteal new bone formation, lesion size, and margins. This information is used to classify the osseous lesion as either aggressive or nonaggressive.[54] MR imaging is used for local evaluation of the tumor at staging, to assess treatment response, and for surveillance for local recurrence. Once MR imaging with contrast of the entire bone has been obtained, the next step in the workup for a suspected bone tumor is either open biopsy or closed biopsy with the decision guided by an experienced orthopedic oncologist.[55] The most common sites of metastases in the primary bone malignancies are the lungs and bones. $^{99m}$Tc-MDP, whole-body MR imaging, or, with increasing frequency, $^{18}$F-FDG PET/CT are used to detect bone metastases. Noncontrast chest CT is used to screen for pulmonary metastases. Several studies in adults have demonstrated the superiority of $^{18}$F-NaF PET/CT compared with $^{99m}$Tc-MDP scan in detecting osseous metastases.[56–60] However, the role of $^{18}$F-NaF PET/CT in primary bone tumors and in the evaluation of osseous metastatic disease in pediatrics is not well established.

Several staging systems are used that are based on both imaging and histologic features.

The American Joint Committee on Cancer staging system[61] for bone tumors includes the following:

- T (tumor): tumor size assessed on MR imaging (may be overestimated due to presence of adjacent bone or soft tissue edema); this was previously classified based on presence of cortical breakthrough into soft tissues
- N (nodes): regional lymph nodes are not usually involved in bone sarcomas, except for in osteosarcoma
- M (metastasis): most common sites for metastasis are lungs and bones

- G (histologic grade): determined by histologic evaluation of representative tissue biopsy specimen; tumors may be classified as low or high grade

A second system used for staging of bone tumors is the "Musculoskeletal Tumor Society Surgical Staging System," also known as the "Enneking staging system," which addresses additional tumor features based on findings on MR imaging.[61,62] These include the following:

- Whether the tumor is encapsulated or not
- Whether the tumor is confined to compartment of origin or extends beyond it
- Whether the tumor is adjacent to or involves the neurovascular bundle

Osteosarcoma (OS), the most common bone sarcoma in the pediatric population, is characterized by the malignant proliferation of osteoid-producing mesenchymal spindle cells. The peak incidence is in the second decade of life. OS has an estimated incidence rate of 4.4 cases per year in 1 million-population aged 0 to 24 years.[63] Approximately 450 patients younger than 25 years are diagnosed with OS each year in the United States. The most common primary sites of OS, in order of frequency, are the femur, the tibia, and the humerus. Rarely, OS may originate in soft tissues or visceral organs, termed extraosseous OS. OS can be diagnosed by core needle biopsy or open surgical biopsy.[48,64]

Although most cases of osteosarcoma are sporadic, certain "hereditary cancer predisposition syndromes" confer heightened susceptibility to OS. These include Li-Fraumeni syndrome, hereditary retinoblastoma, and Rothmund-Thomson syndrome.[65]

At diagnosis, approximately 10% to 20% of patients with OS have metastatic disease, most commonly to lung (85%–90% of metastases) or bone.[66] "Skip lesions" are defined as 2 or more discontinuous lesions in the same bone. A lesion in an adjacent bone across a joint space, should be considered as a hematogenous metastasis and not a skip lesion. Multifocal OS, which has a very poor prognosis, is defined as multiple bone lesions without a clear primary tumor.[64,67]

The typical treatment for OS is neoadjuvant systemic chemotherapy followed by local control with surgical resection of the primary tumor as well as of metastatic disease in the lungs, when possible.[55] The degree of tumor necrosis (TN) in the primary resected mass is assessed and has prognostic value. Patients with ≥90% necrosis have a better prognosis and a lower rate of recurrence in the first 2 years than do patients with less

**Table 1**
**Prognostic factors in osteosarcoma**

| Pretreatment factors | Response to initial therapy factors |
|---|---|
| • Primary tumor site and initial treatment | • Surgical resectability of primary tumor |
| • Size of the primary tumor | • Degree of tumor necrosis |
| • Presence of clinically detectable metastatic disease | |

*Adapted from* Osteosarcoma and malignant fibrous histiocytoma of bone treatment (PDQ(R)): health professional version. 2002. Available at: https://www.cancer.gov/types/bone/patient/osteosarcoma-treatment-pdq.

than 90% necrosis.[64] In contrast to ES, OS is relatively resistant to radiotherapy. Therefore, radiation therapy is reserved for unresectable tumors or when the tumor has been resected with inadequate margins.[64,68]

The 5-year survival rate for OS is approximately 65% to 70% in localized disease but decreases to less than 20% to 30% in patients with metastatic or recurrent disease.[66,68] Patients with isolated pulmonary metastases have a slightly better prognosis that those with additional metastases to other organs.[69,70] Previously identified prognostic factors for OS (**Table 1**) have not been helpful in guiding intensification or deintensification of treatments particularly following initial therapy.[64] As imaging, including [18]F-FDG PET/CT is widely used in the assessment of children with OS, investigators have tried to correlate "radiotracer uptake metrics" with clinical outcomes and determine whether these metrics can be used as biomarkers or surrogates for clinical response and thus for prognostication.

An early review by Brenner and colleagues[71] concluded among other things that, because of an overlap in [18]F-FDG uptake values it is usually not possible to differentiate low-grade or high-grade OS from [18]F-FDG-avid benign lesions such as osteomyelitis or giant cell tumors, thus mandating biopsy for diagnosis.

Harrison and colleagues[52] recently reviewed the literature on the role of [18]F-FDG PET/CT in pediatric sarcomas in general and concluded the following for OS:

- [18]F-FDG PET/CT is an effective tool in delineating the primary tumor and identifying metastatic disease (see **Fig. 1**).[72]
- [18]F-FDG PET/CT is more sensitive than bone scintigraphy in detecting osseous metastases at initial presentation and may replace bone scintigraphy for this indication.[73,74]

- There is a correlation among SUV1, MTV at diagnosis, and change in $SUV_{max}$ with histologic response (ie, TN) and outcomes, including progression-free survival and metastasis-free survival.[75–83] However, to date, none of these metrics have been proven as useful prognostic indicators in determining the need for intensification or deintensification of therapy. Because different imaging metrics have been used by different groups of researchers, consideration of multicenter trials, using a harmonized approach to choosing and evaluating specific radiotracer uptake metrics is needed.
- More studies are needed to evaluate the role of [18]F-FDG PET-CT in detecting local and distant recurrences.[84,85]

Costelloe and colleagues[48] also performed a similar review assessing the role of [18]F-FDG PET/CT in OS and concluded the following:

- The following [18]F-FDG PET/CT radiotracer uptake metrics correlated with clinical outcome at the time of initial diagnosis.
  - SUV1, SUV2, TLG, and MTV correlated significantly with progression-free survival.[79,82]
  - SUV2 and TLG correlated significantly with overall survival.[79]
  - SUV2 and change in SUV correlated significantly with TN.[86]
- [18]F-FDG PET/CT can detect local recurrence and distant osseous metastases.[84,87–89] However, noncontrast chest CT is the preferred modality for the detection and follow-up of lung metastases due to decreased reliability of PET/CT in detecting lung nodules smaller than or equal to 2 cm, as well as lower lobe lesions.[90] This is due to the limitations related to the low-dose free-breathing CT accompanying the PET as well as to the limitations of PET technology itself. The latter includes inaccurate SUV measurements and misregistration of the PET and CT images.[91–95]

The role of [18]F-NaF PET/CT in OS or ES has not been elucidated in children. However, there is early evidence that this tracer may be more sensitive and specific than [18]F-FDG to detect metastases to the lungs or bones in these tumors at diagnosis and restaging and that, further, the use of [18]F-NaF may improve detection of metastases compared with conventional [99m]Tc-MDP imaging in these tumors as well.[32,71,96]

Arvanitis and colleagues,[97] evaluating [18]F-NaF and [18]F-FDG using a transgenetic mouse model of OS, concluded that [18]F-NaF is a sensitive tracer for the detection of pulmonary metastases in this disease and that the combined use of both of these positron agents is a highly sensitive method to noninvasively measure osteosarcoma growth, therapeutic response, and, as importantly, to detect tumor cells that have undergone differentiation and oncogene inactivation.

ES, the second most common bone sarcoma in the pediatric population, is derived from a primordial bone marrow–derived mesenchymal stem cell. A key feature of ES is the presence of a translocation involving the "Ewing Sarcoma Breakpoint Region 1" or EWSR1 gene, located on chromosome 22 band q12, and one of several partner chromosomes. The incidence of ES in the United States is 1 case per 1 million people for all ages and between 9 and 10 cases per 1 million people in patients aged 10 to 19 years.[98] The site of primary disease in ES may be osseous or extraosseous. The most common primary sites for osseous ES are the lower extremities, pelvis, and chest wall; other sites include the upper extremities, spine, hands feet, ribs, and skull. The most common primary sites for extraosseous ES are the trunk, extremities, head and neck, and retroperitoneum.[99]

Pretreatment staging studies for ES include the following:

- Primary site: radiographs followed by MR imaging, when the primary site is in the extremities, or CT, when primary site in not in the extremities
- Noncontrast CT of the chest
- $^{99m}$Tc-MDP bone scan or $^{18}$F-FDG PET/CT to screen for metastatic disease (latter preferred)[55]
- Bone marrow aspiration and biopsy were previously mandated as, unlike OS, ES can metastasize to the bone marrow. According to Reed and colleagues,[55] in patients without metastases identified by $^{18}$F-FDG PET/CT or other imaging studies, the yield of bone marrow aspiration and biopsy is extremely low. Therefore, unless patients are enrolled in a clinical trial, bone marrow aspiration and marrow biopsy may be unnecessary (**Fig. 2**).[55,100,101]

ES may be localized or metastatic at presentation. In localized ES, there is no spread beyond the primary site or regional lymph node involvement on clinical examination or imaging. Continuous extension into adjacent soft tissues is considered localized disease. Five-year event-free survival (EFS) is 73% in localized ES. Approximately 25% of patients have metastatic disease at the time of diagnosis.[98] Standard treatment for ES includes both chemotherapy and local control. Local control is most commonly achieved with

surgery; radiation therapy is reserved for cases when the functional morbidity of surgery is high or when the tumor has been resected with inadequate margins.[55] Approximately 80% of recurrences of ES occur in the first 2 years after the initial diagnosis. The prognosis in recurrent ES is poor, with a 5-year survival of 10% to 15%.[99] The 2 major categories of prognostic factors for patients with ES are summarized in **Table 2**, with details further elucidated in the original publication.

A recent review[52] of the literature regarding the role of $^{18}$F-FDG PET/CT in pediatric ES concluded the following:

- $^{18}$F-FDG PET/CT is useful in detecting bone marrow and skeletal metastases in ES.[102–105]
- $^{18}$F-FDG PET/CT has a lower sensitivity in detecting skull base metastases compared with bone scintigraphy and, therefore, $^{99m}$Tc-MDP bone scintigraphy may be warranted in patients with osseous metastases detected on $^{18}$F-FDG PET/CT to evaluate for skull base metastases that may affect local control measures.[102–105] Although not formally evaluated for this indication, $^{18}$F-NaF may, given its superior imaging characteristics, be an alternative to bone scintigraphy in this situation.
- Correlation between radiotracer uptake metrics, such as SUV1 and SUV2, with TN and clinical outcomes show conflicting results.[76,106–108]
- More studies are needed to evaluate the role of $^{18}$F-FDG PET/CT in detecting local and distant recurrences.

Costelloe and colleagues[48] also reviewed the role of $^{18}$F-FDG PET/CT in ES and concluded the following:

- The following radiotracer uptake metrics correlated with clinical outcome at the time of initial diagnosis:
  - SUV1 and SUV2 correlated significantly with progression-free survival.[106,107,109]
  - SUV1, SUV2, and change in $SUL_{peak}$ correlated significantly with TN and overall survival.[107,109–111]
- $^{18}$F-FDG PET/CT can detect local recurrence and distant osseous metastases (**Fig. 3**); however, noncontrast chest CT is currently the preferred modality for the detection and follow-up of lung metastases for the reasons discussed previously in the section on OS.

### Soft tissue sarcomas

The imaging evaluation of a suspected soft tissue mass may start with ultrasound when there is a

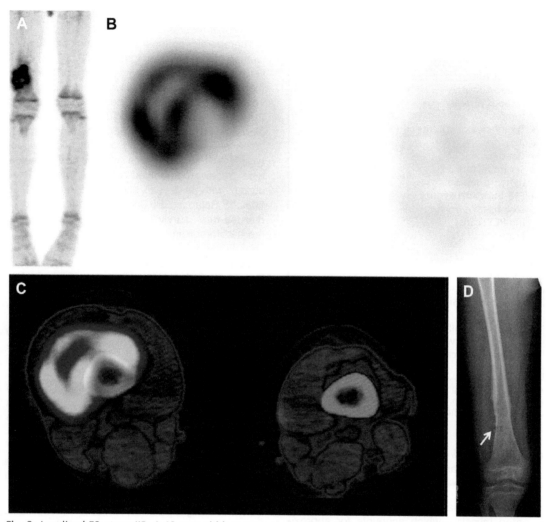

**Fig. 2.** Localized ES, stage IIB. A 12-year-old boy presented with right knee pain and swelling following closed head injury. Initial plain film radiographs (not shown) demonstrated an aggressive osseous lesion on the distal right femoral diaphysis. Anterior MIP image of the lower extremities (*A*), axial PET (*B*), and fused axial PET/CT (*C*) images from a whole-body $^{18}$F-FDG PET/CT demonstrate an $^{18}$F-FDG-avid mass in the distal right femur (SUV$_{max}$ 11.8) with extension into soft tissues. No distant metastatic disease was identified on the torso PET images (not shown). Biopsy was consistent with ES. Postbiopsy anteroposterior radiograph (*D*) of the distal right femur demonstrates the aggressive nature of the osseous lesion with periosteal reaction as well as the biopsy tract (*arrow*). Of note, biopsy of suspect osseous lesions should be performed only after the completion of the MR imaging. The patient was treated with chemotherapy followed by local control surgery, including allograph placement. There was 100% TN on the resected tumor specimen.

suspicion that it may represent specific pathologies, such as a vascular anomaly or a fluid collection including hematoma or abscess. Radiographs may be obtained to differentiate a primary soft tissue lesion from an osseous abnormality with soft tissue extension or to determine the presence of secondary osseous erosion or calcification in a primary soft tissue mass. MR imaging and CT are the 2 main cross-sectional imaging modalities used for local evaluation. MR imaging is the imaging modality of choice for local evaluation of extremity soft tissue tumors. CT or MR imaging may be used for the local evaluation of thoracic, abdominal wall, and retroperitoneal soft tissue sarcomas (**Fig. 4**). Noncontrast chest CT is used to determine the presence of lung metastases. Sentinel lymph node biopsy may also be used as a staging procedure. A needle core or an incisional biopsy, when the former fails, is used to obtain tissue and establish the histologic diagnosis and grade.

Pediatric soft tissue sarcomas, which arise from primitive mesenchymal tissue, account for

**Table 2**
**Prognostic factors in Ewing sarcoma**

| Pretreatment factors | Response to initial therapy factors |
|---|---|
| • Site of tumor | • Amount of viable tumor after chemotherapy |
| • Extraosseous vs osseous primary tumors | • PET uptake after chemotherapy |
| • Tumor size or volume | |
| • Age | |
| • Gender | |
| • Serum lactate dehydrogenase | |
| • F18-fluorodeoxyglucose uptake on staging PET scans | |
| • Presence of metastases | |
| • Previous treatment for cancer | |
| • Cytogenetic factors | |
| • Detectable fusion transcripts in morphologically normal marrow | |
| • Other biological factors | |

*Adapted from* Ewing sarcoma treatment (PDQ(R)): health professional version. 2002. Available at: https://www.cancer.gov/types/bone/hp/ewing-treatment-pdq.

approximately 7% of all childhood tumors in those aged 0 to 14 years, and may be divided into 2 categories[112,113]:

- Rhabdomyosarcoma (RMS): a tumor of striated muscles, which accounts for approximately 50% of soft tissue sarcomas.
- Non-rhabdomyosarcomatous soft tissue sarcomas (NRSTS): a heterogeneous group that includes malignant tumors of connective tissue, peripheral nervous system, smooth muscle, and vascular tissue.[114]

**Rhabdomyosarcoma** The histologic subtypes of RMS include embryonal (57%), alveolar (23%), as well as pleomorphic/anaplastic, mixed type, and spindle cell subtypes, each of which account for less than 2%. The most common primary sites for RMS are head and neck, genitourinary tract, and extremities, with frequencies of occurrence of 25%, 22%, and 18%, respectively.[115]

Between 4% and 28% of cases have metastases at the time of diagnosis. The most common sites of metastatic disease are bone, lung, and distant lymph nodes, with nodal metastases occurring more frequently in those with extremity primary tumors. Survival is lower for those with distant metastases compared with those with local or regional recurrences.[116]

Therapeutic options in RMS include surgery, with en bloc removal of tumor and a cuff of noninvolved tissue, chemotherapy, and/or radiation therapy. EFS in those with low-risk RMS is approximately 90%, whereas it decreases to 65% in those with intermediate-risk disease. Those with high-risk RMS have an EFS of approximately 30% or less depending on histologic subtype.[117–119] Most children with localized disease who receive combined-modality therapy are cured, with a 5-year survival of greater than 70%.[120] Relapses are uncommon after 5 years of disease-free survival; however, relapses are more common in cases with gross residual disease in unfavorable sites after initial surgery and in cases with metastatic disease at diagnosis.[115] Prognostic factors, both clinical and biological, in RMS are summarized in **Table 3**, and the interested reader is referred to the original Web site for further details.[115]

In their recent review of the role of [18]F-FDG PET/CT in pediatric RMSs, Harrison and colleagues[52] concluded the following:

- [18]F-FDG PET/CT is a powerful tool in the initial staging workup, particularly in identifying lymph node and distant metastases in those with RMS (see **Fig. 4**).[121–125]
- On the other hand, the role of [18]F-FDG-PET/CT as a prognostic indicator in RMS remains controversial, mandating further research.

**Non-rhabdomyosarcomatous soft tissue sarcomas** Literature is sparse regarding the role of [18]F-FDG PET/CT in children with NRSTS; however, one of the most widely studied entities in pediatrics is neurofibromatosis. Neurofibromatosis 1 (NF1) is an autosomal dominant phakomatosis that affects 1 in 3500 live births.[126,127] Patients with NF1 may develop benign as well as malignant peripheral nerve sheath tumors. Malignant peripheral nerve sheath tumors (MPNST) are the leading cause of mortality in these patients, with a lifetime risk of developing MPNST ranging between 8% and 13%. Five-year overall survival is 21% to 41% in those who develop MPNST.[128]

Neurofibromas (NFs) are benign peripheral nerve sheath tumors that are inseparable from the normal nerve. According to the most recent World Health Organization (WHO) classification,[129] macroscopically NFs may represent one of the following forms: localized cutaneous, diffuse cutaneous, localized intraneural, plexiform intraneural, and massive diffuse soft tissue plexiform tumor. Most MPNSTs arise from plexiform intraneural

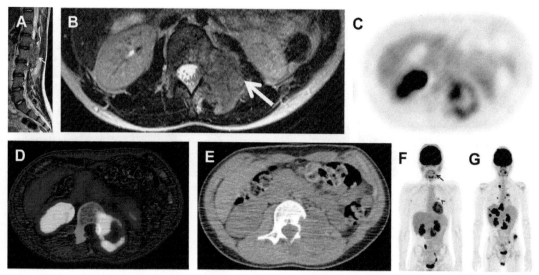

**Fig. 3.** Recurrent ES. At age 15, the patient (same patient as in **Fig. 2**) developed left back pain, swelling in the left lumbar region, and left anterior thigh pain with numbness. Sagittal (*A*) and axial (*B*) T2-weighted MR images of the lumbar spine demonstrate an osseous metastasis at L2, involving the left transverse process and vertebral body, with extension into the left L1-L2 and L2-L3 neural foramina, spinal canal, and left paraspinal muscles (*arrows* in [*A*] and [*B*]). Axial PET (*C*), fused PET-CT (*D*), low-dose CT (*E*) images, and anterior MIP image (*F*) from a whole-body [18]F-FDG PET/CT scan performed for restaging, confirm marked hypermetabolism of the lumbar mass with central necrosis. In addition, there are hypermetabolic metastases involving the left posterior element of C3 (*arrow* in [*F*]) and a left hilar lymph node (*arrowhead* in [*F*]). Anterior MIP image from a whole-body [18]F-FDG PET/ CT scan (*G*) obtained 5 months later, demonstrates disease progression with the development of pleural, pulmonary, right adrenal, and increased number of osseous metastases (greater trochanter of right femur and left iliac wing) despite chemotherapy.

and solitary intraneural NFs and are associated with NF1 in 50% of cases. Malignant transformation may be suspected based on the presence of an enlarging mass, that is, palpable or detected on imaging, and that may be painless or painful.[130]

Several studies have evaluated the role of [18]F-FDG PET/CT in evaluating the transformation of plexiform (NFs) to MPNSTs in adults with NF1.[131–134] In a retrospective study, Tsai and colleagues[135] reviewed the [18]F-FDG PET/CT scans of 20 patients with NF1 who were younger than 21 years and were suspected of having MPNST based on change or progression of symptoms or increased lesion size on MR imaging. A total of 27 FDG-avid lesions in these 21 patients underwent excision or biopsy. NFs were classified as typical neurofibroma, atypical neurofibroma, or MPNST. Atypical neurofibroma was defined as NFs exhibiting nuclear atypia and/or hypercellularity without mitoses or necrosis. MPNSTs were classified as low, intermediate, or high grade depending on degree of tumor differentiation, vascular invasion, necrosis, and number of mitoses. $SUV_{max}$ of plexiform neurofibromas, including typical and atypical types, was significantly different from those of MPNST (2.49, SD = 1.50 vs 7.63, SD = 2.96, p 0.001). A cutoff $SUV_{max}$ value

of 4.0 had a sensitivity and specificity of 100% and 94%, respectively, in distinguishing benign from MPNSTs. These investigators[135] concluded that [18]F-FDG PET/CT may be useful in predicting malignant transformation in peripheral nerve sheath tumors in children with NF1 and that further, there appeared to be a correlation between mean $SUV_{max}$ and tumor grade. **Fig. 5** demonstrates the utility of using [18]F-FDG PET/CT to identify highly metabolic NFs that should be considered for biopsy or resection when malignant transformation is suspected clinically.

Desmoplastic small round blue cell tumor (DSRCT), another NRSTS, is a highly malignant tumor that typically arises in the peritoneal cavity and often presents with widespread metastatic disease. The group at Memorial Sloan Kettering Cancer Center[136] published a retrospective study of 65 patients with DSRCT. Eleven of these patients underwent [18]F-FDG PET/CT imaging at the time of diagnosis, which was found to be extremely effective in identifying all DSRCT sites of disease, with high sensitivity, specificity, and positive and negative predictive values of 96.1%, 98.6%, 98.0%, and 97.1%, respectively. A second, smaller retrospective study from St Jude Children's Research Hospital[137] evaluated 8 pediatric

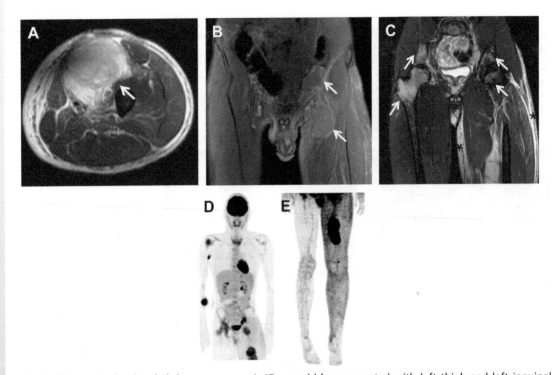

**Fig. 4.** Metastatic alveolar rhabdomyosarcoma. A 17-year-old boy presented with left thigh and left inguinal masses. Axial T1 postcontrast (*A*) MR image of the left thigh demonstrates a heterogeneously enhancing, soft tissue mass in the anterior compartment of the left thigh (*arrow*). Coronal T1 fat-saturated postcontrast (*B*) and coronal STIR (*C*) MR images of the pelvis and upper thighs demonstrate marked conglomerate regional lymphadenopathy in the left inguinal and external iliac regions (*arrows* in [*B*]), with associated venous compression and impaired lymphatic drainage that may be inferred by the presence of subcutaneous edema in the left lower extremity, appreciated as high T2 signal that is not suppressed on STIR sequence (*asterisks* in [*C*]). In addition, bone marrow metastases are present in both femurs and acetabuli (*arrows* in [*C*]). Frontal MIP images of the torso (*D*) and lower extremities (*E*) from a whole-body [18]F-FDG PET/CT scan demonstrate the primary, hypermetabolic soft tissue mass in the left thigh with an $SUV_{max}$ of 7.6 and multiple osseous metastases including the right humeral head, pelvis, right proximal femur, sternum, and vertebrae. The relative lack of clearance of radiotracer from the subcutaneous tissues of the left lower extremity (associated with increased girth) corresponds to the previously described MR findings and is indicative of impaired venous and lymphatic drainage.

patients with histologically proven DSRCT and demonstrated not only that these lesions are [18]F-FDG-avid, but that in follow-up, decrease in or resolution of [18]F-FDG uptake correlated with clinical remission, and finally, that recurrences could be detected with this modality.

It is studies like these and others that allowed Harrison and his colleagues[52] to conclude, based on their review of the literature in pediatric NRSTS that, although [18]F-FDG PET/CT may be a helpful tool in several of the histologic subtypes, more studies are needed to better understand how to optimally incorporate this imaging modality into clinical practice.[136–139]

### Lymphoproliferative neoplasms

**Lymphoma** Lymphomatous involvement of bone may be primary or, more commonly, secondary. In primary lymphoma of bone (PLB), there is either

a single site of bony disease with or without associated regional lymph node involvement, or multifocal bone disease without associated visceral or lymph node involvement (ie, primary multifocal osseous lymphoma). The bony lesion may be associated with cortical destruction or extension via cortical channels as well as a soft tissue mass. In secondary lymphoma of bone, in addition to bony involvement, there is visceral or nonregional lymph node involvement.[140,141] PLB represents 3% to 7% of osseous malignant tumors in all age groups[142] and is more prevalent in adults compared with the pediatric population. Primary bone lymphoma usually occurs in the non-Hodgkin form of the disease, most being large B-cell type. In the Ann Arbor classification, primary bone lymphoma is considered stage E.

Liu[143] reported [18]F-FDG PET/CT findings at staging or restaging in 16 patients with PLB. One

**Table 3**
**Prognostic factors in rhabdomyosarcoma (RMS) and non-rhabdomyosarcoma soft tissue sarcomas (NRSTS)**

| Prognostic factors in RMS | Prognostic factors in NRSTS |
|---|---|
| • Age | • Site of origin |
| • Site of origin | • Tumor size |
| • Tumor size | • Tumor grade |
| • Resectability | • Tumor histology |
| • Histological subtype | • Depth of tumor invasion |
| • PAX3/PAX7-FOXO1 | |
| • Metastases at diagnosis | • Metastases at diagnosis |
| • Lymph node involvement at diagnosis | • Resectability of tumor |
| • Biological characteristics | • Use of radiation therapy |

Adapted from Childhood rhabdomyosarcoma treatment (PDQ(R)): health professional version. 2002. Available at: https://www.cancer.gov/types/soft-tissue-sarcoma/patient/rhabdomyosarcoma-treatment-pdq.

hundred percent (16/16) of lesions were FDG-avid; 93.8% (15/16) demonstrated involvement of the adjacent soft tissues; and in 44% (7/16) an additional 24 bone lesions were detected on [18]F-FDG PET/CT. Wang and colleagues[144] and Park and colleagues[145] also demonstrated that [18]F-FDG PET/CT is a sensitive modality in staging, restaging, and evaluating response to treatment in their patient cohorts of 18 and 19 patients, respectively, with PLB. **Fig. 6** is an example of a case of PLB in which initial anatomic imaging suggested a primary bone sarcoma.

[18]F-FDG PET/CT, which has replaced [67]Gallium citrate in the imaging management of patients with lymphoma, is considered essential for accurate staging, detecting sites of disease not identified by conventional anatomic imaging. [18]F-FDG PET/CT has been shown to change initial staging in up to 23% of children with lymphoma.[146] [18]F-FDG PET/CT is the foundation of widely adopted response criteria used in determining intensification or deintensification of treatment.[147,148]

Chen and colleagues[149] retrospectively reviewed pretreatment [18]F-FDG PET/CT scans from 93 consecutive pediatric patients with non-Hodgkin lymphoma. They compared patterns of [18]F-FDG uptake in bone marrow using SUV measurements at the fifth lumbar vertebra with the results of bone marrow biopsy (BMB) to diagnose the presence or absence of bone marrow involvement. Forty-one of 93 patients were determined to have bone marrow involvement based on a combination of factors that included positive BMB;

confirmation of the focal/multifocal intense FDG uptake pattern with either directed biopsy or targeted MR imaging; or resolution of bone marrow uptake, which matched the treatment response of other lymphoma lesions, on follow-up PET scans. Thirty-nine of 41 were identified by [18]F-FDG PET/CT imaging compared with 23 of 41 by BMB. [18]F-FDG PET/CT had a sensitivity and specificity of 95% and 98%, respectively, compared with 56% and 100% for BMB in the detection of bone marrow involvement. These investigators concluded that [18]F-FDG PET/CT had a high level of accuracy for detecting bone marrow involvement in pediatric NHL, thus eliminating the need for the more invasive BMB procedure in selected patients.

**Leukemia** Leukemia, a malignancy in which hematopoietic stem cells diffusely infiltrate or replace the normal bone marrow, is the most common malignancy in the pediatric population, representing approximately 27% of all pediatric malignancies.[150] Acute lymphocytic leukemia (ALL), the most common form of leukemia in children, represents 21% of all pediatric malignances, and occurs 4 times as frequently as acute myelogenous leukemia (AML), the second most common type of pediatric leukemia. Extramedullary sites of disease involvement, termed myeloid or granulocytic sarcoma or chloromas, are common in the acute myeloid form of pediatric leukemia, occurring in up to 25% of affected children.[151,152] Chloromas are most commonly detected in the head and neck, soft tissues, gastrointestinal system, lymph nodes, peritoneum, or as an extramedullary bony mass. When present, these extramedullary sites of disease are associated with a poor prognosis and, moreover, if left untreated, are fatal within a short period.[153] Extramedullary involvement has also been described in other types of leukemia.[154]

Previously, nuclear medicine imaging was not routinely used in the staging or therapeutic response monitoring of leukemia, but rather, was used as an aide in establishing the diagnosis and to assess for the early and late complications of systemic therapy used to treat this disease. However, extramedullary sites of disease in AML can be difficult to identify by clinical examination or by laboratory assessment, including BMB.[152] More recently, [18]F-FDG PET/CT has been proven helpful in identifying not only suspected but unsuspected sites of extramedullary involvement (**Fig. 7**) and is now recommended by the National Comprehensive Cancer Network (NCCN) guidelines in the staging with acute myeloid leukemia and suspected extramedullary disease.[155–157]

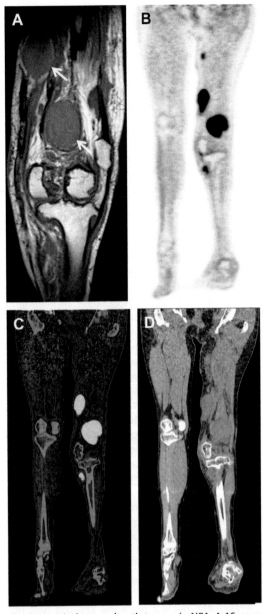

**Fig. 5.** Atypical nerve sheath tumors in NF1. A 16-year-old boy with NF1 presented with several masses in the left lower extremity. Coronal T1 (*A*) MR image demonstrates the 2 largest masses with hypointense T1 signal, in the lower thigh (*arrows*). The masses demonstrated a hyperintense rim on T2-weighted images with a central area of low signal, that is, the "target sign," characteristic for a nerve sheath tumor (not shown). Coronal PET (*B*), fused PET-CT (*C*), and low-dose CT (*D*) images of the bilateral lower extremities, from a whole-body $^{18}$F-FDG PET/CT scan, demonstrate several hypermetabolic nerve sheath tumors. The 2 largest lesions in the left lower thigh have an SUV$_{max}$ of 10.4 and 9 in the superior and inferior lesions, respectively. These were resected and pathology was consistent with atypical neurofibromas, despite the high SUV$_{max}$ value.

## Other neoplasms

**Neuroblastoma (non-metaiodobenzylguanidine avid)** Neuroblastoma (NB), the most common pediatric extracranial soft tissue tumor, comprises 8% of all childhood malignancies.[158] NB has an annual incidence of approximately 10.5 cases per 1 million children.[159] NB most commonly metastasizes to lymph nodes, liver, bone, and bone marrow.[160] Between 50% and 70% of patients with NB present with metastatic disease at diagnosis. Metaiodobenzylguanidine (mIBG), a norepinephrine analog that can be labeled with either $^{131}$I or preferably, $^{123}$I, is more than 90% sensitive and close to 100% specific for the detection of NB, not only in sites of soft tissue involvement but in sites of metastatic disease in bone and bone marrow as well. $^{123}$I-mIBG is currently considered the radiotracer of choice for staging, as well as therapeutic response monitoring in those with NB and, additionally, is used not only as a prognostic indicator in those with high-risk disease but also to determine eligibility for $^{131}$I-mIBG therapy.[161–164] Planar $^{123}$I-mIBG scintigraphy, with SPECT or SPECT-CT, is recommended for these indications.[165]

Most NBs are $^{18}$F-FDG-avid. Moderate $^{18}$F-FDG uptake is seen in mIBG-positive and mIBG-negative NBs with a lower SUVmax of primary tumors in early-stage (I–II) compared with advanced-stage (III–IV) disease (3.03 vs 5.45, respectively, $P$ = .019).[166,167]

$^{123}$I-mIBG is considered superior to $^{18}$F-FDG for a variety of reasons, not the least of which is dosimetry. $^{18}$F-FDG has an inferior diagnostic accuracy in the detection of distant metastases compared with $^{123}$I-mIBG scans due to the superior tumor-to-background contrast and improved detection of bone and bone marrow disease with tumor-specific mIBG scans.[168,169] In addition, the high metabolic activity of normal hematopoietic bone marrow in young children and the intense physiologic brain activity may obscure metastases in the bone marrow and calvarium respectively on $^{18}$F-FDG PET/CT scans.[169,170] However, $^{18}$F-FDG PET/CT is recommended for staging and therapeutic response monitoring in the 10% of patients with NB who are mIBG nonavid or poorly avid (**Fig. 8**).[158]

$^{68}$Gallium DOTATATE is an emerging PET radiotracer showing promise as a scintigraphic agent for the detection and therapeutic response monitoring in somatostatin receptor positive tumors, including NB, particularly those that are mIBG nonavid or poorly avid. $^{68}$Ga-DOTATATE was approved by the FDA for the detection of somatostatin receptor positive neuroendocrine tumors in pediatric and adult patients in 2016. In an early

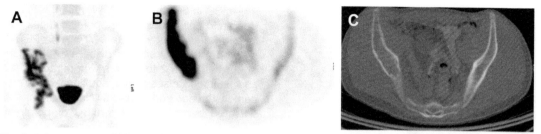

**Fig. 6.** PLB. A 14-year-old boy with newly diagnosed DLBCL, diffuse large B-cell lymphoma of right iliac bone at presentation. Anterior (*A*) MIP image of the lower abdomen and pelvis and axial PET image *(B)* from a whole-body $^{18}$F-FDG PET/CT scan demonstrate FDG-avid involvement of the right ilium, ischium, and pubis mimicking a primary osseous sarcoma. No other sites of FDG-avid disease were identified on whole-body $^{18}$F-FDG PET/CT scan (not shown). Axial CT (*C*) demonstrates a corresponding aggressive, lytic lesion in the right iliac bone.

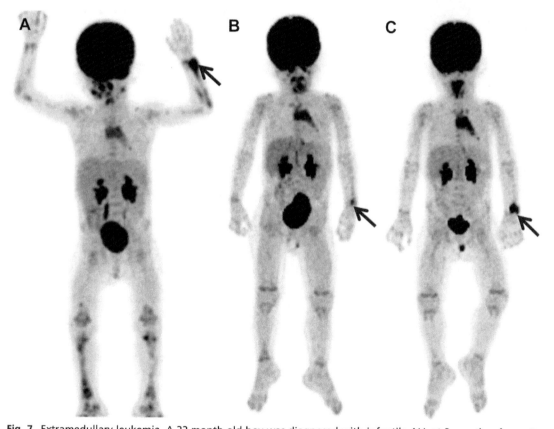

**Fig. 7.** Extramedullary leukemia. A 22-month-old boy was diagnosed with infantile ALL at 3 months of age. Patient had a testicular recurrence at 7 months into therapy and underwent bilateral orchiectomy and chemotherapy followed by unrelated donor bone marrow transplantation at 15 months of age. He subsequently presented with a soft tissue mass in the left forearm consistent with a second, extramedullary site of recurrence. Anterior MIPs from whole-body $^{18}$F-FDG PET/CT scans, at the time of second recurrence (*A*) demonstrate the extramedullary mass in the left forearm (*arrow* in [*A*]) as well as multiple sites of bone marrow disease in the axial and appendicular skeleton (*A*). Sequential subsequent whole-body $^{18}$F-FDG PET/CT scans, at 1 month (*B*) and 2.5 months (*C*) after initial PET/CT scan demonstrate initial decrease in size of the extramedullary mass (*arrow* in [*B*]) in response to blinatumomab, and subsequent increase in size (*arrow* in [*C*]). The forearm lesion was biopsied and was found to be CD19+ ALL on pathology. He subsequently received local radiation to the forearm with resolution of the mass (not shown). $^{18}$F-FDG PET/CT is highly sensitive in detection of extramedullary sites of disease in ALL and AML.

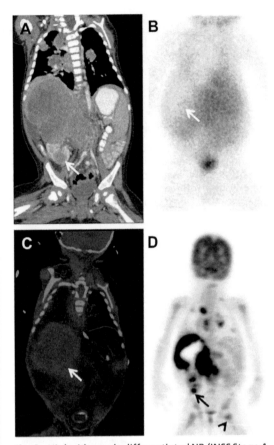

**Fig. 8.** High-risk poorly differentiated NB (INSS Stage 4, INRG SS Stage M), non-MIBG-avid. An 8-month-old boy presented with irritability and right groin mass. Coronal CT image (A) obtained with oral and intravenous contrast, demonstrate a large right suprarenal mass crossing the midline, pulmonary and pleural metastases, mediastinal and hilar lymphadenopathy, and bilateral renal metastases (right renal metastasis depicted with *arrow* in [A], left renal metastasis not shown). The diagnosis of NB was made on bone marrow aspiration and biopsy. [123]I-mIBG scan was performed and the anterior planar (B) as well as coronal fused SPECT/CT images of the chest, abdomen, and pelvis (C) demonstrate that the suprarenal mass (*arrows* in [B] and [C]) metastases seen on CT are not mIBG-avid. Coronal PET image (D) from a whole-body [18]F-FDG PET/CT scan performed after 2 cycles of induction chemotherapy demonstrates that the large right suprarenal mass is centrally necrotic and has a hypermetabolic rim. The mediastinal and hilar lymphadenopathy, the pulmonary and pleural metastases, and the renal metastases are hypermetabolic (*arrow* in [D] depicts metastasis in lower pole of right kidney). Osteomedullary metastases are also present; arrowhead in (D) depicts a left femoral neck metastasis.

study of 8 patients with refractory NB, [68]Ga-DOTATATE demonstrated higher tumor-to-background contrast ratios as well as more lesions than either pretherapy [123]I-mIBG or post-therapy

[131]I-mIBG in 5 of 14 cases.[171] A recent report by Kong and colleagues[172] corroborated these findings. In their study, [68]Ga-DOTATATE PET/CT showed additional sites of disease in 38% (3/8) of children aged 2 to 9 years with refractory NB, and upstaged disease in 1 additional patient by demonstrating bone marrow involvement not detected by diagnostic [123]I-mIBG or posttreatment [131]I-mIBG scans.

There are many advantages of using [68]Ga-DOTATATE PET/CT compared with [123]I-mIBG scans. These include rapid radiotracer uptake allowing acquisition of imaging in less than 90 minutes after radiotracer administration; rapid image acquisition times, often less than 10 minutes, which will shorten sedation times if necessary; noninvasive quantitation for individualized dosimetry estimates for body habitus and tumor burden for subsequent peptide receptor radionuclide therapy. Given these advantages, this agent has the potential to become the preferred molecular imaging modality for pediatric patients with NB.[172,173]

More recently, Abongwa and colleagues[174] published a report on the safety and accuracy results for [68]Ga-DOTA-tyr3-Octreotide (Ga-68-DOTA-TOC) in 26 children and young adults with neuroendocrine tumors who participated in a series of 3 prospective trials; 18 patients were younger than 18 years and 8 patients were between 19 and 29 years old. They reported a sensitivity of 88%, specificity of 100%, positive predictive value of 100%, and negative predictive value of 83% for tumor detection with no significant adverse effects (9 reported grade 1 adverse events).

**Langerhans cell histiocytosis** According to the WHO classification of tumors of bone,[175] Langerhans cell histiocytosis (LCH) is classified as a "tumor of undefined neoplastic nature" that is locally aggressive. LCH is a clonal, likely neoplastic, proliferation of pathologic Langerhans cells. LCH accounts for fewer than 1% of all osseous lesions and may be seen in all ages, although 80% of cases occur in patients younger than 30 years. Male individuals are twice as frequently affected compared with female individuals. Although any bone may be involved, the most frequently involved sites are the skull, particularly the calvarium, femur, pelvis, and mandible. The disease may be polyostotic or monostotic, with monostotic involvement 3 to 4 times more common than the polyostotic form. The most common clinical presentation is pain and swelling at a site of disease.[175]

LCH lesions may show increased or decreased uptake on [99m]Tc-MDP bone scans; bone scan complements plain film skeletal radiographs, as some lesions may be seen on one modality but not another. [18]F-FDG PET-CT has a higher sensitivity and specificity than either of these modalities and is emerging as the imaging modality of choice in LCH (**Fig. 9**). In a preliminary retrospective study performed by Binkovitz and colleagues,[176] [18]F-FDG PET detected all active LCH osseous lesions and successfully differentiated between active and healed lesions after treatment, with treated lesions demonstrating normalization of uptake on [18]F-FDG PET earlier than on bone scintigraphy or plain film radiography. Phillips and colleagues[177] retrospectively reviewed and compared 102 [18]F-FDG PET scans in 44 patients (41 children, 3 adults) with biopsy-proven LCH with 83 corollary imaging studies, including bone scans, MR imaging, CT, or plain films. These investigators concluded that whole-body [18]F-FDG-PET scans detect LCH lesions, disease activity, and early response to therapy in bone and soft tissue lesions, with greater accuracy than other imaging modalities. The

superiority of [18]F-FDG PET to MR imaging in detecting response to therapy was subsequently verified by Mueller and colleagues[178] in a retrospective study comparing 21 [18]F-FDG PET scans with 21 MR imaging scans in 15 patients (age range 4 months to 19 years) with biopsy-proven histiocytosis.

**Osseous metastatic disease** [99m]Tc-MDP bone scintigraphy has, since the inception of its use, been the imaging test of choice for the detection and therapeutic response monitoring of osseous metastatic disease in a variety of malignancies in both adults and children. Recently, a growing body of evidence in adults has demonstrated the superiority of [18]F-NaF PET/CT to [99m]Tc-MDP imaging for this indication, including a meta-analysis by Tateishi and colleagues,[179] which reported sensitivities and specificities of 96% and 98% for disease detection by [18]F-NaF PET/CT.

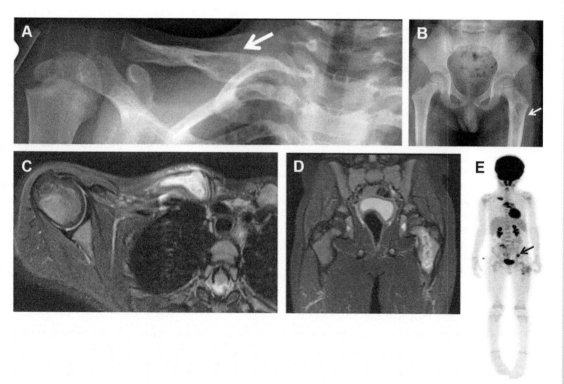

**Fig. 9.** Multisystem LCH. A 5-year-old boy presented with a 16-month history of intermittent right leg pain and 2-month history of right clavicular pain and swelling. Radiographs (*A, B*) demonstrated lytic lesions of the right clavicle (*arrow* in [*A*]) and left proximal femur (*arrow* in [*B*]); these were further evaluated with MR imaging. Axial STIR image of the right clavicle (*C*) and coronal STIR image (*D*) of the pelvis demonstrate homogeneous high-T2 signal in the clavicular lesion and predominantly peripheral high-T2 signal in the left femoral lesion. Both lesions were biopsied and pathology was consistent with LCH. Radiographic skeletal survey (not shown) did not demonstrate additional sites of osseous involvement. Anterior MIP image (*E*) from a whole-body [18]F-FDG PET/CT scan demonstrates that the right clavicular and the left proximal femoral lesion are hypermetabolic; differences in FDG-avidity are probably a reflection of the different chronicities of the lesions. No additional osseous lesions were seen. However, a left, hypermetabolic external iliac lymph node (*arrow* in [*E*]) was also identified and, therefore, the patient had both osseous and lymph node, that is, multisystem, involvement.

Additionally, [18]F-NaF PET/CT was found to be sensitive in the detection of both osteoblastic and osteolytic primary bone lesions in many adult series.[56,60,180,181]

In contradistinction to the adult literature,[56–58,60,181,182] there have been no published studies to date in the pediatric population that evaluate the efficacy of [18]F-NaF PET/CT in the assessment of either primary bone malignancies or osseous metastatic disease.[43]

**Benign osseous lesions** The high image quality of PET combined with the current availability of hybrid CT imaging could aid in the localization and characterization of benign osseous lesions. Although highly sensitive, [18]F-FDG PET/CT has been shown to lack specificity in differentiating benign from malignant bone tumors due to significant overlap in the degree of [18]F-FDG uptake in these entities. Some studies have shown that benign pathologies like giant cell tumor, fibrous dysplasia, chondroma, chondroblastoma, osteoid osteomas, and osteoblastomas occasionally demonstrate [18]F-FDG uptake levels similar or higher to those in malignant lesions.[59,168] Although a cutoff SUV value of 3.7 has been proposed to differentiate benign from malignant bone lesions, sensitivity, specificity, and diagnostic accuracy were found to be only 80%, 63%, and 70%, respectively.[183]

[18]F-NaF has been used in patients with suspected osteoblastoma or osteoid osteoma of either the spine or elsewhere in the skeleton as well as to identify additional lesions in benign osseous diseases with multicentric involvement, such as in LCH. Although many studies have compared the sensitivity, specificity, and accuracy of [18]F-NaF PET/CT with [18]F-FDG PET/CT, [99m]Tc-MDP bone scintigraphy,[56,184–186] or a combination of [18]F-NaF and [18]F-FDG PET/CT,[57,187] the sensitivity, specificity, and accuracy of [18]F-NaF PET or PET/CT in differentiating benign from malignant osseous disease and thus negating the need for diagnostic biopsy or excision has not yet been reported.

# TRAUMA
## Back Pain and Sports-Related Bone Injuries

Evaluation of back pain is the most common indication for [18]F-NaF PET/CT in children and young adults.[40,42,188,189] An important etiology of back pain in young athletes or dancers is injury to the pars interarticularis of the lumbar spine. [18]F-NaF PET/CT detects osseous turnover as an indicator of stress injury or spondylosis, and can potentially do so early in the disease process. Early

identification, combined with early intervention and treatment, can help to prevent progression of stress injury or spondylolysis to a complete fracture. A review of 94 children and young adults undergoing [18]F-NaF PET/CT for back pain demonstrated a cause for back pain in 55% of the patients (52/94). Fifteen patients had 2 or more potential sources of back pain. Diagnoses by [18]F-NaF PET/CT were pars interarticularis or pedicle stress (34%), spinous process injury (16%), vertebral body ring apophyseal injury (14%), stress at a transitional vertebra-sacral articulation (7%) (**Fig. 10**), and sacroiliac joint inflammation/stress (3%).[40] A smaller study of the use of [18]F-NaF PET/CT by Ovadia and colleagues[188] in 15 adolescents with back pain yielded 10 positive cases with diagnoses including 4 cases of spondylolysis, 3 fractures (2 of the transverse process and 1 of the facet), 2 osteoid osteomas, 1 osteitis pubis, 1 sacroiliitis, and 2 herniated disks. Some other processes that may be detected with [18]F-NaF PET in the setting of back pain are facet arthropathy, spinous process fractures, vertebral body compression fractures, and pelvis stress fractures.[189] Higher-quality imaging combined with a shorter imaging times at an equivalent dose makes [18]F-NaF PET/CT a promising alternative to conventional the [99m]Tc-MDP SPECT or SPECT/CT imaging conventionally used for this indication.[19]

Patients who have undergone spinal fusion as treatment for scoliosis can experience postoperative pain related to incomplete bone healing, osseous nonunion, hardware loosening, or infection. [18]F-NaF PET/CT can be used to assess the etiology of back pain in this group of patients by helping to localize the site of abnormal bone turnover when MR or CT might be limited due to hardware artifacts.[43] A study of [18]F-NaF PET/CT in 22 patients with back pain after spinal fusion surgery reported scintigraphic abnormalities in 16 patients. Scintigraphic abnormalities were validated with surgery or clinical follow-up in 15 patients, with only 1 false-positive abnormality identified.[190] Suspected stress injuries at other locations also can be assessed, although benefit over conventional [99m]Tc-MDP bone scan is not clear.

# NONACCIDENTAL TRAUMA

A radiographic skeletal survey is the primary method for identifying fractures in a child with suspected nonaccidental trauma (NAT). Fractures are the second most common injury caused by child abuse.[191] Conventional [99m]Tc-MDP bone scintigraphy has been used occasionally as an alternate complementary imaging study in suspected NAT,

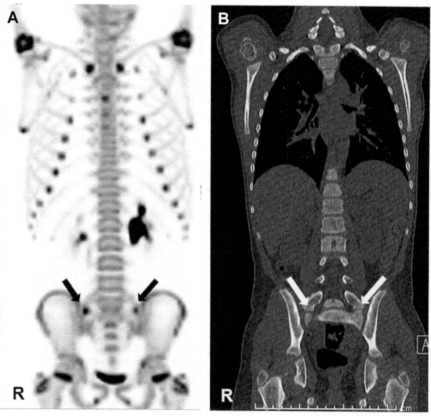

**Fig. 10.** Pseudoarthroses in a lumbosacral transitional vertebrae. A 5-year-old girl presented with back pain. Anterior MIP image (*A*) from an [18]F-NaF PET/CT demonstrates focal bilateral uptake the lumbosacral region (*black arrows*). Coronal CT image in bone window (*B*) demonstrates that these foci of uptake correspond to pseudoarthroses between the transverse processes of a transitional lumbarized S1 vertebra and sacral alae (*white arrows*).

but has been shown to have poor sensitivity for some of the commonly occurring skeletal injuries, including skull fractures and classic metaphyseal lesions (CMLs). Given its greater sensitivity and resolution compared with the [99m]Tc-MDP MDP bone scan, [18]F-NaF PET or PET/CT might be of greater value as a problem-solving tool in cases of suspected or proven child abuse. In a study by Drubach and colleagues[38] of 22 patients younger than 2 with suspected NAT, [18]F-NaF PET was found to be 85% sensitive for the detection of all fractures, 92% sensitive for the detection of thoracic fractures, 93% sensitive for the detection of posterior rib fractures, but only 67% sensitive for the detection of CMLs. [18]F-NaF PET/CT had greater sensitivity in the overall detection of fractures related to child abuse than did the independently reviewed correlative baseline and follow-up skeletal surveys obtained in these same patients, particularly with regard to identification of rib fractures, thus making it an attractive modality in the assessment suspected NAT. However, because of the relatively low sensitivity of

[18]F-NaF PET in the detection of CMLs, a specific fracture in child abuse, initial radiographic evaluation remains necessary (**Fig. 11**).

## INFECTION AND INFLAMMATION
### Osteomyelitis

Almost 50% of cases of osteomyelitis, an infection of bone and bone marrow, occur in children who are younger than 5 years, with boys nearly twice as frequently affected as girls.[192,193] Although acute osteomyelitis typically involves a single site, multifocal involvement can be present in as many as 22% of neonates and 7% of children.[194] The hematogenous spread of bacterial infection is the most frequent cause of acute osteomyelitis in children as opposed to adults in whom osteomyelitis more commonly occurs following direct inoculation of bacteria into bone as a consequence of diabetic foot infections, open fractures, or the surgical treatment of closed injuries.[195]

*Staphylococcus aureus* is the most common etiologic agent identified in culture-positive

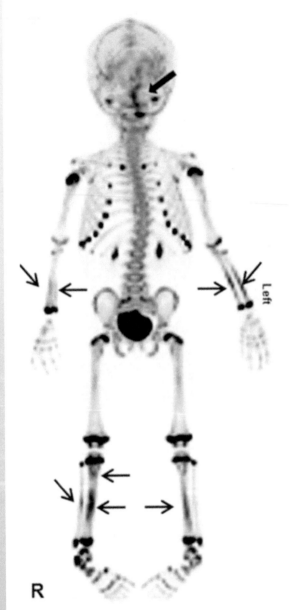

R

Left

**Fig. 11.** NAT. A 15-month-old girl presented with suspected NAT. Anterior MIP image from $^{18}$F-NaF PET/CT demonstrates multiple foci of increased uptake, including linear uptake in the left occipital bone (*thick arrow*), which corresponded to a fracture seen on the preceding skeletal survey (not shown), bilateral radii and ulnas (*thin arrows* on upper extremities); bilateral tibias, and right fibula (*thin arrows* on lower extremities). These are highly concerning for nonaccidental trauma. Many of these fractures had none or subtle correlates on the skeletal survey (not shown). On the skeletal survey, CMLs in multiple extremity bones and left eighth costochondral junction fracture were seen that were occult on the $^{18}$F-NaF PET/CT due to adjacent significant physiologic physeal activity. Radiographic skeletal survey and $^{18}$F-NaF PET/CT scan are complementary in detecting osseous injuries in patients with suspected NAT.

cases of acute osteomyelitis.[196] Unfortunately, the bacteriology as well as the clinical and imaging presentation of acute hematogenous osteomyelitis has changed in the past 2 decades. A recent review of the imaging appearances of osteomyelitis by Jaramillo and colleagues[194] reports an increased incidence of subperiosteal abscess, soft tissue involvement, multifocality, deep venous thrombosis, and pathologic fractures associated with the increased virulence of methicillin-resistant *S aureus*. In addition, *Kingella kingae* has emerged as a more commonly seen pathogen.[194,196]

In children, the metaphysis or the metaphyseal equivalents are the primary sites of infection due to their increased vascularity. Metaphyseal equivalents include the junction of bone and cartilage in a flat bone, round bone, or the periphery of a secondary ossification center.[197] In radiology, it is classically taught that in children younger than 18 months, transphyseal bridging vessels allow the spread of the infection to the epiphysis and joint space; likewise, physeal closure in late adolescence reestablishes this vascular connection and once again renders the adjacent joint cavity susceptible to infection as is commonly seen in adults with osteomyelitis. Gilbertson-Dahdal and colleagues[198] retrospectively reviewed the MR imaging studies of 32 pediatric patients aged 2 to 16 years with clinically suspected osteomyelitis. In 81% of the patients, transphyseal extension of infection into the epiphysis was detected. Therefore, it may be concluded that transphyseal extension of pyogenic osteomyelitis is more common than is classically taught.

According to Jaramillo and colleagues,[194] 3 questions need to be addressed with imaging. These include the presence or absence of osteomyelitis, the site of involvement and multifocality, and whether associated complications of acute osteomyelitis are present. The imaging approach typically starts with a radiograph and is followed by either a 2-phase or 3-phase $^{99m}$Tc-MDP bone scan or contrast-enhanced MR imaging. The bone scan is often the initial study obtained to confirm the diagnosis of suspected osteomyelitis and to provide whole-body assessment for multifocal disease involvement.[199] Although the $^{99m}$Tc-MDP bone scan exposes the child to ionizing radiation, it is often more readily available, less expensive, and less frequently requires the use of sedation as compared with MR imaging. On the other hand, MR imaging does not expose the patient to ionizing radiation and is particularly useful when the site of infection is known, when vertebral or pelvic osteomyelitis is suspected, or if there is no response to antibiotics after 48 hours

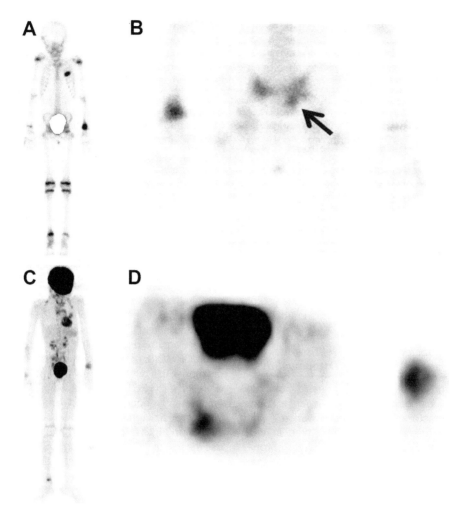

**Fig. 12.** CRMO. A 7-year-old girl with suspected ES. Anterior whole-body (*A*) and post-void, posterior spot images of the pelvis (*B*) from a $^{99m}$Tc-MDP bone scan demonstrate increased uptake in a left rib, the left distal radial metaphysis, right sacrum (*arrow* in [*B*]), and the right distal tibial metaphysis. The radial lesion was consistent with CRMO on biopsy. Anterior MIP (*C*) and axial (*D*) image from a whole-body $^{18}$F-FDG PET/CT scan demonstrate that all lesions are FDG-avid. Note normal physiologic sites of uptake including thymus and brown fat in the supraclavicular regions that should not be confused with pathology.

of treatment, particularly if complications are suspected. In some institutions, MR imaging is the initial imaging modality of choice for suspected osteomyelitis and if MR imaging is not available, then a combination of bone scintigraphy and ultrasound are used to detect osseous and extraosseous complications, including subperiosteal and soft tissue abscesses, joint effusion, or deep venous thrombosis.[194]

$^{18}$F-FDG PET/CT has been shown to be highly sensitive (100%) and specific (86%–96%) for acute uncomplicated osteomyelitis in adults.[200,201] $^{18}$F-FDG uptake has also been reported in children with osteomyelitis. However, due to cost, radiation exposure, and the need for sedation in the young child, $^{18}$F-FDG PET/CT is of limited utility in the diagnosis of acute osteomyelitis compared with the combination of physical examination, altered laboratory markers, and $^{99m}$Tc-MDP bone scan.[18]

Signore and colleagues[21] reviewed the literature regarding the use of $^{18}$F-FDG PET/CT in the evaluation of osteomyelitis or soft tissue infections in the pediatric population and concluded that although there have been no large pediatric studies performed, $^{18}$F-FDG PET/CT can be useful to detect sites of suspected occult infection, a role that has shown promise in adults. Warmann and colleagues[202] demonstrated that $^{18}$F-FDG PET/CT also may be of value in distinguishing reparative activity from residual infection and be preferable to MR imaging in this regard.

On the other hand, [18]F-FDG PET/CT is the imaging modality of choice in adults with chronic osteomyelitis, where sensitivity, specificity, and accuracy of 100%, 88%, and 93%, respectively, have been reported by de Winter and colleagues.[203] Reported specificity of [18]F-FDG PET/CT for chronic osteomyelitis is higher than that of MR imaging, as well as of conventional scintigraphic techniques, such as [99m]Tc-MDP bone scan, [67]Ga scan, or radiolabeled white blood cell imaging.[204,205]

[68]Ga can be used in the imaging of infection and inflammation in both preclinical and clinical settings.[44] Nanni and colleagues[206] evaluated 40 [68]Ga-citrate PET/CT scans in 31 adult patients with suspected osteomyelitis or discitis and reported an overall diagnostic accuracy of 90%, sensitivity of 100%, specificity of 76%, positive predictive value of 85%, and negative predictive value of 100% for the diagnosis of these 2 entities. To date, no pediatric studies evaluating the use of [68]Ga-citrate in osteomyelitis have been published.

### Chronic Nonbacterial Osteomyelitis and Chronic Recurrent Multifocal Osteomyelitis

According to Hofmann and colleagues,[207] chronic nonbacterial osteomyelitis (CNO) is an autoimmune inflammatory bone disorder with a "wide clinical spectrum ranging from mild, time-limited, monofocal bone inflammation to severe, chronically active or recurrent multifocal bone inflammation." The most severe presentations in this spectrum are referred to as chronic recurrent multifocal osteomyelitis (CRMO). Familial/monogenic and sporadic forms of CNO have been described.[207] CNO is primarily seen in children, typically in the 9-year to 14-year age group, with a marked female predominance. The most commonly involved sites are the metaphyses of the distal femur, proximal and distal tibia, distal fibula, and clavicle. The spine, pelvis, and epiphyseal equivalents in thorax also may be involved. Spinal involvement may result in vertebra plana. The metaphyseal lesions may cross into the adjacent epiphysis. The disease process may be monostotic or polyostotic; the latter may be symmetric or asymmetrical.[207–209]

The underlying etiology is autoimmune and no infectious agent is identified on bone biopsy. On histology, chronic nonspecific inflammation is seen. CNO is often diagnosed after the exclusion of other diseases, such as neoplasm and infection. Although CNO typically has a relapsing and remitting course, it may be self-limited in some cases.[207–209] Treatment options include analgesics, nonsteroidal anti-inflammatory agents, corticosteroids, and bisphosphonates.[208] CNO is now considered by some to be a part of the SAPHO syndrome spectrum (synovitis, acne, pustulosis, hyperostosis, and osteitis).[208–210]

On radiographs, the main imaging findings are hyperostosis with cortical bone hypertrophy, resultant cortical thickening, bone expansion, and narrowing of the medullary canal; and osteitis with inflammation of the medullary canal and resultant sclerotic and lytic areas. Fluid-sensitive MR imaging sequences, such as short TI inversion recovery (STIR), initially demonstrate bone marrow edema in the metaphysis, with possible epiphyseal extension. Additional findings may include hyperostosis, periosteal reaction, and inflammation in the adjacent soft tissues. Fluid-sensitive MR imaging sequences may also be used to detect involvement in subclinical sites of disease. In comparison with MR imaging, [99m]Tc-MDP whole-body bone scintigraphy has several shortcomings in these patients, namely the use of ionizing radiation and obscuration of the juxtaphyseal lesions by the normal physiologic uptake in the adjacent growth plates.[208]

There are few reports of the use of [18]F-FDG PET/CT in CRMO. Liu[211] reported a case in a 45-year-old man with a destructive rib lesion in 2016. In children, [18]F-FDG PET/CT evaluation of CNO[22,212] has inadvertently occurred when anatomic imaging suggested a diagnosis of primary bone malignancy such as in **Fig. 12**. There also have been reports of use the use of [18]F-FDG imaging in SAPHO to determine distribution of the disease and differentiate active from inactive lesions.[210] Newer agents, such as NaF and [68]Ga, may prove useful for both CRMO and SAPHO, particularly to determine response to therapy.

## SUMMARY

Although more work needs to be done to ultimately determine the role of [18]F-FDG PET/CT as a surrogate biomarker in children with bone and soft tissue tumors, this radiotracer has gained wide acceptance in the detection and therapeutic response monitoring of these diseases. [18]F-FDG PET/CT is used to a lesser degree in the evaluation and monitoring of bone infections in children with the exception of chronic osteomyelitis and, perhaps, CRMO. Resurgence of interest in [18]F-NaF PET/CT as well as the development of [68]Ga-labeled tracers pose exciting new opportunities for use in musculoskeletal imaging applications in children.

## REFERENCES

1. Muehe AM, Theruvath AJ, Lai L, et al. How to provide gadolinium-free PET/MR cancer staging of

children and young adults in less than 1 h: the Stanford approach. Mol Imaging Biol 2017;48: 1920.

2. Daldrup-Link H. How PET/MR can add value for children with cancer. Curr Radiol Rep 2017;5(3): 1920.

3. Shammas A, Lim R, Charron M. Pediatric FDG PET/CT: physiologic uptake, normal variants, and benign conditions. Radiographics 2009;29(5):1467–86.

4. Grant FD. Normal variations and benign findings in pediatric 18F-FDG-PET/CT. PET Clin 2014;9(2): 195–208.

5. Siegel JA, Pennington CW, Sacks B. Subjecting radiologic imaging to the linear no-threshold hypothesis: a non sequitur of non-trivial proportion. J Nucl Med 2017;58(1):1–6.

6. Preston DL, Cullings H, Suyama A, et al. Solid cancer incidence in atomic bomb survivors exposed in utero or as young children. J Natl Cancer Inst 2008; 100(6):428–36.

7. Brenner D, Elliston C, Hall E, et al. Estimated risks of radiation-induced fatal cancer from pediatric CT. AJR Am J Roentgenol 2001;176(2):289–96.

8. Jafari ME, Daus AM. Applying image gently SM and image wisely SM in nuclear medicine. Health Phys 2013;104(2 Suppl 1):S31–6.

9. Gelfand MJ, Parisi MT, Treves ST. Pediatric radiopharmaceutical administered doses: 2010 North American consensus guidelines. J Nucl Med 2011;52(2):318–22.

10. Lassmann M, Biassoni L, Monsieurs M, et al. The new EANM paediatric dosage card. Eur J Nucl Med Mol Imaging 2007;34(5):796–8.

11. Lassmann M, Treves ST. Pediatric radiopharmaceutical administration: harmonization of the 2007 EANM paediatric dosage card (Version 1.5.2008) and the 2010 North American Consensus guideline. Eur J Nucl Med Mol Imaging 2014;41(8):1636.

12. Treves ST, Gelfand MJ, Fahey FH, et al. Update of the North American consensus guidelines for pediatric administered radiopharmaceutical activities. J Nucl Med 2016;57(12):15N–8N.

13. Dosage Card - EANM. Available at: http://www.eanm.org/publications/dosage-card/. Accessed February 25, 2018.

14. Gelfand MJ, Lemen LC. PET/CT and SPECT/CT dosimetry in children: the challenge to the pediatric imager. Semin Nucl Med 2007;37(5):391–8.

15. Parisi MT, Bermo MS, Alessio AM, et al. Optimization of pediatric PET/CT. Semin Nucl Med 2017; 47(3):258–74.

16. Gallagher BM, Fowler JS, Gutterson NI, et al. Metabolic trapping as a principle of radiopharmaceutical design: some factors responsble for the biodistribution of [18F] 2-deoxy-2-fluoro-D-glucose. J Nucl Med 1978; 19(10):1154–61.

17. Parisi MT. Functional imaging of infection: conventional nuclear medicine agents and the expanding role of 18-F-FDG PET. Pediatr Radiol 2011;41(7): 803–10.

18. Basu S, Chryssikos T, Moghadam-Kia S, et al. Positron emission tomography as a diagnostic tool in infection: present role and future possibilities. Semin Nucl Med 2009;39(1):36–51.

19. Drubach LA. Nuclear medicine techniques in pediatric bone imaging. Semin Nucl Med 2017;47(3): 190–203.

20. Grant FD, Drubach LA, Treves ST. 18)F-Fluorodeoxyglucose PET and PET/CT in pediatric musculoskeletal malignancies. PET Clin 2010;5(3): 349–61.

21. Signore A, Glaudemans AWJM, Gheysens O, et al. Nuclear medicine imaging in pediatric infection or chronic inflammatory diseases. Semin Nucl Med 2017;47(3):286–303.

22. Parisi MT, Otjen JP, Stanescu AL, et al. Radionuclide imaging of infection and inflammation in children: a review. Semin Nucl Med 2018;48(2):148–65.

23. Servaes S. Imaging infection and inflammation in children with (18)F-FDG PET and (18)F-FDG PET/CT. J Nucl Med Technol 2011;39(3):179–82.

24. del Rosal T, Goycochea WA, Mendez-Echevarria A, et al. (1)(8)F-FDG PET/CT in the diagnosis of occult bacterial infections in children. Eur J Pediatr 2013; 172(8):1111–5.

25. Depas G, Decortis T, Francotte N, et al. F-18 FDG PET in infectious diseases in children. Clin Nucl Med 2007;32(8):593–8.

26. Grant FD, Gelfand MJ, Drubach LA, et al. Radiation doses for pediatric nuclear medicine studies: comparing the North American consensus guidelines and the pediatric dosage card of the European Association of Nuclear Medicine. Pediatr Radiol 2015;45(5):706–13.

27. Alessio AM, Kinahan PE, Manchanda V, et al. Weight-based, low-dose pediatric whole-body PET/CT protocols. J Nucl Med 2009;50(10):1570–7.

28. Blau M, Nagler W, Bender MA. Fluorine-18: a new isotope for bone scanning. J Nucl Med 1962;3: 332–4.

29. Thrall JH. Technetium-99m labeled agents for skeletal imaging. CRC Crit Rev Clin Radiol Nucl Med 1976;8(1):1–31.

30. Davis MA, Jones AL. Comparison of 99mTc-labeled phosphate and phosphonate agents for skeletal imaging. Semin Nucl Med 1976;6(1): 19–31.

31. Hawkins RA, Choi Y, Huang SC, et al. Evaluation of the skeletal kinetics of fluorine-18-fluoride ion with PET. J Nucl Med 1992;33(5):633–42.

32. Hoh CK, Hawkins RA, Dahlbom M, et al. Whole body skeletal imaging with [18F]fluoride ion and PET. J Comput Assist Tomogr 1993;17(1):34–41.

33. Weber DA, Greenberg EJ, Dimich A, et al. Kinetics of radionuclides used for bone studies. J Nucl Med 1969;10(1):8–17.

34. Costeas A, Woodard HQ, Laughlin JS. Depletion of 18F from blood flowing through bone. J Nucl Med 1970;11(1):43–5.

35. Blake GM, Park-Holohan SJ, Cook GJ, et al. Quantitative studies of bone with the use of 18F-fluoride and 99mTc-methylene diphosphonate. Semin Nucl Med 2001;31(1):28–49.

36. Grant FD, Fahey FH, Packard AB, et al. Skeletal PET with 18F-fluoride: applying new technology to an old tracer. J Nucl Med 2008;49(1):68–78.

37. Ohnona J, Michaud L, Balogova S, et al. Can we achieve a radionuclide radiation dose equal to or less than that of 99mTc-hydroxymethane diphosphonate bone scintigraphy with a low-dose 18F-sodium fluoride time-of-flight PET of diagnostic quality? Nucl Med Commun 2013;34(5): 417–25.

38. Drubach LA, Johnston PR, Newton AW, et al. Skeletal trauma in child abuse: detection with 18F-NaF PET. Radiology 2010;255(1):173–81.

39. Segall G, Delbeke D, Stabin MG, et al. SNM practice guideline for sodium 18F-fluoride PET/CT bone scans 1.0. J Nucl Med 2010;51(11):1813–20.

40. Lim R, Fahey FH, Drubach LA, et al. Early experience with fluorine-18 sodium fluoride bone PET in young patients with back pain. J Pediatr Orthop 2007;27(3):277–82.

41. Drubach LA, Sapp MV, Laffin S, et al. Fluorine-18 NaF PET imaging of child abuse. Pediatr Radiol 2008;38(7):776–9.

42. Drubach LA. Pediatric bone scanning: clinical indication of (18)F NaF PET/CT. PET Clin 2012;7(3): 293–301.

43. Grant FD. (1)(8)F-fluoride PET and PET/CT in children and young adults. PET Clin 2014;9(3): 287–97.

44. Vorster M, Maes A, Wiele CV de, et al. Gallium-68 PET: a powerful generator-based alternative to infection and inflammation imaging. Semin Nucl Med 2016;46(5):436–47.

45. Shamim SA, Kumar A, Kumar R. PET/computed tomography in neuroendocrine tumor: value to patient management and survival outcomes. PET Clin 2015;10(3):411–21.

46. Kilian K. 68)Ga-DOTA and analogs: current status and future perspectives. Rep Pract Oncol Radiother 2014;19(Suppl):S13–21.

47. Poeppel TD, Binse I, Petersenn S, et al. 68Ga-DOTATOC versus 68Ga-DOTATATE PET/CT in functional imaging of neuroendocrine tumors. J Nucl Med 2011;52(12):1864–70.

48. Costelloe CM, Chuang HH, Daw NC. PET/CT of osteosarcoma and Ewing sarcoma. Semin Roentgenol 2017;52(4):255–68.

49. Li Y-J, Dai Y-L, Cheng Y-S, et al. Positron emission tomography (18)F-fluorodeoxyglucose uptake and prognosis in patients with bone and soft tissue sarcoma: a meta-analysis. Eur J Surg Oncol 2016; 42(8):1103–14.

50. Im H-J, Bradshaw T, Solaiyappan M, et al. Current methods to define metabolic tumor volume in positron emission tomography: which one is better? Nucl Med Mol Imaging 2018;52(1):5–15.

51. Wahl RL, Jacene H, Kasamon Y, et al. From RECIST to PERCIST: evolving considerations for PET response criteria in solid tumors. J Nucl Med 2009;50(Suppl 1):122S–50S.

52. Harrison DJ, Parisi MT, Shulkin BL. The role of (18) F-FDG-PET/CT in pediatric sarcoma. Semin Nucl Med 2017;47(3):229–41.

53. Grimer RJ, Hogendoorn P, Vanel D. Tumours of bone: introduction. In: CDM F, Bridge JA, Hogendoorn P, et al, editors. WHO classification of tumours of soft tissue and bone. 4th edition. Lyon (France): International Agency for Research on Cancer; 2013. p. 244–7.

54. Miller TT. Bone tumors and tumorlike conditions: analysis with conventional radiography. Radiology 2008;246(3):662–74.

55. Reed DR, Hayashi M, Wagner L, et al. Treatment pathway of bone sarcoma in children, adolescents, and young adults. Cancer 2017;123(12): 2206–18.

56. Even-Sapir E, Metser U, Flusser G, et al. Assessment of malignant skeletal disease: initial experience with 18F-fluoride PET/CT and comparison between 18F-fluoride PET and 18F-fluoride PET/CT. J Nucl Med 2004;45(2):272–8.

57. Iagaru A, Mittra E, Mosci C, et al. Combined 18F-fluoride and 18F-FDG PET/CT scanning for evaluation of malignancy: results of an international multicenter trial. J Nucl Med 2013;54(2): 176–83.

58. Bortot DC, Amorim BJ, Oki GC, et al. (1)(8)F-Fluoride PET/CT is highly effective for excluding bone metastases even in patients with equivocal bone scintigraphy. Eur J Nucl Med Mol Imaging 2012; 39(11):1730–6.

59. Damle NA, Bal C, Bandopadhyaya GP, et al. The role of 18F-fluoride PET-CT in the detection of bone metastases in patients with breast, lung and prostate carcinoma: a comparison with FDG PET/CT and 99mTc-MDP bone scan. Jpn J Radiol 2013;31(4):262–9.

60. Jadvar H, Desai B, Conti PS. Sodium 18F-fluoride PET/CT of bone, joint, and other disorders. Semin Nucl Med 2015;45(1):58–65.

61. Jawad MU, Scully SP. In brief: classifications in brief: Enneking classification: benign and malignant tumors of the musculoskeletal system. Clin Orthop Relat Res 2010;468(7):2000–2.

62. Enneking WF. A system of staging musculoskeletal neoplasms. Clin Orthop Relat Res 1986; 204:9–24.

63. Mirabello L, Troisi RJ, Savage SA. Osteosarcoma incidence and survival rates from 1973 to 2004: data from the surveillance, epidemiology, and end results program. Cancer 2009;115(7):1531–43.

64. Osteosarcoma and Malignant Fibrous Histiocytoma of Bone Treatment (PDQ®)–Health Professional Version was originally published by the National Cancer Institute. Updated June 11, 2018. Available at https://www.cancer.gov/types/bone/hp/osteosarcoma-treatment-pdq. Accessed February 25, 2018.

65. Ripperger T, Bielack SS, Borkhardt A, et al. Childhood cancer predisposition syndromes: a concise review and recommendations by The Cancer Predisposition Working Group of the Society for Pediatric Oncology and Hematology. Am J Med Genet A 2017;173(4):1017–37.

66. Brown HK, Schiavone K, Gouin F, et al. Biology of bone sarcomas and new therapeutic developments. Calcif Tissue Int 2018;102(2):174–95.

67. Kager L, Zoubek A, Kastner U, et al. Skip metastases in osteosarcoma: experience of the cooperative osteosarcoma study group. J Clin Oncol 2006;24(10):1535–41.

68. Harrison DJ, Geller DS, Gill JD, et al. Current and future therapeutic approaches for osteosarcoma. Expert Rev Anticancer Ther 2018;18(1):39–50.

69. Kushner BH, Meyers PA. How effective is dose-intensive/myeloablative therapy against Ewing's sarcoma/primitive neuroectodermal tumor metastatic to bone or bone marrow? The Memorial Sloan-Kettering experience and a literature review. J Clin Oncol 2001;19(3):870–80.

70. Paulussen M, Ahrens S, Craft AW, et al. Ewing's tumors with primary lung metastases: survival analysis of 114 (European Intergroup) Cooperative Ewing's Sarcoma Studies patients. J Clin Oncol 1998;16(9):3044–52.

71. Brenner W, Bohuslavizki KH, Eary JF. PET imaging of osteosarcoma. J Nucl Med 2003;44(6): 930–42.

72. Quartuccio N, Treglia G, Salsano M, et al. The role of Fluorine-18-Fluorodeoxyglucose positron emission tomography in staging and restaging of patients with osteosarcoma. Radiol Oncol 2013; 47(2):97–102.

73. Byun BH, Kong C-B, Lim I, et al. Comparison of (18)F-FDG PET/CT and (99 m)Tc-MDP bone scintigraphy for detection of bone metastasis in osteosarcoma. Skeletal Radiol 2013;42(12): 1673–81.

74. Hurley C, McCarville MB, Shulkin BL, et al. Comparison of (18) F-FDG-PET-CT and bone scintigraphy for evaluation of osseous metastases in newly diagnosed and recurrent osteosarcoma. Pediatr Blood Cancer 2016;63(8):1381–6.

75. Hamada K, Tomita Y, Inoue A, et al. Evaluation of chemotherapy response in osteosarcoma with FDG-PET. Ann Nucl Med 2009;23(1):89–95.

76. Denecke T, Hundsdorfer P, Misch D, et al. Assessment of histological response of paediatric bone sarcomas using FDG PET in comparison to morphological volume measurement and standardized MRI parameters. Eur J Nucl Med Mol Imaging 2010;37(10):1842–53.

77. Byun BH, Kong C-B, Lim I, et al. Combination of 18F-FDG PET/CT and diffusion-weighted MR imaging as a predictor of histologic response to neoadjuvant chemotherapy: preliminary results in osteosarcoma. J Nucl Med 2013;54(7): 1053–9.

78. Hongtao L, Hui Z, Bingshun W, et al. 18F-FDG positron emission tomography for the assessment of histological response to neoadjuvant chemotherapy in osteosarcomas: a meta-analysis. Surg Oncol 2012;21(4):e165–70.

79. Costelloe CM, Macapinlac HA, Madewell JE, et al. 18F-FDG PET/CT as an indicator of progression-free and overall survival in osteosarcoma. J Nucl Med 2009;50(3):340–7.

80. Hawkins DS, Conrad EU3, Butrynski JE, et al. [F-18]-fluorodeoxy-D-glucose-positron emission tomography response is associated with outcome for extremity osteosarcoma in children and young adults. Cancer 2009;115(15):3519–25.

81. Frezza AM, Beale T, Bomanji J, et al. Is [F-18]-fluorodeoxy-D-glucose positron emission tomography of value in the management of patients with craniofacial bone sarcomas undergoing neoadjuvant treatment? BMC Cancer 2014;14(1):23.

82. Byun BH, Kong C-B, Park J, et al. Initial metabolic tumor volume measured by 18F-FDG PET/CT can predict the outcome of osteosarcoma of the extremities. J Nucl Med 2013;54(10):1725–32.

83. Kong C-B, Byun BH, Lim I, et al. (1)(8)F-FDG PET SUVmax as an indicator of histopathologic response after neoadjuvant chemotherapy in extremity osteosarcoma. Eur J Nucl Med Mol Imaging 2013;40(5):728–36.

84. Chang KJ, Kong C-B, Cho WH, et al. Usefulness of increased 18F-FDG uptake for detecting local recurrence in patients with extremity osteosarcoma treated with surgical resection and endoprosthetic replacement. Skeletal Radiol 2015;44(4):529–37.

85. Quartuccio N, Fox J, Kuk D, et al. Pediatric bone sarcoma: diagnostic performance of (1)(8)F-FDG PET/CT versus conventional imaging for initial staging and follow-up. AJR Am J Roentgenol 2015; 204(1):153–60.

86. Byun BH, Kim SH, Lim SM, et al. Prediction of response to neoadjuvant chemotherapy in

osteosarcoma using dual-phase (18)F-FDG PET/CT. Eur Radiol 2015;25(7):2015–24.

87. Arush MWB, Israel O, Postovsky S, et al. Positron emission tomography/computed tomography with 18fluoro-deoxyglucose in the detection of local recurrence and distant metastases of pediatric sarcoma. Pediatr Blood Cancer 2007;49(7):901–5.

88. Dancheva Z, Bochev P, Chaushev B, et al. Dual-time point 18FDG-PET/CT imaging may be useful in assessing local recurrent disease in high grade bone and soft tissue sarcoma. Nucl Med Rev Cent East Eur 2016;19(1):22–7.

89. Sharma P, Khangembam BC, Suman KCS, et al. Diagnostic accuracy of 18F-FDG PET/CT for detecting recurrence in patients with primary skeletal Ewing sarcoma. Eur J Nucl Med Mol Imaging 2013;40(7):1036–43.

90. Mortensen J. Assessing nodules detected in lung cancer screening: the value of positron emission tomography. Eur Respir J 2015;45(2):314–6.

91. Goerres GW, Kamel E, Heidelberg T-NH, et al. PET-CT image co-registration in the thorax: influence of respiration. Eur J Nucl Med Mol Imaging 2002;29(3):351–60.

92. Hashimoto Y, Tsujikawa T, Kondo C, et al. Accuracy of PET for diagnosis of solid pulmonary lesions with 18F-FDG uptake below the standardized uptake value of 2.5. J Nucl Med 2006;47(3):426–31.

93. Kim SK, Allen-Auerbach M, Goldin J, et al. Accuracy of PET/CT in characterization of solitary pulmonary lesions. J Nucl Med 2007;48(2):214–20.

94. Lupi A, Zaroccolo M, Salgarello M, et al. The effect of 18F-FDG-PET/CT respiratory gating on detected metabolic activity in lung lesions. Ann Nucl Med 2009;23(2):191–6.

95. Osman MM, Cohade C, Nakamoto Y, et al. Respiratory motion artifacts on PET emission images obtained using CT attenuation correction on PET-CT. Eur J Nucl Med Mol Imaging 2003;30(4):603–6.

96. Schirrmeister H, Guhlmann A, Elsner K, et al. Sensitivity in detecting osseous lesions depends on anatomic localization: planar bone scintigraphy versus 18F PET. J Nucl Med 1999;40(10):1623–9.

97. Arvanitis C, Bendapudi PK, Tseng JR, et al. (18)F and (18)FDG PET imaging of osteosarcoma to non-invasively monitor in situ changes in cellular proliferation and bone differentiation upon MYC inactivation. Cancer Biol Ther 2008;7(12):1947–51.

98. Esiashvili N, Goodman M, Marcus RBJ. Changes in incidence and survival of Ewing sarcoma patients over the past 3 decades: Surveillance Epidemiology and End Results data. J Pediatr Hematol Oncol 2008;30(6):425–30.

99. Ewing Sarcoma Treatment (PDQ®)–Health Professional Version was originally published by the National Cancer Institute. Updated August 17, 2018. Available at https://www.cancer.gov/types/bone/hp/ewing-treatment-pdq. Accessed February 25, 2018.

100. Kopp LM, Hu C, Rozo B, et al. Utility of bone marrow aspiration and biopsy in initial staging of Ewing sarcoma. Pediatr Blood Cancer 2015;62(1):12–5.

101. Anderson PM. Futility versus utility of marrow assessment in initial Ewing sarcoma staging workup. Pediatr Blood Cancer 2015;62(1):1–2.

102. Volker T, Denecke T, Steffen I, et al. Positron emission tomography for staging of pediatric sarcoma patients: results of a prospective multicenter trial. J Clin Oncol 2007;25(34):5435–41.

103. Franzius C, Sciuk J, Daldrup-Link HE, et al. FDG-PET for detection of osseous metastases from malignant primary bone tumours: comparison with bone scintigraphy. Eur J Nucl Med 2000;27(9):1305–11.

104. Newman EN, Jones RL, Hawkins DS. An evaluation of [F-18]-fluorodeoxy-D-glucose positron emission tomography, bone scan, and bone marrow aspiration/biopsy as staging investigations in Ewing sarcoma. Pediatr Blood Cancer 2013;60(7):1113–7.

105. Treglia G, Salsano M, Stefanelli A, et al. Diagnostic accuracy of (1)(8)F-FDG-PET and PET/CT in patients with Ewing sarcoma family tumours: a systematic review and a meta-analysis. Skeletal Radiol 2012;41(3):249–56.

106. Hawkins DS, Schuetze SM, Butrynski JE, et al. [18F]Fluorodeoxyglucose positron emission tomography predicts outcome for Ewing sarcoma family of tumors. J Clin Oncol 2005;23(34):8828–34.

107. Raciborska A, Bilska K, Drabko K, et al. Response to chemotherapy estimates by FDG PET is an important prognostic factor in patients with Ewing sarcoma. Clin Transl Oncol 2016;18(2):189–95.

108. Gaston LL, Di Bella C, Slavin J, et al. 18F-FDG PET response to neoadjuvant chemotherapy for Ewing sarcoma and osteosarcoma are different. Skeletal Radiol 2011;40(8):1007–15.

109. Salem U, Amini B, Chuang HH, et al. (18)F-FDG PET/CT as an indicator of survival in Ewing sarcoma of bone. J Cancer 2017;8(15):2892–8.

110. Hwang JP, Lim I, Kong C-B, et al. Prognostic value of SUVmax measured by pretreatment fluorine-18 fluorodeoxyglucose positron emission tomography/computed tomography in patients with Ewing sarcoma. Heymann D, ed. PLoS One 2016;11(4):e0153281.

111. Hyun OJ, Luber BS, Leal JP, et al. Response to early treatment evaluated with 18F-FDG PET and PERCIST 1.0 predicts survival in patients with Ewing sarcoma family of tumors treated with a monoclonal antibody to the insulinlike growth factor 1 receptor. J Nucl Med 2016;57(5):735–40.

112. Pappo AS, Dirksen U. Rhabdomyosarcoma, Ewing sarcoma, and other round cell sarcomas. J Clin Oncol 2018;36(2):168–79.

113. Pappo AS, Pratt CB. Soft tissue sarcomas in children. Cancer Treat Res 1997;91:205–22.

114. Childhood Soft Tissue Sarcoma Treatment (PDQ®)–Health Professional Version was originally published by the National Cancer Institute. Updated April 2, 2018. Available at https://www.cancer.gov/types/soft-tissue-sarcoma/hp/child-soft-tissue-treatment-pdq. Accessed February 25, 2018.

115. Childhood Rhabdomyosarcoma Treatment (PDQ®)–Health Professional Version was originally published by the National Cancer Institute. Updated April 4, 2018. Available at https://www.cancer.gov/types/soft-tissue-sarcoma/hp/rhabdomyosarcoma-treatment-pdq. Accessed February 25, 2018.

116. Kim JR, Yoon HM, Koh K-N, et al. Rhabdomyosarcoma in children and adolescents: patterns and risk factors of distant metastasis. AJR Am J Roentgenol 2017;209(2):409–16.

117. Walterhouse DO, Pappo AS, Meza JL, et al. Shorter-duration therapy using vincristine, dactinomycin, and lower-dose cyclophosphamide with or without radiotherapy for patients with newly diagnosed low-risk rhabdomyosarcoma: a report from the Soft Tissue Sarcoma Committee of the Children's Oncology Group. J Clin Oncol 2014;32(31):3547–52.

118. Arndt CAS, Stoner JA, Hawkins DS, et al. Vincristine, actinomycin, and cyclophosphamide compared with vincristine, actinomycin, and cyclophosphamide alternating with vincristine, topotecan, and cyclophosphamide for intermediate-risk rhabdomyosarcoma: Children's Oncology Group study D9803. J Clin Oncol 2009;27(31):5182–8.

119. Breneman JC, Lyden E, Pappo AS, et al. Prognostic factors and clinical outcomes in children and adolescents with metastatic rhabdomyosarcoma—a report from the Intergroup Rhabdomyosarcoma Study IV. J Clin Oncol 2003;21(1):78–84.

120. Crist WM, Anderson JR, Meza JL, et al. Intergroup rhabdomyosarcoma study-IV: results for patients with nonmetastatic disease. J Clin Oncol 2001;19(12):3091–102.

121. Federico SM, Spunt SL, Krasin MJ, et al. Comparison of PET-CT and conventional imaging in staging pediatric rhabdomyosarcoma. Pediatr Blood Cancer 2013;60(7):1128–34.

122. Eugene T, Corradini N, Carlier T, et al. (1)(8)F-FDG-PET/CT in initial staging and assessment of early response to chemotherapy of pediatric rhabdomyosarcomas. Nucl Med Commun 2012;33(10):1089–95.

123. Norman G, Fayter D, Lewis-Light K, et al. An emerging evidence base for PET-CT in the management of childhood rhabdomyosarcoma: systematic review. BMJ Open 2015;5(1):e006030.

124. Dharmarajan KV, Wexler LH, Gavane S, et al. Positron emission tomography (PET) evaluation after initial chemotherapy and radiation therapy predicts local control in rhabdomyosarcoma. Int J Radiat Oncol Biol Phys 2012;84(4):996–1002.

125. Casey DL, Wexler LH, Fox JJ, et al. Predicting outcome in patients with rhabdomyosarcoma: role of [(18)f]fluorodeoxyglucose positron emission tomography. Int J Radiat Oncol Biol Phys 2014;90(5):1136–42.

126. Listernick R, Charrow J. Neurofibromatosis-1 in childhood. Adv Dermatol 2004;20:75–115.

127. National Institutes of Health Consensus Development Conference Statement: neurofibromatosis. Bethesda, Md., USA, July 13-15, 1987. Neurofibromatosis 1988;1(3):172–8.

128. Widemann BC. Current status of sporadic and neurofibromatosis type 1-associated malignant peripheral nerve sheath tumors. Curr Oncol Rep 2009;11(4):322–8.

129. Antonescu CR, Brems H, Legius E, et al. Neurofibroma (including variants). In: Fletcher C, Bridge JA, Hogendoorn P, et al, editors. WHO classification of tumours of soft tissue and bone. 4th edition. Lyon (France): International Agency for Research on Cancer; 2013. p. 174–6.

130. Nielsen GP, Antonescu CR, Lothe RA. Malignant peripheral nerve sheath tumor. In: Fletcher C, Bridge JA, Hogendoorn P, et al, editors. WHO classification of tumours of soft tissue and bone. 4th edition. Lyon (France): International Agency for Research on Cancer; 2013. p. 187–9.

131. Treglia G, Taralli S, Bertagna F, et al. Usefulness of whole-body fluorine-18-fluorodeoxyglucose positron emission tomography in patients with neurofibromatosis type 1: a systematic review. Radiol Res Pract 2012;2012(5):431029.

132. Combemale P, Valeyrie-Allanore L, Giammarile F, et al. Utility of 18F-FDG PET with a semiquantitative index in the detection of sarcomatous transformation in patients with neurofibromatosis type 1. Scarpa A, ed. PLoS One 2014;9(2):e85954.

133. Benz MR, Czernin J, Dry SM, et al. Quantitative F18-fluorodeoxyglucose positron emission tomography accurately characterizes peripheral nerve sheath tumors as malignant or benign. Cancer 2010;116(2):451–8.

134. Khiewvan B, Macapinlac HA, Lev D, et al. The value of (1)(8)F-FDG PET/CT in the management of malignant peripheral nerve sheath tumors. Eur J Nucl Med Mol Imaging 2014;41(9):1756–66.

135. Tsai LL, Drubach L, Fahey F, et al. [18F]-Fluorodeoxyglucose positron emission tomography in children with neurofibromatosis type 1 and

plexiform neurofibromas: correlation with malignant transformation. J Neurooncol 2012;108(3):469–75.

136. Arora VC, Price AP, Fleming S, et al. Characteristic imaging features of desmoplastic small round cell tumour. Pediatr Radiol 2013;43(1):93–102.

137. Ostermeier A, McCarville MB, Navid F, et al. FDG PET/CT imaging of desmoplastic small round cell tumor: findings at staging, during treatment and at follow-up. Pediatr Radiol 2015;45(9):1308–15.

138. Herrmann K, Benz MR, Czernin J, et al. 18F-FDG-PET/CT imaging as an early survival predictor in patients with primary high-grade soft tissue sarcomas undergoing neoadjuvant therapy. Clin Cancer Res 2012;18(7):2024–31.

139. Chang KJ, Lim I, Park JY, et al. The role of (18)F-FDG PET/CT as a prognostic factor in patients with synovial sarcoma. Nucl Med Mol Imaging 2015;49(1):33–41.

140. Beal K, Allen L, Yahalom J. Primary bone lymphoma: treatment results and prognostic factors with long-term follow-up of 82 patients. Cancer 2006;106(12):2652–6.

141. Ostrowski ML, Unni KK, Banks PM, et al. Malignant lymphoma of bone. Cancer 1986;58(12):2646–55.

142. Bowman WE, Cooper KL, Unni KK, et al. Malignant lymphoma of bone. Orthopedics 1982;5(1):77–85.

143. Liu Y. The role of 18F-FDG PET/CT in staging and restaging primary bone lymphoma. Nucl Med Commun 2017;38(4):319–24.

144. Wang L-J, Wu H-B, Wang M, et al. Utility of F-18 FDG PET/CT on the evaluation of primary bone lymphoma. Eur J Radiol 2015;84(11):2275–9.

145. Park YH, Kim S, Choi S-J, et al. Clinical impact of whole-body FDG-PET for evaluation of response and therapeutic decision-making of primary lymphoma of bone. Ann Oncol 2005;16(8):1401–2.

146. Kanoun S, Cottereau A-S, Berriolo-Riedinger A, et al. "Staging, restaging and treatment response assessment" in lymphomas: what we should know. J Nucl Med 2018;59(4):714–5.

147. Cheson BD. PET/CT in lymphoma: current overview and future directions. Semin Nucl Med 2018;48(1):76–81.

148. Barrington SF, Mikhaeel NG, Kostakoglu L, et al. Role of imaging in the staging and response assessment of lymphoma: consensus of the International Conference on Malignant Lymphomas Imaging Working Group. J Clin Oncol 2014;32(27):3048–58.

149. Chen S, Wang S, He K, et al. PET/CT predicts bone marrow involvement in paediatric non-Hodgkin lymphoma and may preclude the need for bone marrow biopsy in selected patients. Eur Radiol 2018;28(7):2942–50.

150. Linabery AM, Ross JA. Trends in childhood cancer incidence in the U.S. (1992-2004). Cancer 2008;112(2):416–32.

151. Stove HK, Sandahl JD, Abrahamsson J, et al. Extramedullary leukemia in children with acute myeloid leukemia: a population-based cohort study from the Nordic Society of Pediatric Hematology and Oncology (NOPHO). Pediatr Blood Cancer 2017;64(12). https://doi.org/10.1002/pbc.26520.

152. Paydas S, Zorludemir S, Ergin M. Granulocytic sarcoma: 32 cases and review of the literature. Leuk Lymphoma 2006;47(12):2527–41.

153. Almond LM, Charalampakis M, Ford SJ, et al. Myeloid sarcoma: presentation, diagnosis, and treatment. Clin Lymphoma Myeloma Leuk 2017;17(5):263–7.

154. Zhang S, Wang W, Kan Y, et al. Extramedullary infiltration of acute lymphoblastic leukemia in multiple organs on FDG PET/CT. Clin Nucl Med 2018;43(3):217–9.

155. Stolzel F, Rollig C, Radke J, et al. 1)8)F-FDG-PET/CT for detection of extramedullary acute myeloid leukemia. Haematologica 2011;96(10):1552–6.

156. Elojeimy S, Luana Stanescu A, Parisi MT. Use of 18F-FDG PET-CT for detection of active disease in acute myeloid leukemia. Clin Nucl Med 2016;41(3):e137–40.

157. NCCN clinical practice guidelines in oncology. Available at: https://www.nccn.org/professionals/physician_gls/pdf/aml.pdf. Accessed February 17, 2018.

158. Sharp SE, Gelfand MJ, Shulkin BL. Pediatrics: diagnosis of neuroblastoma. Semin Nucl Med 2011;41(5):345–53.

159. London WB, Castleberry RP, Matthay KK, et al. Evidence for an age cutoff greater than 365 days for neuroblastoma risk group stratification in the Children's Oncology Group. J Clin Oncol 2005;23(27):6459–65.

160. DuBois SG, Kalika Y, Lukens JN, et al. Metastatic sites in stage IV and IVS neuroblastoma correlate with age, tumor biology, and survival. J Pediatr Hematol Oncol 1999;21(3):181–9.

161. Parisi MT, Eslamy H, Park JR, et al. (1)(3)(1)I-metaiodobenzylguanidine theranostics in neuroblastoma: historical perspectives; practical applications. Semin Nucl Med 2016;46(3):184–202.

162. Yanik GA, Parisi MT, Naranjo A, et al. Validation of post-induction Curie scores in high risk neuroblastoma. A Children's Oncology Group (COG) and SIOPEN group report on SIOPEN/HR-NBL1. J Nucl Med 2018;59(3):502–8.

163. Yanik GA, Parisi MT, Shulkin BL, et al. Semiquantitative mIBG scoring as a prognostic indicator in patients with stage 4 neuroblastoma: a report from the Children's oncology group. J Nucl Med 2013;54(4):541–8.

164. Brisse HJ, McCarville MB, Granata C, et al. Guidelines for imaging and staging of neuroblastic

tumors: consensus report from the International Neuroblastoma Risk Group Project. Radiology 2011;261(1):243–57.

165. Biermann M, Schwarzlmuller T, Fasmer KE, et al. Is there a role for PET-CT and SPECT-CT in pediatric oncology? Acta Radiol 2013;54(9):1037–45.

166. Chawla M, Kumar R, Agarwala S, et al. Role of positron emission tomography-computed tomography in staging and early chemotherapy response evaluation in children with neuroblastoma. Indian J Nucl Med 2010;25(4):147–55.

167. Choi YJ, Hwang HS, Kim HJ, et al. (18)F-FDG PET as a single imaging modality in pediatric neuroblastoma: comparison with abdomen CT and bone scintigraphy. Ann Nucl Med 2014;28(4):304–13.

168. Shulkin BL, Mitchell DS, Ungar DR, et al. Neoplasms in a pediatric population: 2-[F-18]-fluoro-2-deoxy-D-glucose PET studies. Radiology 1995;194(2):495–500.

169. Sharp SE, Shulkin BL, Gelfand MJ, et al. 123I-MIBG scintigraphy and 18F-FDG PET in neuroblastoma. J Nucl Med 2009;50(8):1237–43.

170. Papathanasiou ND, Gaze MN, Sullivan K, et al. 18F-FDG PET/CT and 123I-metaiodobenzylguanidine imaging in high-risk neuroblastoma: diagnostic comparison and survival analysis. J Nucl Med 2011;52(4):519–25.

171. Gains JE, Bomanji JB, Fersht NL, et al. 177Lu-DOTATATE molecular radiotherapy for childhood neuroblastoma. J Nucl Med 2011;52(7):1041–7.

172. Kong G, Hofman MS, Murray WK, et al. Initial experience with gallium-68 DOTA-octreotate PET/CT and peptide receptor radionuclide therapy for pediatric patients with refractory metastatic neuroblastoma. J Pediatr Hematol Oncol 2016;38(2):87–96.

173. Hofman MS, Lau WFE, Hicks RJ. Somatostatin receptor imaging with 68Ga DOTATATE PET/CT: clinical utility, normal patterns, pearls, and pitfalls in interpretation. Radiographics 2015;35(2):500–16.

174. Abongwa C, Mott S, Schafer B, et al. Safety and accuracy of (68)Ga-DOTATOC PET/CT in children and young adults with solid tumors. Am J Nucl Med Mol Imaging 2017;7(5):228–35.

175. DeYoung B, Egeler RM, Rollins BJ. Langerhans cell histiocytosis. In: WHO Press, editor. WHO classification of tumours of soft tissue and bone. Lyon (France): International Agency for Research on Cancer; 2013. p. 356–7.

176. Binkovitz LA, Olshefski RS, Adler BH. Coincidence FDG-PET in the evaluation of Langerhans' cell histiocytosis: preliminary findings. Pediatr Radiol 2003;33(9):598–602.

177. Phillips M, Allen C, Gerson P, et al. Comparison of FDG-PET scans to conventional radiography and bone scans in management of Langerhans cell histiocytosis. Pediatr Blood Cancer 2009;52(1):97–101.

178. Mueller WP, Coppenrath E, Pfluger T. Nuclear medicine and multimodality imaging of pediatric neuroblastoma. Pediatr Radiol 2013;43(4):418–27.

179. Tateishi U, Morita S, Taguri M, et al. A meta-analysis of (18)F-Fluoride positron emission tomography for assessment of metastatic bone tumor. Ann Nucl Med 2010;24(7):523–31.

180. Bhargava P, Hanif M, Nash C. Whole-body F-18 sodium fluoride PET-CT in a patient with renal cell carcinoma. Clin Nucl Med 2008;33(12):894–5.

181. Even-Sapir E. (1)(8)F-fluoride PET/computed tomography imaging. PET Clin 2014;9(3):277–85.

182. Iagaru A. 18F-Fluoride PET in the assessment of malignant bone disease. J Nucl Med 2015;56(10):1476–7.

183. Shin DS, Shon O-J, Han D-S, et al. The clinical efficacy of (18)F-FDG-PET/CT in benign and malignant musculoskeletal tumors. Ann Nucl Med 2008;22(7):603–9.

184. Fonager RF, Zacho HD, Langkilde NC, et al. Diagnostic test accuracy study of (18)F-sodium fluoride PET/CT, (99m)Tc-labelled diphosphonate SPECT/CT, and planar bone scintigraphy for diagnosis of bone metastases in newly diagnosed, high-risk prostate cancer. Am J Nucl Med Mol Imaging 2017;7(5):218–27.

185. Fonager RF, Zacho HD, Langkilde NC, et al. (18)F-fluoride positron emission tomography/computed tomography and bone scintigraphy for diagnosis of bone metastases in newly diagnosed, high-risk prostate cancer patients: study protocol for a multicentre, diagnostic test accuracy study. BMC Cancer 2016;16:10.

186. Fonager RF, Zacho HD, Langkilde NC, et al. Prospective comparative study of (18)F-sodium fluoride PET/CT and planar bone scintigraphy for treatment response assessment of bone metastases in patients with prostate cancer. Acta Oncol 2018;57(8):1063–9.

187. Iagaru A, Mosci C, Dick DW, et al. Combined 18F-fluoride and 18F-FDG PET/CT: a response based on actual data from prospective studies. Eur J Nucl Med Mol Imaging 2013;40(12):1922–4.

188. Ovadia D, Metser U, Lievshitz G, et al. Back pain in adolescents: assessment with integrated 18F-fluoride positron-emission tomography-computed tomography. J Pediatr Orthop 2007;27(1):90–3.

189. Drubach LA, Connolly SA, Palmer EL3. Skeletal scintigraphy with 18F-NaF PET for the evaluation of bone pain in children. AJR Am J Roentgenol 2011;197(3):713–9.

190. Quon A, Dodd R, Iagaru A, et al. Initial investigation of (1)(8)F-NaF PET/CT for identification of vertebral sites amenable to surgical revision after spinal

fusion surgery. Eur J Nucl Med Mol Imaging 2012; 39(11):1737–44.

191. Loder RT, Feinberg JR. Orthopaedic injuries in children with nonaccidental trauma: demographics and incidence from the 2000 kids' inpatient database. J Pediatr Orthop 2007;27(4):421–6.

192. Grammatico-Guillon L, Maakaroun Vermesse Z, Baron S, et al. Paediatric bone and joint infections are more common in boys and toddlers: a national epidemiology study. Acta Paediatr 2013;102(3): e120–5.

193. van Schuppen J, van Doorn MMAC, van Rijn RR. Childhood osteomyelitis: imaging characteristics. Insights Imaging 2012;3(5):519–33.

194. Jaramillo D, Dormans JP, Delgado J, et al. Hematogenous osteomyelitis in infants and children: imaging of a changing disease. Radiology 2017; 283(3):629–43.

195. Pineda C, Vargas A, Rodriguez AV. Imaging of osteomyelitis: current concepts. Infect Dis Clin North Am 2006;20(4):789–825.

196. Peltola H, Paakkonen M. Acute osteomyelitis in children. N Engl J Med 2014;370(4):352–60.

197. Nixon GW. Hematogenous osteomyelitis of metaphyseal-equivalent locations. AJR Am J Roentgenol 1978;130(1):123–9.

198. Gilbertson-Dahdal D, Wright JE, Krupinski E, et al. Transphyseal involvement of pyogenic osteomyelitis is considerably more common than classically taught. AJR Am J Roentgenol 2014;203(1):190–5.

199. Dartnell J, Ramachandran M, Katchburian M. Haematogenous acute and subacute paediatric osteomyelitis: a systematic review of the literature. J Bone Joint Surg Br 2012;94(5):584–95.

200. Strobel K, Stumpe KDM. PET/CT in musculoskeletal infection. Semin Musculoskelet Radiol 2007; 11(4):353–64.

201. Palestro CJ. FDG-PET in musculoskeletal infections. Semin Nucl Med 2013;43(5):367–76.

202. Warmann SW, Dittmann H, Seitz G, et al. Follow-up of acute osteomyelitis in children: the possible role of PET/CT in selected cases. J Pediatr Surg 2011; 46(8):1550–6.

203. de Winter F, van de Wiele C, Vogelaers D, et al. Fluorine-18 fluorodeoxyglucose-position emission tomography: a highly accurate imaging modality for the diagnosis of chronic musculoskeletal infections. J Bone Joint Surg Am 2001;83-A(5):651–60.

204. Chacko TK, Zhuang H, Nakhoda KZ, et al. Applications of fluorodeoxyglucose positron emission tomography in the diagnosis of infection. Nucl Med Commun 2003;24(6):615–24.

205. Meller J, Koster G, Liersch T, et al. Chronic bacterial osteomyelitis: prospective comparison of (18)F-FDG imaging with a dual-head coincidence camera and (111)In-labelled autologous leucocyte scintigraphy. Eur J Nucl Med Mol Imaging 2002; 29(1):53–60.

206. Nanni C, Errani C, Boriani L, et al. 68Ga-citrate PET/CT for evaluating patients with infections of the bone: preliminary results. J Nucl Med 2010; 51(12):1932–6.

207. Hofmann SR, Kapplusch F, Girschick HJ, et al. Chronic Recurrent Multifocal Osteomyelitis (CRMO): presentation, pathogenesis, and treatment. Curr Osteoporos Rep 2017;15(6):542–54.

208. Greenwood S, Leone A, Cassar-Pullicino VN. SAPHO and recurrent multifocal osteomyelitis. Radiol Clin North Am 2017;55(5):1035–53.

209. Alshammari A, Usmani S, Elgazzar AH, et al. Chronic recurrent multifocal osteomyelitis in children: a multidisciplinary approach is needed to establish a diagnosis. World J Nucl Med 2013; 12(3):120–3.

210. Schaub S, Sirkis HM, Kay J. Imaging for synovitis, acne, pustulosis, hyperostosis, and osteitis (SAPHO) syndrome. Rheum Dis Clin North Am 2016; 42(4):695–710.

211. Liu Y. Chronic nonbacterial osteomyelitis with FDG avid rib destruction and extensive lymphadenopathy. Clin Nucl Med 2016;41(9):730–1.

212. Parisi MT, Iyer RS, Stanescu AL. Nuclear medicine applications in pediatric musculoskeletal diseases: the added value of hybrid imaging. Semin Musculoskelet Radiol 2018;22(1):25–45.

# Hot Topics of Research in Musculoskeletal Imaging
## PET/MR Imaging, MR Fingerprinting, Dual-energy CT Scan, Ultrashort Echo Time

Soheil Kooraki, MD[a], Majid Assadi, MD[b],
Ali Gholamrezanezhad, MD, FEBNM, DABR[c],*

## KEYWORDS

• MR imaging • Musculoskeletal imaging • PET • Tumor

## KEY POINTS

• The practical role of various novel imaging techniques remain unclear for musculoskeletal applications.
• Ultrashort echo time sequence is capable of imaging the deepest layers of the cartilage.
• PET/MR imaging might dedicate to imaging of degenerative joint disease, inflammatory and infectious arthritis, pain-related neural activity, and assessment of muscle function.
• Dual-energy CT scan have been used for quantification of mono-sodium urate crystals, however several other applications require more extensive research.

## INTRODUCTION

The ever-changing world of technology has evolved the concept of medical imaging. Musculoskeletal imaging has highly taken advantage of the advancements. Imaging modalities, which were once used for obtaining anatomic information, now can be used for obtaining functional, metabolic, and even biochemical data. Moreover, the introduction of new hybrid imaging systems has enabled the simultaneous anatomic/metabolic imaging. The practical role of several novel imaging methods remains unclear in the musculoskeletal system. The authors aim to present the current applications of 4 novel imaging methods, including magnetic resonance fingerprinting (MRF), ultrashort echo time (UTE) sequence, hybrid PET/MR, and dual-energy CT scan (DECT) in musculoskeletal radiology. Their main objective is to highlight current research topics and discuss the possible future research directions.

## MAGNETIC RESONANCE FINGERPRINTING

Conventional MR imaging is theoretically aimed to produce a single echo of a constant signal at a single time point using a fixed set of radio frequency (RF) pulses and flip angles. However, the signal acquisition process may be contaminated by the fact that applying multiple RF pulses in a particular sequence may result in other spins and stimulated echoes at undesired times. Conventionally, these undesired echoes are refocused or spoiled to help the single target signal reaching a steady state, from which images can be made. These conventional pulse sequences and the acquired images typically provide qualitative data with various weightings or contrasts that reflect a

---

[a] Department of Radiology, Shariati Hospital, Tehran University of Medical Sciences, Tehran, Iran; [b] The Persian Gulf Nuclear Medicine Research Center, Bushehr University of Medical Sciences, Bushehr, Iran; [c] Department of Diagnostic Radiology, Keck School of Medicine, University of Southern California (USC), 1520 San Pablo Street, Suite L1600, Los Angeles, CA 90033, USA
* Corresponding author.
E-mail addresses: gholamre@med.usc.edu; a.gholamrezanezhad@yahoo.com

PET Clin 14 (2019) 175–182
https://doi.org/10.1016/j.cpet.2018.08.014

particular tissue parameter (eg, T1 relaxation, T2 relaxation).

MRF is a novel and promising approach to non-invasively investigate tissue properties (such as T1, T2, and off-resonance B0) by providing weighted measurements or images from which several quantitative tissue relationships are simultaneously obtained.[1–3] MRF technique was first developed in the departments of Radiology and Biomedical engineering of Case Western Reserve University, as well as University Hospitals of Cleveland.[1] MRF consists of the creation of a time series evolution by changing acquisition parameters, such as flip angle and TR, in a pseudorandom manner. This time series of measurements are subsequently "matched" or compared against simulation and a precalculated "dictionary."[2] The output is a quantitative map that is generated by analyzing temporally and spatially acquired incoherent signals. The main difference of MRF with conventional MR imaging is producing signal dynamics instead of a constant signal.[4]

As a noninvasive tool, MRF has been suggested to quantitatively analyze complex tissue alterations that can represent early indicators of diseases. It has been suggested that MRF may increase the sensitivity and specificity of conventional MR imaging and can be used to identify specific materials or tissues within the target organ. Therefore, optimization of the acquisition parameters and clinical applications of MRF has become a hot research topic.

The advent of various techniques of MR imaging has revolutionized the diagnostic management of musculoskeletal disorders.[5] However, limitations of MR imaging for musculoskeletal disorders have been widely appreciated. For example, the diagnostic accuracy of contrast-enhanced MR imaging in differentiating benign from malignant bone tumors is only about 80%, with many nontumoral conditions mimicking osseous neoplasms. In post-treatment settings, differentiation of posttherapy necrosis and local recurrence can be challenging in some instances, because neovascularity in necrotic areas, the presence of vascularized granulation tissue, or reactive hyperemia can all cause contrast enhancement that may be mistaken for residual/recurrent neoplastic tissue.[6]

Recently there has been a growing interest in exploring various clinical applications of MRF; however, studies on the possible application of MRF for musculoskeletal disorders are limited. Technical challenges have to be overcome to optimize MRF for different indications.

The authors' aim in this section is to discuss current trends of MRF and whether this technology can be extended to musculoskeletal imaging.

Prior studies on animal models of bone and soft tissue tumors support the authors' hypothesis regarding the potential role of MRF in the evaluation of bone tumors. Witzel and colleagues[7] conducted an experimental MR imaging study using a rat model of osteosarcoma. The tumor was distinctly delineated from adjacent normal-appearing bone when the tumor volume was between 0.3 and 7.5 cm$^2$. They found a significant correlation between increased tumor volume and increment in T1 and T2 relaxation times. T1 relaxation times slightly reduced with tumors greater than 5 cm$^3$, whereas T2 relaxation times remained unchanged in tumors above 2.5 cm$^3$. Histologic evolutions and variability in water content were found to contribute to the variations of relaxation times. In a study on the bone marrow (BM) of B16 melanoma tumor-bearing mice versus healthy control, the mean T2 relaxation time of infiltrated BM was found to be significantly longer than that of normal BM (41 ms vs 28 ms). T2 relaxation time was suggested as an indicator of early bone metastases.[8] Preclinical in vivo MRF has been sensitive to known pathology in animal tumor models.[9]

Although no prior clinical study has directly evaluated the value of MRF for musculoskeletal applications, several studies have been performed on the clinical impact of this technique in various human conditions. Blank and colleagues[10] studied the role of MRF-derived relaxometry in a small group of patients with brain glioma. MRF-derived relaxation time successfully distinguished tumor from nonneoplastic normal white matter. In addition, MRF-derived T1 and T2 values were significantly higher in high-grade neoplasms compared with low-grade ones. They observed relaxation time of peritumoral vasogenic edema to be significantly different from relaxation times in both neoplastic tissue and normal healthy white matter.

Quantitative differentiation of prostate cancer from normal peripheral zone has been successfully performed by using MRF relaxometry measures.[11] Another clinical study on 6 patients with 20 focal liver lesions as well as 8 asymptomatic individuals found that T1 and T2 values in metastatic liver lesions of breast adenocarcinoma is significantly different from perilesional hepatic parenchyma and normal hepatic parenchyma of healthy volunteers.[12] Moreover, MRF has also been used in the noninvasive assessment of tissue blood volume and oxygenation map.[13]

The authors' hypothesis in the value of MRF for the evaluation of musculoskeletal neoplastic diseases is further supported by prior publications showing T1 mapping of BM being helpful in the detection of BM infiltrates in patients with lymphoma and also for the evaluation of response to treatment. In this setting, elevated marrow T1 values suggest neoplastic involvement, whereas normalization of T1 values in the posttransplant/postchemotherapy period suggests response to treatment.[14–16] Although sarcomatous tissues show changes in their relaxometry parameters, relaxation times of normal tissue in the course of chemotherapy for bone sarcoma are not affected by the treatment.[17] Quantitative MR imaging before BM biopsy may also reduce false-negative biopsy results.[15]

More recently, quantitative MR mapping techniques have been used for evaluation of the biochemical changes in articular cartilage. This might be valuable in the imaging of knee injury, cartilage degeneration, and postoperative changes.[18] In a study of T1 and T2 relaxation times in 84 synovial fluids obtained from various rheumatologic diseases, the T1/T2 ratio was more sensitive for differentiation of inflammatory and noninflammatory arthropathies, in comparison with the isolated T1 or T2 relaxation times. In particular, high values of T1/T2 ratio were detected in patients with septic arthritis.[19]

In summary, the studies on the possible capabilities of MRF in musculoskeletal imaging are preliminary. Clinical studies are required to evaluate the power of this technique in musculoskeletal imaging.

## ULTRASHORT ECHO TIME SEQUENCE

The osteochondral junction is a complex tissue structure of 100 to 200 μm thick with essential functions relating to the structural stability, proper nutrition, and repair of the articular cartilage.[20] Conventional MR sequences are inadequate at visualization of the osteochondral junction, mainly due to the intrinsic ultrashort T2 relaxation time of osteochondral structure. Ultrashort time echo (UTE) imaging is a technique to isolate the signal from the osteochondral junction. Ultrashort echo time is capable of imaging the deepest layer of the articular cartilage, calcified and uncalcified cartilage, and also cartilaginous endplates.

Although the role of UTE sequences for chondral and osteochondral junction imaging has been established for several years, published clinical studies are limited, and vendor-specific sequences have not yet been validated and optimized for clinical applications.

Bae and collegues[21] used a 3-Tesla (T) magnet to investigate the value of UTE imaging in the evaluation of 5 cadaveric patellar cartilage-bone interfaces in naturally occurring and experimentally prepared human cartilage-bone specimens. They found that all patellar segments demonstrate a high-intensity linear signal near the osteochondral junction. This signal was not visible on fat-suppressed protein density or T1-weighted sequences. The high signal intensity was only visible in samples containing cartilaginous parts and not in those containing only bone. These findings showed that the high signal of human articular joints in UTE comes from the deepest layer of the cartilage, without contribution of subchondral bone to the signal.

Du and colleagues[22] aimed at imaging zone of calcified cartilage (ZCC) with UTE. In their study, a dual inversion recovery UTE (DIR-UTE) sequence was used on phantoms and also in 6 cadaveric patellae using a clinical 3-T GE MR scanner. The results showed that DIR-UTE is a noninvasive method for high-resolution imaging of ZCC. Moreover, this imaging is useful for the assessment of the biochemical structure of ZCC and bone-cartilage interfaces.

In a clinical study by Ma and colleagues,[23] 7 healthy volunteers and 1 patient with suspected tear of the lateral meniscus were evaluated by using a double-echo pulse sequence and 3D UTE MR imaging. Multiplanar reconstruction followed by subtraction of the primary double-echo images increased the image signal-to-noise ratio. The study findings suggested that double-pulse sequence MR imaging with 3D UTE might display the short T2 components, such as deep chondral layer and osteochondral junction. In another preliminary study, Goto and colleagues[24] found UTE sequence to be useful in imaging of the deep layers of the knee cartilage.

The main limitations of previous studies include small sample size and/or investigation on nonhuman or cadaveric tissues, which might lead to different results from in vivo imaging. The added value of UTE imaging in clinical decision-making of musculoskeletal radiology is not clear yet. Additional studies are required to fully understand the implications of MR changes of the osteochondral junction for the assessment of the joints, especially knee joint.

In summary, UTE is found to be valuable for imaging of osteochondral junction in small studies. Further studies are required to better establish the use of this technique in joint imaging.

## PET/MR IMAGING

The introduction of integrated PET/MR imaging has been highly promising, because MR imaging provided structural, anatomic, and functional data, whereas PET allows quantification of metabolic measures. PET has the ability to assess the earliest metabolic changes at a molecular level in many of musculoskeletal disorders. Therefore, PET/MR imaging can provide a comprehensively combined anatomic, functional, and metabolic view in a single imaging section.[25,26]

Because PET/MR imaging is an emerging method for musculoskeletal imaging, the potentials of this modality remain in the realm of research. This part aims to talk about the current status of PET/MR imaging in musculoskeletal disorders. PET/MR imaging can be used for a variety of oncologic and nononcologic musculoskeletal conditions. A variety of nononcologic disorders have been studied by this method on preliminary studies.[27] Several hot-trending studies will be discussed in here.

Early studies have shown that PET/MR imaging might be more sensitive for detecting subchondral bone changes before structural abnormalities on MR imaging. In a study of 22 individuals with knee pain, Kogan and colleagues[28] used PET/MR imaging for characterization of degenerative joint disease. All kinds of subchondral lesions had significantly higher SUVmax in comparison with normal-appearing bone on MR imaging. Overall, 172 areas with high uptake volumes of interest were visualized on PET with fludeoxyglucose (FDG-PET), with only 63% of them showing signal abnormality on MR imaging. These findings showed superiority of PET/MR imaging over PET or MR imaging alone for early detection of metabolic and morphologic abnormalities in degenerative joint disease.

There is considerable potential for combined PET/MR imaging for assessment of infectious and inflammatory disease. PET is highly sensitive for early disease activity in patients suffering from rheumatoid arthritis (RA), whereas MR imaging can provide high-resolution structural changes in the course of the disease. Miese and colleagues[29] are the first to perform [18]F FDG-PET/ MR imaging of hand for assessment of disease status in early RA. They found increased FDG uptake in areas with synovitis and tenovaginitis corresponding to the contrast-enhancing areas on MR imaging.

Fahnert and colleagues[30] investigated the role of combined PET/MR imaging in 30 patients suspected for spondylodiscitis. MR imaging had a sensitivity and specificity of 50% and 71%, respectively. However, when PET data were added sensitivity and specificity were significantly increased to 100% and 80%, respectively. It is suggested that PET/MR imaging might be valuable in improving the diagnostic accuracy of imaging in diabetic foot and also in differentiating diabetic foot from other conditions such as Charcot joint.[31] However, no clinical studies have been carried out in this area.

Pain is the most common cause of medical seeks. There is a growing interest on imaging of pain-related neural activity. Studies in both rat and human models have shown increased FDG uptake in injured nerves causing neuropathy. On the other hand, MR imaging has been useful when looking for peripheral nerve inflammation, nerve entrapment, and tracking of macrophages with small particles of iron oxide.[32] The experience of Biswal and colleagues[33] with FDG-PET/MR imaging on 6 patients with neuropathic pain showed focal increased FDG uptake in areas of affected nerves.

The fascinating study of Haddock and colleagues[34] on the application of PET/MR imaging in muscle function included 10 active young men while repeated knee extension and hand gripping exercise. There was a significant correlation between FDG uptake and increased muscle T2 values. Alterations in muscle T2 might be considered as a marker of glucose uptake.

On the other hand, theoretically, PET/MR imaging might dedicate to imaging of musculoskeletal oncologic conditions. PET/MR imaging provides a measure of a tumor's biological behavior including cellularity, detailed chemical content, and vascularity.[35] Several technical issues need to be considered. Most importantly, PET/MR imaging protocols need to be defined separately for each malignancy type.

A few case studies have proposed potential for PET/MR imaging in the staging of bone/soft tissue malignancies.[34] However, Platzek and colleagues[36] evaluated the power of FDG-PET/MR imaging for the staging of bone and soft tissue sarcoma in 29 patients and did not find any superiority for PET/MR imaging over conventional imaging. In a study of 41 patients with suspected soft tissue sarcoma recurrence, Erfanian and colleagues[37] found significantly higher accuracy for hybrid PET/MR imaging compared with MR imaging alone. Also, PET/MR imaging was more confident in delineating malignant lesions.

PET/MR imaging is reported to be helpful in workup of patients with diffuse myelomatous disease.[38] In a study on 24 individuals with multiple myeloma, Shortt and colleagues[39] used PET and MR imaging for the measurement of disease activity in comparison with BM biopsy as the gold standard. Combined PET/MR imaging had a higher specificity compared with MR imaging or PET scan alone and led to a positive predictive value of 100%. Compared with PET/CT, PET/MR imaging is limited in the characterization of rib and skull lesions; however, it is superior to PET/CT for identification of intramedullary lesions.[38]

In summary, PET/MR imaging seems to be valuable in imaging of a subset of tumoral and nontumoral musculoskeletal conditions. Rather than possible oncologic applications, PET/MR imaging might dedicate to imaging of degenerative joint disease, inflammatory and infectious arthritis, pain-related neural activity, and assessment of muscle function.

## DUAL-ENERGY CT SCAN

Dual Energy CT scan (DECT), and spectral CT scan are trending imaging technologies, which has shown substantial beneficial diagnostic effects during the last decade. These techniques allow clinicians to discriminate various elements in the body based on their biochemical composition.

Spectral CT scan is acquired using the entire spectrum of energy levels and then during post-processing steps, any energy levels might be chosen. Dual-energy scanners use 2 separate x-ray tubes for acquiring images at 2 different energy levels. Each X-ray has a different energy level. The biochemical composition is determined by x-ray absorption of the target tissue/substance related to the atomic number and material density.[40,41] The raw data then require considerable postprocessing to produce clinically practical images. The most common method is to obtain spectral information from comparison of different low-voltage and high-voltage reconstructed image voxels. Then several types of algorithms can be used to generate the desired image. One common type of algorithm provides a color-coded map of a specific material or substance.[42] The potentials of DECT for musculoskeletal imaging seem highly fascinating. Dual-energy CT scan has been used for quantification of urate crystals in gout, imaging of tendons and ligaments, bone densitometry, detection of BM edema, and reduction of metal artifact. In this section, various clinical uses of DECT and promising future research directions are discussed.

DECT was primarily used for identification of urate depositions in the kidney.[43] Several studies have shown DECT to be highly sensitive and specific for mapping monosodium urate (MSU) deposits in individuals with gout. DECT scan allows differentiation of low-molecular-weight uric acid from high-molecular-weight calcium.[40] DECT might be 4 times effective than clinical examination in finding urate depositions.[44] Bongartz and colleagues[45] studied the diagnostic accuracy of DECT on 40 patients with gout, 41 patients with other types of joint diseases, and a third group consisting of 30 patients with suspected gout and negative synovial fluid analysis. The study showed

sensitivity and specificity of 90% and 83%, respectively, for DECT in the diagnosis of gout; however, lower sensitivity was achieved in those with the recent-onset disease. DECT showed MSU deposits in 14 individuals of the third group, pointing toward the diagnostic value of the technique in suspected individuals who have a negative synovial fluid analysis. Moreover, studies have shown DECT to be capable of estimating the gouty tophi volumes, which might help clinicians in monitoring the effects of urate-lowering therapies.[44,46]

MR imaging is the gold standard for the imaging of ligaments and tendons. DECT is capable of imaging tendons and ligaments due to high hydroxylysine and hydroxyproline content in the collagen of these structures.[47] Several studies have investigated the value of DECT in imaging of ligament and tendon, yielding controversial results; however, most have reported higher accuracy of MR imaging compared with DECT. Dual-energy CT scan might be useful only when there is a contraindication for MR imaging. Fickert and colleagues[48] compared the power of DECT and MR imaging for the diagnosis of induced anterior cruciate ligament (ACL) injury in a porcine knee joint model. They found higher sensitivity and specificity for MR imaging in those with complete ACL rupture. There are sparse research data about the possible role of DECT for characterization of tendons.

DECT scan has also been attempted for mapping bone density distribution in the lumbar vertebrae. Wesarg and colleagues[49] found localized bone density in DECT to be a better correlate of local force measurements, compared with bone density in dual-energy X-ray absorptiometry (DXA). Later, in a clinical in vivo study, Wichmann and colleagues[50] assessed quantification of bone density distribution in 160 lumbar vertebrae of 40 patients. The study showed that creating a phantomless DECT-based bone densitometry map is practical in a postprocessing station. This can further allow creating a color-coded 3-dimensional model of trabecular bone density distribution in lumbar spine. However, according to the obtained data, no significant correlation was observed between DECT and DXA values. The investigators justified that DXA measures BMD of both cortical and trabecular bones, whereas DECT quantifies only trabecular bone density. It is not clear whether patients with osteoporosis might benefit from this technique or not. One main drawback of DECT is the high radiation dose compared with DXA, which limits its current use in BMD.

DECT is useful for demonstrating BM edema by creating virtual noncalcium images (VNCa). VNCa subtracts calcium signal from bone, allowing evaluation of the BM signal. The images can be produced in a grayscale overly, color-coded or 3-dimensional fashion, depending on user preference.[51,52] Bierry and colleagues[53] examined 20 patients with trauma-related nontumoral vertebral compression fracture by DECT and found out a negative predictive value of higher than 97% for DECT, showing the high value of DECT to rule out recent vertebral fracture. Another clinical study on 25 patients with radiographically occult hip fractures showed a sensitivity and specificity of 90% and 40%, respectively, for VNCa DECT in proper diagnosis of the fracture; however, they did not use MR imaging as the gold standard. Thomas and colleagues[54] examined the accuracy of DECT versus regular CT scan and MR imaging for BM lesion detection in 32 individuals with multiple myeloma or monoclonal gammopathy of unknown significance. DECT was superior to regular CT scan for detection of BM infiltration; however, compared with MR imaging as the gold standard, it had lower sensitivity. DECT might be helpful in other skeletal traumatic settings as well. Darezz and colleagues[55] used VNCa DECT for visualization of acute scaphoid fracture in 3 patients, of whom 2 had normal radiography and conventional CT scan. It is not clear if DECT is capable of discriminating pathologic from osteoporotic vertebral fracture. Besides, one potential bias of VNCa DECT imaging is that the marrow fat increases with age and it can interfere with the quantitative evaluation.

There is also growing evidence about the value of DECT in reducing metal artifact. Bamberg and colleagues[56] showed that DECT allows significant reduction in metal artifact and increment in diagnostic value. They reported superior diagnostic quality in 27 out of 31 patients in comparison with conventional CT scan. Lee and colleagues[57] used DECT with metal artifact reduction software (MARS) in phantoms and 26 patients with metallic hardware. They suggested that MARS could improve visualization of the prosthesis; however, caution must be taken, because MARS might not be powerful in metal artifact reduction of titanium prosthesis.

In summary, rather than the practical use of DECT for quantification of MSU crystals, other promising applications need extensive research before implementing into routine practice.

## SUMMARY

There is a rapidly growing interest in application of novel imaging techniques for characterization of various musculoskeletal disorders. Although some techniques are already used for several musculoskeletal disorders, ongoing research is required to validate others. The authors presented current research trends and possible future research directions. There are considerable potentials in MRF, UTE, PET/MR, and DECT for characterization of various musculoskeletal disorders. Ongoing research is required for evaluation and validation of these interesting techniques.

## REFERENCES

1. Ma D, Gulani V, Seiberlich N, et al. Magnetic resonance fingerprinting. Nature 2013;495(7440):187–92.
2. Cauley SF, Setsompop K, Ma D, et al. Fast group matching for MR fingerprinting reconstruction. Magn Reson Med 2015;74(2):523–8.
3. Bottomley PA, Foster TH, Argersinger RE, et al. A review of normal tissue hydrogen NMR relaxation times and relaxation mechanisms from 1-100 MHz: dependence on tissue type, NMR frequency, temperature, species, excision, and age. Med Phys 1984;11(4):425–48.
4. Jerecic R, Griswold M, Jiang Y, et al. Magnetic resonance fingerprinting (MRF) with echo splitting. Siemens AG Case Western Reserve University; 2014.
5. Alizai H, Chang G, Regatte RR. MRI of the musculoskeletal system: advanced applications using high and ultrahigh field MRI. Semin Musculoskelet Radiol 2015;19(4):363–74.
6. Nascimento D, Suchard G, Hatem M, et al. The role of magnetic resonance imaging in the evaluation of bone tumours and tumour-like lesions. Insights Imaging 2014;5(4):419–40.
7. Witzel JG, Bohndorf K, Prescher A, et al. Osteosarcoma of the nude rat. A model for experimental magnetic resonance imaging studies of bone tumors. Invest Radiol 1992;27(3):205–10.
8. Gauvain KM, Garbow JR, Song SK, et al. MRI detection of early bone metastases in b16 mouse melanoma models. Clin Exp Metastasis 2005;22(5):403–11.
9. Gao Y, Chen Y, Ma D, et al. Preclinical MR fingerprinting (MRF) at 7 T: effective quantitative imaging for rodent disease models. NMR Biomed 2015;28(3):384–94.
10. de Blank P, Badve C, Ma D, et al. Characterization of tumor grade and extent using magnetic resonance fingerprinting: initial results. Neuro Oncol 2016;18(Supple 3):iii166.
11. Badve C YA, Pahwa S, et al. Quantitative differentiation of prostate cancer from normal peripheral zone using Magnetic Resonance Fingerprinting (MRF) and diffusion mapping. Proceedings of the 23th Annual Meeting of ISMRM. Toronto, Ontario, Canada. Abstract # 38482015.
12. Chen Y, Jiang Y, Pahwa S, et al. MR fingerprinting for rapid quantitative abdominal imaging. Radiology 2016;279(1):278–86.
13. Christen T, Pannetier NA, Ni WW, et al. MR vascular fingerprinting: a new approach to compute cerebral

blood volume, mean vessel radius, and oxygenation maps in the human brain. Neuroimage 2014;89: 262–70.

14. Smith SR, Williams CE, Edwards RH, et al. Quantitative magnetic resonance imaging in autologous bone marrow transplantation for Hodgkin's disease. Br J Cancer 1989;60(6):961–5.

15. Smith SR, Williams CE, Edwards RH, et al. Quantitative magnetic resonance studies of lumbar vertebral marrow in patients with refractory or relapsed Hodgkin's disease. Ann Oncol 1991;2(Suppl 2):39–42.

16. Smith SR, Roberts N, Percy DF, et al. Detection of bone marrow abnormalities in patients with Hodgkin's disease by T1 mapping of MR images of lumbar vertebral bone marrow. Br J Cancer 1992; 65(2):246–51.

17. Holscher HC, van der Woude HJ, Hermans J, et al. Magnetic resonance relaxation times of normal tissue in the course of chemotherapy: a study in patients with bone sarcoma. Skeletal Radiol 1994; 23(3):181–5.

18. Wang L, Regatte RR. T(1)rho MRI of human musculoskeletal system. J Magn Reson Imaging 2015; 41(3):586–600.

19. Teyssier R, Colson F, Teyssier M. In vitro differentiation of inflammatory and non-inflammatory states of the synovial fluid by magnetic protonic relaxation. C R Seances Soc Biol Fil 1987;181(6):645–50 [in French].

20. Bae WC, Biswas R, Chen K, et al. UTE MRI of the osteochondral junction. Curr Radiol Rep 2014;2(2):35.

21. Bae WC, Dwek JR, Znamirowski R, et al. Ultrashort echo time MR imaging of osteochondral junction of the knee at 3 T: identification of anatomic structures contributing to signal intensity. Radiology 2010; 254(3):837–45.

22. Du J, Carl M, Bae WC, et al. Dual inversion recovery ultrashort echo time (DIR-UTE) imaging and quantification of the zone of calcified cartilage (ZCC). Osteoarthritis Cartilage 2013;21(1):77–85.

23. Ma L, Meng Q, Chen Y, et al. Preliminary use of a double-echo pulse sequence with 3D ultrashort echo time in the MRI of bones and joints. Exp Ther Med 2013;5(5):1471–5.

24. Goto H, Fujii M, Iwama Y, et al. Magnetic resonance imaging (MRI) of articular cartilage of the knee using ultrashort echo time (uTE) sequences with spiral acquisition. J Med Imaging Radiat Oncol 2012; 56(3):318–23.

25. Lee IS, Jin YH, Hong SH, et al. Musculoskeletal applications of PET/MR. Semin Musculoskelet Radiol 2014;18(2):203–16.

26. Kogan F, Broski SM, Yoon D, et al. Applications of PET-MRI in musculoskeletal disease. J Magn Reson Imaging 2018;48(1):27–47.

27. Gholamrezanezhad A, Basques K, Batouli A, et al. Clinical nononcologic applications of PET/CT and PET/MRI in musculoskeletal, orthopedic, and rheumatologic imaging. AJR Am J Roentgenol 2018; 210(6):W245–63.

28. Kogan F, Fan AP, McWalter EJ, et al. PET/MRI of metabolic activity in osteoarthritis: a feasibility study. J Magn Reson Imaging 2017;45(6):1736–45.

29. Miese F, Scherer A, Ostendorf B, et al. Hybrid 18F-FDG PET-MRI of the hand in rheumatoid arthritis: initial results. Clin Rheumatol 2011;30(9): 1247–50.

30. Fahnert J, Purz S, Jarvers JS, et al. Use of simultaneous 18F-FDG PET/MRI for the detection of spondylodiskitis. J Nucl Med 2016;57(9):1396–401.

31. Glaudemans AW, Quintero AM, Signore A. PET/MRI in infectious and inflammatory diseases: will it be a useful improvement? Eur J Nucl Med Mol Imaging 2012;39(5):745–9.

32. Kogan F, Fan AP, Gold GE. Potential of PET-MRI for imaging of non-oncologic musculoskeletal disease. Quant Imaging Med Surg 2016;6(6):756–71.

33. Biswal S, Behera D, Yoon DH, et al. [18F]FDG PET/MRI of patients with chronic pain alters management: early experience. EJNMMI Phys 2015; 2(Suppl 1):A84.

34. Haddock B, Holm S, Poulsen JM, et al. Assessment of muscle function using hybrid PET/MRI: comparison of (18)F-FDG PET and T2-weighted MRI for quantifying muscle activation in human subjects. Eur J Nucl Med Mol Imaging 2017;44(4):704–11.

35. Werner MK, Schmidt H, Schwenzer NF. MR/PET: a new challenge in hybrid imaging. AJR Am J Roentgenol 2012;199(2):272–7.

36. Platzek I, Beuthien-Baumann B, Schramm G, et al. FDG PET/MR in initial staging of sarcoma: initial experience and comparison with conventional imaging. Clin Imaging 2017;42:126–32.

37. Erfanian Y, Grueneisen J, Kirchner J, et al. Integrated 18F-FDG PET/MRI compared to MRI alone for identification of local recurrences of soft tissue sarcomas: a comparison trial. Eur J Nucl Med Mol Imaging 2017;44(11):1823–31.

38. Broski SM, Goenka AH, Kemp BJ, et al. Clinical PET/MRI: 2018 update. AJR Am J Roentgenol 2018; 211(2):295–313.

39. Shortt CP, Gleeson TG, Breen KA, et al. Whole-Body MRI versus PET in assessment of multiple myeloma disease activity. AJR Am J Roentgenol 2009;192(4): 980–6.

40. Nicolaou S, Liang T, Murphy DT, et al. Dual-energy CT: a promising new technique for assessment of the musculoskeletal system. AJR Am J Roentgenol 2012;199(5 Suppl):S78–86.

41. Khanduri S, Goyal A, Singh B, et al. The utility of dual energy computed tomography in musculoskeletal imaging. J Clin Imaging Sci 2017;7:34.

42. Johnson TR. Dual-energy CT: general principles. AJR Am J Roentgenol 2012;199(5 Suppl):S3–8.

43. Graser A, Johnson TR, Bader M, et al. Dual energy CT characterization of urinary calculi: initial in vitro and clinical experience. Invest Radiol 2008;43(2): 112–9.

44. Choi HK, Al-Arfaj AM, Eftekhari A, et al. Dual energy computed tomography in tophaceous gout. Ann Rheum Dis 2009;68(10):1609–12.

45. Bongartz T, Glazebrook KN, Kavros SJ, et al. Dual-energy CT for the diagnosis of gout: an accuracy and diagnostic yield study. Ann Rheum Dis 2015; 74(6):1072–7.

46. Mallinson PI, Coupal TM, McLaughlin PD, et al. Dual-energy CT for the musculoskeletal system. Radiology 2016;281(3):690–707.

47. Johnson TR, Krauss B, Sedlmair M, et al. Material differentiation by dual energy CT: initial experience. Eur Radiol 2007;17(6):1510–7.

48. Fickert S, Niks M, Dinter DJ, et al. Assessment of the diagnostic value of dual-energy CT and MRI in the detection of iatrogenically induced injuries of anterior cruciate ligament in a porcine model. Skeletal Radiol 2013;42(3):411–7.

49. Wesarg S, Kirschner M, Becker M, et al. Dual-energy CT-based assessment of the trabecular bone in vertebrae. Methods Inf Med 2012;51(5):398–405.

50. Wichmann JL, Booz C, Wesarg S, et al. Dual-energy CT-based phantomless in vivo three-dimensional bone mineral density assessment of the lumbar spine. Radiology 2014;271(3):778–84.

51. Wang CK, Tsai JM, Chuang MT, et al. Bone marrow edema in vertebral compression fractures: detection with dual-energy CT. Radiology 2013;269(2): 525–33.

52. Petritsch B, Kosmala A, Weng AM, et al. Vertebral compression fractures: third-generation dual-energy CT for detection of bone marrow edema at visual and quantitative analyses. Radiology 2017;284(1): 161–8.

53. Bierry G, Venkatasamy A, Kremer S, et al. Dual-energy CT in vertebral compression fractures: performance of visual and quantitative analysis for bone marrow edema demonstration with comparison to MRI. Skeletal Radiol 2014;43(4):485–92.

54. Thomas C, Schabel C, Krauss B, et al. Dual-energy CT: virtual calcium subtraction for assessment of bone marrow involvement of the spine in multiple myeloma. AJR Am J Roentgenol 2015;204(3): W324–31.

55. Dareez NM, Dahlslett KH, Engesland E, et al. Scaphoid fracture: bone marrow edema detected with dual-energy CT virtual non-calcium images and confirmed with MRI. Skeletal Radiol 2017; 46(12):1753–6.

56. Bamberg F, Dierks A, Nikolaou K, et al. Metal artifact reduction by dual energy computed tomography using monoenergetic extrapolation. Eur Radiol 2011; 21(7):1424–9.

57. Lee YH, Park KK, Song HT, et al. Metal artefact reduction in gemstone spectral imaging dual-energy CT with and without metal artefact reduction software. Eur Radiol 2012;22(6):1331–40.

# Future Perspective of the Application of Positron Emission Tomography-Computed Tomography-MR Imaging in Musculoskeletal Disorders

Andrea Angelini, MD, PhD[a], Paolo Castellucci, MD[b], Francesco Ceci, MD, PhD[c,d],*

## KEYWORDS

- Fluorodeoxyglucose-positron emission tomography/computed tomography (18F-FDG-PET/CT)
- 18F-FDG-PET/MRI • Sarcoma • Staging • Therapy assessment • PET-guided biopsy

## KEY POINTS

- Fluorodeoxyglucose-positron emission tomography/computed tomography (18F-FDG-PET/CT) is useful in sarcomas diagnosis, grading, staging, biopsy guidance, monitoring response to therapy, restaging for recurrence, and prognosis.
- 18F-FDG-PET/MRI combines the high spatial resolution of MRI in the study of soft tissue, with the functional analysis provided by PET imaging, which allows the tumor characterization.
- 18F-FDG-PET/MRI has the advantage of reduced radiation dose, which is important in pediatric patients.

## INTRODUCTION

Computed tomography (CT) and MRI are the preferred anatomically based imaging modalities in the evaluation of musculoskeletal tumors. In recent years, positron emission tomography (PET) with 18F-fluorodeoxy-glucose (18F-FDG) has been used increasingly to provide complementary information for various indications, especially in sarcomas.[1] In fact, this functional imaging technology can differentiate between benign and malignant lesions based on the metabolic activity. A further advantage is that the acquisition of PET data is not affected by metal implants and is frequently used in patients treated with limb-salvage surgery. Owing to the low spatial resolution and anatomic localization capability of PET technology, the addition of a hybrid partner with high soft tissue and contrast resolution has led to the development of PET/CT and PET/MRI

Disclosure Statement: The authors declare no commercial associations that might pose conflict of interest in connection with this article.

[a] Department of Orthopedics and Orthopedic Oncology, University of Padova, Via 8 Febbraio 1848, 2, 35122 Padova, Italy; [b] Nuclear Medicine, Azienda Ospedaliero-Universitaria di Bologna, University of Bologna, Via massarenti 9, 40138, Bologna, Italy; [c] Department of Molecular and Medical Pharmacology, Ahmanson Translational Imaging Division, University of California at Los Angeles (UCLA), 200 Medical Plaza, Suite B114, Los Angeles CA 90095, USA; [d] Department of Medical and Surgical Sciences, University of Bologna, Bologna, Italy
* Corresponding author. Nuclear Medicine, Ronald Regan UCLA Medical Center, 200 UCLA Medical Plaza, Suite B114, Los Angeles, CA.
E-mail address: fceci@mednet.ucla.edu

PET Clin 14 (2019) 183–191
https://doi.org/10.1016/j.cpet.2018.08.012
1556-8598/19/© 2018 Elsevier Inc. All rights reserved.

systems.[2] These combined systems enable fast and accurate full-body evaluation, increasing diagnostic and clinical relevant data from the imaging studies.

During the last decade, 18F-FDG-PET/CT has been shown to be useful in sarcoma detection and grading,[3] staging[4] biopsy guidance,[5] monitoring response to therapy,[6] restaging for recurrence,[7] and determining prognosis.[8]

More recent studies investigated the feasibility and efficacy of PET/MRI in sarcomas, showing excellent agreement and promising results compared with the currently preferred imaging methods.[9,10] PET/MRI is a hybrid imaging modality that combines the high resolution of MRI in the study of soft-tissue lesions and the peculiarities of PET imaging that allow the characterization of tissues using either receptorial or metabolic radiopharmaceuticals. In bone and soft-tissue sarcoma, MRI is mostly used for local staging and detection of local relapse. In pediatric patients, the use of MRI associated to PET, instead of CT, could largely reduce the radiation exposure. Moreover, the simultaneous use of PET and MRI could be considered a sort of 1 stop shop with the intent to reduce the number of cumulative studies during staging and follow0up. Summarizing the use of PET MRI in sarcoma patients could lead to many advantages such as a reduction in exposure to ionizing radiation, a reduction in the number of investigations performed during the clinical history of the disease, and the complementary information provided by the 2 techniques allowing a characterization of the tissue either from the anatomic or functional point of view.[9–11]

## INITIAL DIAGNOSIS AND STAGING

Osteosarcoma and Ewing sarcoma are the most common primary malignant tumors of bone, especially in children and young adults. They can metastasize to the lungs or other areas of bone (either distant bones, or in certain cases, within the same bone as skip lesions). Metastatic bone carcinomas, multiple myeloma, and chondrosarcoma are the most frequent bone malignancies in adults. Standard staging includes imaging of the primary tumor via plain radiographs and CT/ MRI and pulmonary assessment for lung metastases via chest CT. Bone scan is useful to screen for skeletal metastases. Staging is the most researched area for PET scanning in sarcoma. FDG PET imaging has been shown to be helpful as part of initial staging, especially combining the anatomic detail of CT or MRI with the ability to assess metabolic activity.

Several studies have confirmed the role of 18F-FDG-PET/CT as an effective tool to delineate the primary tumor.[12] Usually high-grade tumors are metabolically active showing a high standardized uptake value (SUV) value,[3] but sometimes they may have a low metabolic activity (p.e. necrotic areas). On the other hand, every highly metabolically active area should not be necessarily considered a malignant entity.[13] In a retrospective study of 212 bone and soft tissue sarcomas, Charest and colleagues[14] found that all lesions with an SUV value greater than 6.5 were high grade although many high-grade sarcomas had an SUV less than 6.5. The SUV value of the 77 cases of high-grade soft tissue sarcomas was 11.8 plus or minus 8.3, and the intensity was lower mainly in liposarcomas, leiomiosarcomas, and fibrosarcomas, whereas concerning bone sarcomas, the mean SUVmax of chondrosarcomas was 5.6.[14] Other authors found a correlation between a SUV value greater than 7.5 and histologic findings of increased mitosis rate and cellularity.[15] SUV can thus give an estimation of tumor grade before biopsy, but PET/CT does not replace biopsy of the lesion and histologic examination by a pathologist to determine the grade.

PET/CT is also a reliable imaging technique to detect occult distant bone metastases in osteosarcoma or bone involvement at diagnosis in patients with metastatic carcinoma or multiple myelomas.[12,16] A retrospective analysis of more than 117 cases of bone and soft tissue sarcoma showed high accuracy in the detection of additional distant metastases when FDG-PET/CT was combined with conventional imaging modalities.[8] In a multicenter study on 46 pediatric patients affected by Ewing sarcoma or osteo/rhabdomyosarcoma, Denecke and colleagues[1] reported that FDG-PET and conventional imaging were equally accurate for detecting the primary tumor (100% accuracy), whereas PET was superior in assessing lymph node involvement and bone localizations. Similarly, a high sensitivity for the detection of distant lesions on initial staging was shown with FDG-PET in a retrospective study of 212 patients with sarcoma.[14] Multiple studies have found the same benefit from the use of 18F-FDG-PET/CT in staging of patients with Ewing sarcoma.[1,17,18] A meta-analysis confirmed the use of 18F-FDG-PET/CT in identifying skeletal metastases, with some limitations regarding skull-based lesions and small pulmonary nodules.[18] Considering the superiority in sensitivity and accuracy, the increased use of combined PET/CT compared with traditional 99mTc bone scintigraphy is more than a future perspective.[12,19–21] The accuracy of 18F-FDG-PET/CT compared with chest CT in screening for pulmonary metastatic disease in sarcomas is still debated. There have been multiple studies demonstrating higher sensitivity of CT for detection of pulmonary metastases compared with PET alone[22] The combined PET/CT analysis provides both metabolic and anatomic data. It should be noted that the CT component is usually not optimized for imaging of the lungs, as it is not performed during a breath-hold following inspiration. In a small study of patients with osteosarcoma with pulmonary nodules identified on chest CT, 18F-FDG-PET/CT was found to have high sensitivity, specificity, and positive and negative predictive values (90.3%, 87.5%, 87.5%, and 90.3%, respectively) in determining benign versus malignant lesions.[23] Angelini and colleagues[7] reported that the performance of 18F-FDG-PET/CT to detect lung metastases in osteosarcoma resulted in sensitivity, specificity, accuracy, positive, and negative predictive values of 80%, 100%, 92%, 100%, and 88%, respectively. Other studies reported a low positive predictive value of PET/CT versus conventional CT scan for evaluation of nodal or lung metastases.[1,18,24] Considering that the lung is the most common site of metastases in sarcomas, the contradictory results in the detection of pulmonary nodules should be considered a limitation (**Fig. 1**).

The applications of PET/MRI in initial staging of sarcoma patients have been studied by Platzek and colleagues.[9] They studied 29 patients with sarcoma at presentation with the aim of comparing the results of PET/MRI with conventional imaging (CT and MRI alone). Weighted kappa ($\kappa$) was used to assess the agreement between the 2 methods. The accuracy of PET/MRI and conventional imaging for distant metastases was compared using receiver operating characteristic (ROC) analysis. According to this study, there were not statistically significant differences in T and M stage between PET/MRI and conventional modalities in all patients ($\kappa = 1$). For N stage, the results were the same in all but 1 patient ($\kappa = 0.65$). The authors concluded that there is an excellent agreement between hybrid PET/MRI and CT and MRI alone in initial staging of sarcoma.

The literature is limited and unclear regarding the use of 18F-FDG-PET/CT in the staging of soft tissue sarcomas, as well as for prognostication and therapeutic response monitoring. This is largely because of the wide variety of extremely rare histologic subtypes grouped under the same classification. Moreover, most soft tissue masses have nonspecific imaging features, with attenuation similar to skeletal muscle at CT evaluation, low-to-intermediate signal on T1-weighted images, and intermediate-to-high signal on T2-weighted images.[25] In most of the cases, high-grade tumors may include fat, calcifications, fibrous tissue, cystic areas with acute-to-subacute hemorrhage, and necrosis. For example, lesions such as myxoid liposarcomas are typically non-FDG avid.[26] FDG-PET/CT is not routinely utilized for evaluation of indeterminate soft tissue masses, because it does not have the ability to differentiate benign tumors from low- or intermediate-grade sarcomas,.[3] Good results have been reported in the use of 18F-FDG-PET/CT for initial staging workup of pediatric rhabdomyosarcoma.[27,28] This imaging modality seems to be more effective in documenting lymph node, bone, and bone marrow disease compared with conventional imaging techniques,[27] reducing the indication of bone scintigraphy and bone marrow biopsies.[29]

More studies need to be performed to better understand how best to incorporate the FDG PET as an imaging modality into clinical practice for evaluation of soft tissue sarcomas.[29] A possible advantage for soft tissue sarcoma imaging could be represented by the superior soft tissue contrast of MRI combined with its multiparametric imaging capabilities. Diffusion-weighted MRI or MR spectroscopy may potentially be correlated with metabolic data derived from the PET component, opening new perspectives in noninvasive assessment of sarcomas. The advantage of PET/MR is represented by decreased radiation burden in younger patients, potentially preventing secondary radiation-induced malignancies.

## POSITRON EMISSION TOMOGRAPHY-GUIDED BIOPSY

Metabolic imaging is helpful in planning and guiding biopsy. FDG-PET has been shown to identify the most metabolically active area within a sarcoma that can be used for accurate sampling.[30,31] Sarcomas are usually large malignant lesions that can be heterogeneous, often with areas of necrosis. If these areas are sampled, the diagnosis is subject to sampling error, and there is a risk of tumor grade underestimation.[32] Hain and colleagues[30] evaluated the use of FDG-PET guided biopsy in patients with a suspected soft tissue sarcoma. The histology of the biopsy site of the 8 malignant lesions confirmed that site as the area with most pleiomorphism and highest mitotic index within the sarcoma. However, the routine use of PET-guided biopsy is not yet well established and should be considered when conventional CT/ultrasound-guided biopsy results are inconclusive. Future perspectives may be represented by PET/MRI-guided biopsy.

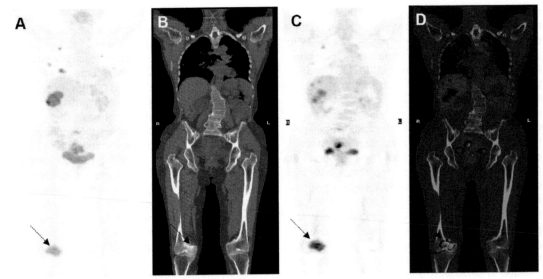

**Fig. 1.** 24-year-old woman affected by osteosarcoma of the right femur at presentation. 18F-FDG PET/CT showed the primary lesion in the right femur (*dotted arrow*) and multiple bone, liver, and lung metastases. (*A*) Maximum intensity projection (MIP) images, (*B*) CT images; (*C*) PET images; (*D*) fused images.

The PET/MRI may represent a future perspective in guided biopsy of soft tissue sarcomas. In fact, the higher definition of soft tissue features may have a significant role in tissue sampling planning.[33]

## RESPONSE TO THERAPY

The assessment of response to therapy is a field where PET/CT can provide added value. The role of 18F-FDG PET/CT in predicting response to chemotherapy in bone sarcomas[6,34] and soft-tissue sarcomas[35] has been investigated in numerous studies with contradictory results,[36] because of extreme heterogeneity of histotypes and limited case series. The importance of histologic response to neoadjuvant chemotherapy as a prognostic factor in bone sarcomas is well known.[37] Cheon and colleagues[38] found that the MRI-based tumor volume change, used in combination with FDG SUV pre-/post-therapy data, was associated with the histologic response. The ratio between SUVmax as measured on 18F-FDG-PET/CT at diagnosis and following neoadjuvant chemotherapy has been found to predict histologic response.[39] Dimitrakopoulou-Strauss and colleagues[34] used multiparameter FDG kinetic analysis to confirm the association between the tumor FDG metabolic rate and the histologic response. Several studies have correlated the metabolic response via 18F-FDG-PET/CT with good histologic response following neoadjuvant chemotherapy in patients with osteosarcoma.[40]

Palmerini and colleagues[6] reported SUV at baseline, associated with histologic/radiological response, as an independent prognostic factor on survival analyzing 32 patients with osteosarcoma and 45 with Ewing sarcoma.

Therapeutic response in soft tissue sarcomas is based on size criteria, even if evaluating the tumor volume reduction is not particularly helpful.[41] However, many soft tissue sarcomas may actually increase in size in response to effective therapy because of increased necrosis and fluid accumulation. FDG-PET has been considered for therapeutic response to chemotherapy by assessing the change in FDG avidity. Benz and colleagues[42] reported a 35% or greater reduction FDG uptake after the first cycle of chemotherapy analyzing 50 patients with high-grade soft tissue sarcomas (100% sensitivity and 67% specificity in predicting histopathologic response). Similar results were reported on 42 patients with resectable biopsy-proven soft tissue sarcomas who underwent an FDG-PET before and after therapy, with a 100% sensitivity and 71% specificity for assessment of histopathologic response with reduction in FDG uptake.[41] The authors showed that the difference between the SUV before and after therapy (SUV-diff) values was more accurate for assessing the response than either the presence of substantial tumor necrosis or the response evaluation criteria in solid tumors (RECIST).[41]

PET/MRI in response assessment after chemotherapy was so far poorly investigated: twelve patients with sarcoma who underwent FDG PET/MRI were included in the study by Schuler and colleagues.[43] According to Choi criteria for MRI, therapy response was classified as stable disease in 6/12 patients (50%) and as partial remission in 6/12 patients (50%). In conclusion, response assessment using Choi criteria based on contrast-enhanced MRI in comparison to FDG PET imaging only demonstrates slight correlation in sarcoma patients.

## PROGNOSTIC VALUE

In patients with sarcoma, prognostic factors are important to define the best therapeutic approach and schedule follow-up examinations. Tumor type (bone vs soft tissue sarcomas), site (extremity vs trunk), tumor volume, metastasis at diagnosis, surgical margins, and histologic response to chemotherapy are recognized as significant prognostic factors in the planning of treatment for sarcomas. As histologic response is a strong predictor of outcome in primary bone tumors, it suggests that reduction in metabolic activity on 18F-FDG-PET/CT following surgery and chemotherapy may predict outcome as well. Many published reports focused on the association between tumor FDG uptake and tumor necrosis in sarcomas.[36,39] Several studies have shown 18F-FDG-PET/CT to be an independent predictor of outcome in osteosarcoma,[44,45] even if others reported opposite results.[46]

A significant association between the tumor SUV and several histopathologic parameters (including tumor grade, tumor cellularity, mitotic figure counts, and overexpression of p53) has been reported in a large series of well-characterized soft tissue and bone tumors.[15] Furthermore, SUVmax and FDG heterogeneous distribution seem to be able to distinguish between higher-risk patients and lower-risk patients.[47] A correlation between pretherapy SUVmax and event-free survival has been reported in synovial sarcoma[48] and Ewing sarcoma, with a trend in patients with osteosarcoma.[6] Instead of SUV, Ye and colleagues[49] reported that in patients with osteosarcoma it was possible to discriminate between responders and nonresponders on the basis of PET results through the measurement of tumor-to-background ratio (TBR), considered significantly better than SUV. However, the interobserver variability of TBR seems to be high compared with SUV analysis.[42] Identification of patients who are more likely to have a less favorable histologic response to neoadjuvant chemotherapy is a potential clinical application, because such patients would be candidates for more aggressive front-line chemotherapy.

## DETECTION OF RECURRENCE

18F-FDG-PET/CT is important for restaging after surgery in detecting sarcoma recurrence. Recent data have clearly demonstrated a role in patients with osteosarcoma.[7,12] Angelini and colleagues[7] performed a study to investigate the diagnostic accuracy of 18F-FDG-PET/CT in osteosarcoma patients suspicious for disease recurrence after adequate surgical therapy. Analyzing 37 cases, they found an overall high sensitivity (91%), specificity (75%), and accuracy (89%) with 18F-FDG-PET/CT that justified its use to confirm or rule out relapses in patients with clinical/imaging suspicion. Arush and colleagues[50] reported that FDG-PET scan was useful for the correct interpretation of suspected recurrences at conventional imaging findings. In fact, the presence of a metallic implant/prosthesis, asymmetrical weigh bearing, imaging changes after chemotherapy, and eventual presence of callous formation or scar tissues makes interpretation of routinely imaging studies difficult in these patients.[1,51,52] Another study[51] demonstrated that although FDG uptake can persist at the surgical site in patients with osteosarcoma of the extremity for over 3 years following surgical resection, an increased change in SUVmax over time is associated with high risk of local recurrence, suggesting a role for 18F-FDG-PET/CT in screening patients for risk of local recurrence. In fact, recurrent tumors are usually more aggressive and FDG avid; thus metabolic alterations may precede the appearance of morphologically detectable lesions. An additional role of PET/MRI includes the possibility to differentiate between postoperative fibrosis or inflammation and residual or recurrent tumor after surgery. With the prolonged survival and the increasing efficiency of current chemotherapy regimens, the correct evaluation of disease response and post-treatment changes during follow-up is becoming more important.

18F-FDG-PET/CT shows valuable results not only for detecting local relapses, but also for lung metastases, even if the added value is still debated.[53] In a recent study examining the use of 18F-FDG-PET/CT in osteosarcoma and Ewing sarcoma, although the examination could identify pulmonary metastases in some cases, the sensitivity was less than that for chest CT, with a relatively high rate of false negatives.[12] Angelini and colleagues[7] reported a good accuracy in detecting relapses also for lung nodules; nevertheless, chest CT should remain the imaging of choice to investigate lungs.

Further advantage is that 18F-FDG-PET/CT is a whole-body imaging method that could be useful

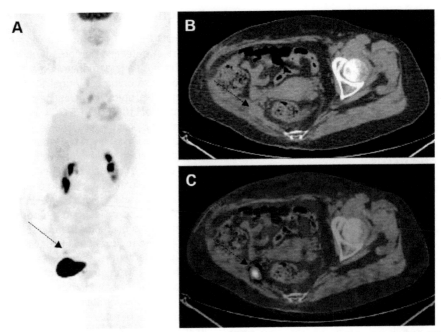

**Fig. 2.** 34-year-old woman affected by chondro-sarcoma of the right pelvis. Surgery 2 years before 18F-FDG PET/ CT. PET images showed an area of faint uptake in the right pelvis consistent with a local relapse after biopsy (*dotted arrow*). (*A*) MIP images; (*B*) CT images; (*C*) fused images.

in order to detect unexpected distant metastases.[7,50] In fact, in the presence of more than 1 site of relapse, the treatment strategy should be modified (**Fig. 2**).

The use of PET/MRI in the detection of local recurrences of soft tissue sarcomas has been investigated by Erfanian and colleagues,[54] who compared the diagnostic accuracy of PET/MRI and MRI alone after resection of the primary tumors. The authors studied with 18F-FDG-PET/ MRI 41 patients with clinically suspected tumor relapse of soft tissue sarcoma. MRI and PET/MRI were independently interpreted by 2 experienced physicians. The diagnostic confidence in each reading for the identification of malignant lesions was determined. Histopathological verification and follow-up imaging were applied for standard of reference. According to the gold standard, the presence of relapse was assessed in 27 of 41 patients. Sensitivity, specificity, positive predictive value, negative predictive value, and accuracy for the detection of local tumor recurrence were 82%, 86%, 92%, 71%, and 83% for MRI, and 96%, 79%, 90%, 92%, and 90% for PET/MRI ($P$>.05), respectively. Moreover, it is interesting to point out that PET/MRI showed significantly higher confidence levels ($P$<.05) for the determination of malignant lesions. The authors concludeed that 18F-FDG PET/MRI is an excellent imaging method in the evaluation of recurrent soft tissue sarcoma and seems to be superior to MRI alone.

## SUMMARY

In summary, robust data support the routine use of 18F-FDG-PET either using CT or MRI in patients with sarcoma. The applications range from diagnosis and staging to restaging, prognosis, and assessment of response to therapies. However, there is not a clear schedule of its use in the therapeutic management of these malignant neoplasm, and there is not a homogeneous consensus considering its evaluation in different histotypes. In the future, the application of PET-CT-MRI in sarcoma may increase accuracy in all of these applications. Further studies should be performed in order to discriminate between the 18F-FDG uptake of neoplastic tissue and that of nonmalignant diseases such as inflammatory or infectious processes including osteomyelitis, arthropathies, and postsurgical/traumatic inflammation. Other fields that require further analyses are the optimal timing and cut-off values for prediction of response or outcome that are not clearly defined at today. The extensive use of PET/MRI will reduce radiation dose, which is of great importance, particularly in pediatric in patients. There is need of a wide learning curve, however, and studies on the correct evaluation of this new imaging technique from all the members of the multidisciplinary oncologic team. In the authors' opinion ,PET/CT-MRI should be considered an innovative noninvasive procedure that will change the approach on musculoskeletal malignant neoplasms.

## REFERENCES

1. Denecke T, Steffen I, Misch D, et al. Positron emission tomography for staging of pediatric sarcoma patients: results of a prospective multicenter trial. J Clin Oncol 2007;25:5435–41.
2. Kempf-Bielack B, Bielack SS, Jürgens H, et al. Osteosarcoma relapse after combined modal- ity therapy: an analysis of unselected patients in the Cooperative Osteosarcoma Study Group (COSS). J Clin Oncol 2005;23:559–68.
3. Bastiaannet E, Groen H, Jager PL, et al. The value of FDG-PET in the detection, grading and response to therapy of soft tissue and bone sarcomas; a systematic review and meta-analysis. Cancer Treat Rev 2004;30:83–101.
4. Roberge D, Vakilian S, Alabed YZ, et al. FDG PET/CT in initial staging of adult soft-tissue sarcoma. Sarcoma 2012;2012:960194.
5. Park JH, Park EK, Kang CH, et al. Intense accumulation of 18F-FDG, not enhancement on MRI, helps to guide the surgical biopsy accurately in soft tissue tumors. Ann Nucl Med 2009;23(10):887–9. Park 2009.
6. Palmerini E, Colangeli M, Nanni C, et al. The role of FDG PET/CT in patients treated with neoadjuvant chemotherapy for localized bone sarcomas. Eur J Nucl Med Mol Imaging 2017;44(2):215–23.
7. Angelini A, Ceci F, Castellucci P, et al. The role of 18F-FDG PET/CT in the detection of osteosarcoma recurrence. Eur J Nucl Med Mol Imaging 2017; 44(10):1712–20.
8. Tateishi U, Yamaguchi U, Seki K, et al. Glut-1 expression and enhanced glucose metabolism are associated with tumour grade in bone and soft tissue sarcomas: a prospective evaluation by [18F]fluorodeoxyglucose positron emission tomog- raphy. Eur J Nucl Med Mol Imaging 2006;33:683–91.
9. Platzek I, Beuthien-Baumann B, Schramm G, et al. FDG PET/MR in initial staging of sarcoma: initial experience and comparison with conventional imaging. Clin Imaging 2017;42:126–32.
10. Partovi S, Chalian M, Fergus N, et al. Magnetic resonance/positron emission tomography (MR/PET) oncologic applications: bone and soft tissue sarcoma. Semin Roentgenol 2014;49(4):345–52.
11. Andersen KF, Jensen KE, Loft A. PET/MR imaging in musculoskeletal disorders. PET Clin 2016;11(4): 453–63.
12. Quartuccio N, Treglia G, Salsano M, et al. The role of Fluorine-18- Fluorodeoxyglucose positron emission tomography in staging and restaging of patients with osteosarcoma. Radiol Oncol 2013;47(2): 97–102.
13. Ioannidis JP, Lau J. 18F-FDG PET for the diagnosis and grading of soft-tissue sarcoma: a meta-analysis. J Nucl Med 2003;44:717–24.
14. Charest M, Hickeson M, Lisbona R, et al. FDG PET/CT imaging in primary osseous and soft tissue sarcomas: a retrospective review of 212 cases. Eur J Nucl Med Mol Imaging 2009;36(12):1944–51.
15. Folpe AL, Lyles RH, Sprouse JT, et al. (F-18) fluorodeoxyglucose positron emission tomography as a predictor of pathologic grade and other prognostic variables in bone and soft tissue sarcoma. Clin Can Cancer Res 2000;6:1279–87.
16. Terpos E, Dimopoulos MA, Moulopoulos LA. The role of imaging in the treatment of patients with multiple myeloma in 2016. Am Soc Clin Oncol Educ Book 2016;35:e407–17.
17. Newman EN, Jones RL, Hawkins DS. An evaluation of [F-18]-fluoro- deoxy-D-glucose positron emission tomography, bone scan, and bone marrow aspiration/biopsy as staging investigations in Ewing sarcoma. Pediatr Blood Cancer 2013;60(7):1113–7.
18. Treglia G, Salsano M, Stefanelli A, et al. Diagnostic accuracy of 18F-FDG- PET and PET/CT in patients with Ewing sarcoma family tumours: a systematic review and a meta-analysis. Skeletal Radiol 2012; 41(3):249–56.
19. Byun BH, Kong CB, Lim I, et al. Comparison of (18) F-FDGPET/CT and (99m) Tc-MDP bone scintigraphy for detection of bone metastasis in osteosarcoma. Skeletal Radiol 2013;42(12):1673–81.
20. Hurley C, McCarville MB, Shulkin BL, et al. Comparison of (18)F-FDG- PET-CT and bone scintigraphy for evaluation of osseous metastases in newly diagnosed and recurrent osteosarcoma. Pediatr Blood Cancer 2016;63(8):1381–6.
21. Lecouvet FE, Talbot JN, Messiou G, et al, EORTC Imaging Group. Monitoring the response of bone metastases to treatment with magnetic resonance imaging and nuclear medicine techniques: a review and position statement by the European Organisation for Research and Treatment of Cancer imaging group. Eur J Cancer 2014;50:2519–31.
22. Roberge D, Hickeson M, Charest M, et al. Initial McGill experience with fluorodeoxyglucose PET/CT staging of soft-tissue sarcoma. Curr Oncol 2010; 17:18–22.
23. Cistaro A, Lopci E, Gastaldo L, et al. The role of 18F-FDGPET/CT in the metabolic characterization of lung nodules in pediatric patients with bone sarcoma. Pediatr Blood Cancer 2012;59(7):1206–10.
24. Fuglo HM, Jorgensen SM, Loft A, et al. The diagnostic and prognostic value of 18F-FDG PET/CT in the initial assessment of high-grade bone and soft tissue sarcoma. A retrospective study of 89 patients. Eur J Nucl Med Mol Imaging 2012;39(9):1416–24.
25. Walker EA, Salesky JS, Fenton ME, et al. Magnetic resonance imaging of malignant soft tissue

neoplasms in the adult. Radiol Clin North Am 2011; 49:1219–34, vi.

26. Amini B, Jessop AC, Ganeshan DM, et al. Contemporary imaging of soft tissue sarcomas. J Surg Oncol 2015;111(5):496–503.

27. Federico SM, Spunt SL, Krasin MJ, et al. Comparison of PET-CT and conventional imaging in staging pediatric rhabdomyosarcoma. Pediatr Blood Cancer 2013;60(7):1128–34.

28. Norman G, Fayter D, Lewis-Light K, et al. An emerging evidence base for PET-CT in the management of childhood rhabdomyosarcoma: a systematic review. BMJ Open 2015;5(1):1–8.

29. Harrison DJ, Parisi MT, Shulkin BL. The role of [18]F-FDG-PET/CT in pediatric sarcoma. Semin Nucl Med 2017;47(3):229–41.

30. Hain SF, O'Doherty MJ, Bingham J, et al. Can FDG PET be used to successfully direct preoperative biopsy of soft tissue tumors? Nucl Med Commun 2003;24(11):1139–43.

31. Kobayashi K, Bhargava P, Raja S, et al. Image-guided biopsy: what the interventional radiologist needs to know about PET/CT. Radiographics 2012; 32(5):1483–501.

32. Klaeser B, Mueller MD, Schmid RA, et al. PET-CT-guided interventions in the management of FDG-positive lesions in patients suffering from solid malignancies: initial experiences. Eur Radiol 2009; 19(7):1780–5.

33. Skubitz KM, D'Adamo DR. Sarcoma. Mayo Clin Proc 2007;82:1409–32.

34. Dimitrakopoulou-Strauss A, Strauss LG, Egerer G, et al. Impact of dynamic 18F-FDG PET on the early prediction of therapy outcome in patients with high-risk soft-tissue sarcomas after neoadjuvant chemotherapy: a feasibility study. J Nucl Med 2010;51(4):551–8.

35. Rakheja R, Makis W, Tulbah R, et al. Necrosis on FDG PET/CT correlates with prognosis and mortality in sarcomas. AJR Am J Roentgenol 2013;201(1): 170–7.

36. Iagaru A, Masamed R, Chawla SP, et al. F-18 FDG PET and PET/CT evaluation of response to chemotherapy in bone and soft tissue sarcomas. Clin Nucl Med 2008;33(1):8–13.

37. Palmerini E, Staals EL, Ferrari S, et al. Diagnosis and prognosis for the Ewing family of tumors. Expert Opin Med Diagn 2009;3(4):445–52.

38. Cheon GJ, Kim MS, Lee JA, et al. Prediction model of chemotherapy response in osteosarcoma by 18F-FDG PET and MRI. J Nucl Med 2009;50(9): 1435–40.

39. Hamada K, Tomita Y, Inoue A, et al. Evaluation of chemotherapy response in osteosarcoma with FDG-PET. Ann Nucl Med 2009;23(1):89–95.

40. Kong CB, Byun BH, Lim I, et al. 18F-FDG PET SUV-max as an indicator of histopathologic re-sponse after neoadjuvant chemotherapy in extremity osteosarcoma. Eur J Nucl Med Mol Imaging 2013;40(5): 728–36.

41. Evilevitch V, Weber WA, Tap WD, et al. Reduction of glucose metabolic activity is more accurate than change in size at predicting histopathologic response to neoadjuvant therapy in high-grade soft-tissue sarcomas. Clin Cancer Res 2008;14: 715–20.

42. Benz MR, Evilevitch V, Allen-Auerbach MS, et al. Treatment monitoring by 18F-FDG PET/CT in patients with sarcomas: interobserver variability of quantitative parameters in treatment-induced changes in histopathologically responding and non responding tumors. J Nucl Med 2008;49(7): 1038–46.

43. Schuler MK, Platzek I, Beuthien-Baumann B, et al. (18)F-FDG PET/MRI for therapy response assessment in sarcoma: comparison of PET and MR imaging results. Clin Imaging 2015;39(5):866–70.

44. Costelloe CM, Macapinlac HA, Madewell JE, et al. 18F-FDG PET/CT as an indicator of progression-free and overall survival in osteosarcoma. J Nucl Med 2009;50(3):340–7.

45. Frezza AM, Beale T, Bomanji J, et al. Is [F-18]-fluorodeoxy-D-glucose positron emission tomography of value in the management of patients with craniofacial bone sarcomas undergoing neoadjuvant treatment? BMC Cancer 2014;14:23.

46. Hawkins DS, Conrad EU 3rd, Butrynski JE, et al. [F-18]-fluorodeoxy-D-glucose-positron emission tomography response is associated with outcome for extremity osteosarcoma in children and young adults. Cancer 2009;115(15):3519–25.

47. Eary JF, O'Sullivan F, O'Sullivan J, et al. Spatial hetero-geneity in sarcoma 18F-FDG uptake as a predictor of patient outcome. J Nucl Med 2008; 49(12):1973–9.

48. Lisle JW, Eary JF, O'Sullivan J, et al. Risk assessment based on FDG-PET imaging in patients with synovial sarcoma. Clin Orthop Relat Res 2009; 467(6):1605–11.

49. Ye Z, Zhu J, Tian M, et al. Response of osteogenic sarcoma to neoadjuvant therapy: evaluated by 18F-FDG-PET. Ann Nucl Med 2008;22(6):475–80.

50. Arush MW, Israel O, Postovsky S, et al. Positron emission tomography/computed tomography with 18fluoro-deoxyglucose in the detection of local recurrence and distant metastases of pediatric sarcoma. Pediatr Blood Cancer 2007;49(7):901–5.

51. Chang KJ, Kong CB, Cho WH, et al. Usefulness of increased 18F-FDG uptake for detecting local recurrence in patients with extremity osteo-sarcoma treated with surgical resection and endoprosthetic replacement. Skeletal Radiol 2015;44(4):529–37.

52. Abdoli M, Dierckx RA, Zaidi H. Metal artifact reduction strategies for improved attenuation correction in

hybrid PET/CT imaging. Med Phys 2012;39: 3343–60.

53. London K, Stege C, Cross S, et al. 18F-FDG PET/CT compared to conventional imaging modalities in pediatric primary bone tumors. Pediatr Radiol 2012;42: 418–30.

54. Erfanian Y, Grueneisen J, Kirchner J, et al. Integrated 18F-FDG PET/MRI compared to MRI alone for identification of local recurrences of soft tissue sarcomas: a comparison trial. Eur J Nucl Med Mol Imaging 2017;44(11): 1823–31.

# Moving?

## Make sure your subscription moves with you!

To notify us of your new address, find your **Clinics Account Number** (located on your mailing label above your name), and contact customer service at:

**Email: journalscustomerservice-usa@elsevier.com**

**800-654-2452** (subscribers in the U.S. & Canada)
**314-447-8871** (subscribers outside of the U.S. & Canada)

**Fax number: 314-447-8029**

**Elsevier Health Sciences Division**
**Subscription Customer Service**
**3251 Riverport Lane**
**Maryland Heights, MO 63043**

*To ensure uninterrupted delivery of your subscription, please notify us at least 4 weeks in advance of move.

ELSEVIER